Aesthetic Gynecology Rejuvenation

Aesthetic Gynecology is a fast-growing market amid much new demand from patients since gynecological defects can have a considerable impact on their quality of life. This fully illustrated text provides an authoritative guide from international experts on the anatomical, functional, and medical aspects, details the surgical treatments, and documents the clinical and procedural points arising.

Alexander Bader, MD, of the Bader Medical Institute of London is the President of the European Society of Aesthetic Gynecology ESAG. He has performed over 5000 operations worldwide and has operated on patients from more than 45 different countries, with over 15 years of experience. Dr Bader is the pioneer of Cosmetic Gynecology as we know it today in Europe. For the last 10 years, he has been one of the most highly respected teachers on the topic and his dedication and commitment to the topic has inspired hundreds of surgeons to follow in his footsteps.

Aesthetic Gynecology Rejuvenation

Edited by
Alexander Bader
Bader Medical Institute
London, UK

CRC Press
Taylor & Francis Group
Boca Raton London New York

CRC Press is an imprint of the
Taylor & Francis Group, an **informa** business

First edition published 2024
by CRC Press
2385 NW Executive Center Drive, Suite 320, Boca Raton FL 33431

and by CRC Press
4 Park Square, Milton Park, Abingdon, Oxon, OX14 4RN

CRC Press is an imprint of Taylor & Francis Group, LLC

ISBN: 978-0-367-37290-3 (hbk)
ISBN: 978-1-032-61996-5 (pbk)
ISBN: 978-0-429-35307-9 (ebk)

DOI: 10.1201/9780429353079

Typeset in Times
by MPS Limited, Dehradun

Printed in the UK by Severn, Gloucester on responsibly sourced paper

MIX
Paper | Supporting responsible forestry
FSC® C022174

Videos can be accessed via Support Material: https://resourcecentre.routledge.com/books/9780367372903

Contents

Preface

Female genital reshaping surgery is one of the most in-demand aesthetic procedures nowadays. The complex of these procedures is frequently named Aesthetic or Cosmetic Gynecology, and the surgeons performing these procedures, mainly gynecologists, call themselves aesthetic or cosmetic gynecologists.

The background demand arises with the women's desire to improve the appearance of that particular and sensitive part of their body. A few decades ago, it was almost impossible to consider even opening such a discussion among medical professionals; however, as with everything else, evolution comes from a need, and genital reshaping can be a real need due to malformation of the shape, length, or width of tissues. On the other hand, it can also be a luxury need to allow a better appearance in the eye of the patient herself. Whatever the motivations behind female genital reshaping surgery, there is one fact that we cannot ignore, which is the impact of these procedures on a woman's self-esteem, confidence, and general psychological status.

The examination of the shape of the genitalia seems to be an ancient habit, and people have admired their bodies for as long as we know; even those of the Stone Age reflected this in their art. The body shape has long been reflected in art, including the genitalia. Visiting any Greek archaeological museum will allow the visitor to immediately realise how perfectly symmetrical the statues of bodies are, including the shape of the genitalia. You will never see or notice asymmetrical labia or a hypertrophic clitoris, or a bulgy and wrinkled clitoral hood skin; the female genitalia was perfectly shaped. Observing the genitalia is also our daily habit. It became more popular with the revolution of intimate area shaving. People started realizing what they had there and started to have an opinion on how this might look, based on their personal views. The liberation of sexual discussions in the Western world, especially in the media, is one of the factors behind this evolution. The liberation of sexual behaviour between couples is also an essential factor.

The above factors motivated many healthcare professionals, especially gynecologists, to explore the topic. Plastic surgeons played an essential role in introducing the topic to the audience since they were the first specialists to discuss and perform some procedures to reshape the external female genitalia. Today, excluding this service from a gynecology practise seems almost impossible; patients' awareness is very high, and they know what is needed or what they wish to have. Since the topic is in high demand, special attention should be given to the psychological relationship with genital reshaping – from the psychological background in how patients might perceive the shape of the genitalia to what would be the impact of having a procedure performed there.

This book shares some important and impressive historical background related to female genitalia reshaping. The book mainly focuses on specific field techniques and finally includes the psychological aspects.

To my students and trainees, I always like to say: "Aesthetic Surgery is an art and Aesthetic Gynecology belongs to it".

Alexander Bader, MD, FAAOCG

Contributors

Elvira Brătilă
Obstetrics and Gynecology Department
"Carol Davila" University of Medicine and Pharmacy
and
Obstetrics and Gynecology Department
"Prof. Dr. Panait Sirbu" Clinical Obstetrics and Gynecology Hospital
Bucharest, Romania

Claudio Catalisano
Rigenera Clinic
Milan, Italy

Diana-Elena Coamdasu
Obstetrics and Gynecology Department
"Carol Davila" University of Medicine and Pharmacy
and
Obstetrics and Gynecology Department
"Prof. Dr. Panait Sirbu" Clinical Obstetrics and Gynecology Hospital
Bucharest, Romania

Mario Goisis
London Aesthetic Academy
UK

Stelios Kiosses
Harvard University Extension School
Cambridge, Massachusetts, USA
and
Edison Education
Stoke on Trent, UK

Piotr Kolczewski
Pomeranian Medical University
Szczecin, Poland

Rafal Kuzlik
SaskaMed Clinic
Warsaw, Poland

Sophie Menkes
Centre de Médecine Esthétique et Régénérative
Clinique Nescens
Genolier, Switzerland

Diana Mihai
Obstetrics and Gynecology Department
"Carol Davila" University of Medicine and Pharmacy
and
Obstetrics and Gynecology Department
"Prof. Dr. Panait Sirbu" Clinical Obstetrics and Gynecology Hospital
Bucharest, Romania

Dawid Serafin
Plastic Gynecology Center
Serafin Clinic
Gliwice, Poland

Video Access

Videos can be accessed via Support Material:

https://resourcecentre.routledge.com/books/9780367372903

1 History and Background of Aesthetic Gynecology

Elvira Brătilă and Diana Mihai

WHEN DID WOMEN BECOME INTERESTED IN IMPROVING THEIR GENITAL APPEARANCE?

It is obvious nowadays that women are paying more attention to their intimate parts – on the one hand, to the anatomy, and on the other hand, to the functionality of the vulvovaginal area – but let us see when this interest started. It is difficult to date exactly the interest from the patients, of course, but as for doctors we found evidence of interviews, books and medical conferences about clitoral surgery, circumcision, vaginoplasty and labiaplasty in the United States since the 1890s [1].

We include here publications showing interest of the doctors to enhance female sexual pleasure. Also, the African culture had an interest in genital surgery that goes away back in time but those procedures were meant to mutilate women and destroy any sexual interest. Aesthetic Gynecology techniques concentrate on providing women better aspect and functionality, but history shows us that in the 1960s a doctor started to offer patients this type of surgery, even if they did not request it, as he considered the female genitalia as "structurally inadequate" for intercourse.

A famous malpractice case is Dr. James C. Burt, who performed even without consent, experimental genital surgery, promoting it as an enhancement of the sexual life of women [2]. The Ohio gynecologist circumcised and "realigned" the vagina of about 2000 women over 22 years, but these experiments led many times to severe complications. He even released in 1975 his book called *The Surgery of Love*, which claimed his surgery would turn women into "horny little mice" as "the difference between rape and rapture is salesmanship" [3].

Even if the approach of the "Love Doctor" was not ethical, this shows that the interest in Aesthetic Gynecology existed and was increasing. In 1978 the first paper was published that mentioned a medical labiaplasty in the *European Journal of Obstetrics and Gynecology*, which was referred to as "Benign Enlargement of the Labia Minora" [4], and then in 1984, the first aesthetic labiaplasty was discussed in the *Plastic Reconstructive Surgery Journal* [5].

After these, the medical literature starts gradually to have more and more papers on vulva-perineoplasty, cosmetic vaginal surgery, vaginal rejuvenation, labiaplasty and all Aesthetic Gynecology procedures, including the psychological aspects involved in this medical field [6]. This is because women have different ideal body image and try to fit in a physical prototype they create. This is nothing new; women always have been preoccupied by their look, weight, and height. The new thing was that this prototype started to include the intimate area as well. Due to the internet they had access to other naked women and to analyze the "perfect genital area". In 1997, Fredrickson and Roberts published the Objectification Theory in the *Psychology of Women Quarterly* [7].

This is important to mention because, as an Aesthetic Gynecology specialist, you must understand the patients will come to you and request different interventions, and you must understand also that many of them will have different mentality than from you are used to in obstetrics and gynecology. Most patients will have rational and logical requests, of course, but some will need psychological guidance – and in order to identify them, you should be aware of the Objectification Theory [8].

This states that repeated personal physical inspection and evaluation as well as repeated comparison with other women will give females the perspective of an observer of their bodies. This means women will eventually come to regard themselves as "objects", or a collection of parts, that must be "fixed" in order to be then used by others. The important thing is that this self-objectification will determine real health sequelae [9,10].

The recommendation is to talk to your patient and try to find out the answer to the question: "Why do you want this aesthetic genital procedure?" In other words, gynecologists involved in this emerging field have to develop this new intuition and to understand that a person will perceive the body image as a multidimensional construction, and will have a reaction to this image taking into account affective (e.g., shame, dysphoria), cognitive (e.g., discontent, desire for change), and behavioural (e.g., avoidance, concealment) aspects [11,12].

WHAT WERE THE MOST COMMON ASPECTS THE WOMEN WERE UNHAPPY WITH AND WHAT HAS BEEN THE MOST COMMON AESTHETIC GYNECOLOGY PROCEDURE?

With Aesthetic Gynecology, we can improve many areas of the vulva-vaginal area: the shape or size of the labia, the

DOI: 10.1201/9780429353079-1

diameter and the laxity of the vagina, the clitoral hood, the hymen and scars after delivery or perineoplasty and so on. The most demanded genital surgical procedure was and still is labiaplasty. This procedure had an accelerated increase all over the world, especially after the explosion of the internet and the availability of magazines and pictures with naked women. For example, in the United Kingdom, the National Health Service reported a 200% increase in labiaplasties performed between 1998 and 2008 [13].

In the United States, the number of patients requesting labiaplasty in 2005 was 793, increasing to 1030 in 2006, while in 2013 the number was 5070, with a 44% increase from 2012. In 2014, already the number was 7535, representing a 49% increase. Similar trends have been documented in other Western countries, including Australia [8,14].

The American Society for Aesthetic Plastic Surgery statistics show that the demand for labiaplasty in 2017 increased by 217.3% from 2012 (about 11,000 procedures in 2017), the majority of labiaplasties being performed in the age group 19–34 years old (with an increase of 55.3%), and the next age group as number of procedures being 35–50 years old (with an increase of 34.2%) [15].

Most of the women requesting labiaplasty complain of enlarged labia minora, that protrudes beyond labia majora, labia asymmetry and dark-coloured skin. Existing medical conditions such as labial hypertrophy and congenital adrenal hyperplasia, can cause discomfort or pain during sports or wearing tight clothes as well as intercourse impairment. However, most patients requested labiaplasty in order to improve their self-esteem and sexual satisfaction [8].

Many times, women express anxiety in their intimate life due to the fact that the labia minora are larger than the labia majora. Nevertheless, female patients have marital problems that have nothing to do with their genital aspect but think that with a perfect vulvovaginal area they will gain a perfect relationship as well. It may sound strange, but it is more frequent than you would think. So all the international societies of Cosmetic Gynecology highlight the importance of having a deep conversation with your patient in order to establish realistic goals, to increase patient satisfaction and to reduce complication rates.

There are many techniques for labiaplasty, which have been continuously debated over the years in order to establish which one is the best. In order to achieve best results, do not follow the "trends" of labiaplasty, but choose the technique that is best for each patient, as every patient is different: deepithelialized reduction, linear incision, composite reduction, wedge reduction, W-plasty excision or Z-plasty [16].

WHAT WERE AND WHEN WERE THE FIRST AESTHETIC GYNECOLOGY PROCEDURES REPORTED?

Aesthetic Gynecology procedures or vaginal rejuvenation techniques refer to surgical and non-surgical treatments performed for three reasons:

1. Improve genital anatomy (reduce the width of the vagina, tighten the vulvovaginal area, improve visually the aesthetic genital aspect and restore the pelvic anatomy)
2. Improve genital functionality (enhance sex life, treat dyspareunia, anorgasmia, urinary incontinence, vaginal atrophy, prolaps)
3. Improve psychological symptoms such as shame, depression and fear of intimacy

The non-surgical treatments developed later, once modern technology developed of course. The surgical procedures, though, are more than a thousand years old and were first described as methods to suture vaginal lacerations post-delivery, by Trotula, in 1050 AD in *Treatments for Women* [14,17].

Having this in mind, we can understand that actually Aesthetic Gynecology procedures have always been present in the life of the obstetrician when resolving delivery complications and in the life of the gynecologist when repairing the vulva-vaginal area after cancers of malformations and later in the life of the uro-gynecologist when restoring the pelvic anatomy and treating urinary incontinence and prolaps. Aesthetic Gynecology comprises all these fields, but the modern aspect is that it combines all these techniques, having in the centre the functional and psychological well-being of the female patient.

So, Cosmetic Gynecology, as a state of art, requires a deeper understanding of the woman, including anatomy, functionality and psychology. This is the goal we are moving toward today, even if at first it was mainly about restoring the aesthetic visual aspect, as we found in medical literature, when in 1984 the *Journal of Plastic Reconstructive Surgery* begins to mention the term "cosmetic vaginal surgery". Perineoplasty, vaginoplasty consist in the repair of the vaginal entrance, with the reformation of the perineal body, improving sexual satisfaction and aesthetic aspect but also defecation and urinary symptoms if present and if performed correctly [16].

Vaginal rejuvenation and Cosmetic Gynecology raised a lot of controversy worldwide, due to lack of standardized nomenclature and because some doctors had more commercial and marketing interests than medical. For example, in 2007, the American College of Obstetricians and Gynecologists (ACOG) stated these "are not accepted surgical practises, as there is paucity of data supporting their safety and efficacy, despite potential complications, such as infection, dyspareunia, scarring, and altered sensation". In 2013, a similar ethical opinion paper was released by the Royal College of Obstetricians and Gynecologists (RCOG), followed by the Royal Australian and New Zealand College of Obstetricians and Gynecologists (RANZCOG) and the Society of Obstetricians and Gynecologists of Canada (SOGC) [14].

Articles came out against this background, reporting outcomes to clarify the current scenario. In 2017, for example, Giussy Barbara et al. realized a review of

Pubmed literature from January 2000 and September 2016 on vaginal rejuvenation procedures, concluding that "Vaginal rejuvenation is described as a safe and effective surgical procedure for the enhancement of sexual functioning in women with an acquired sensation of vaginal laxity and consequent sexual dissatisfaction" but also stating that the doctor must have an extensive discussion with the patient in order to avoid unrealistic expectations and that psychological and sexological counselling should be recommended to all patients before procedures [14]. As presented earlier in this chapter, we agree and support these recommendations as well as the need for more strong data and multicentre randomized controlled studies [18].

WHEN DID THE TREATMENT WITH PRP START BEING USED IN AESTHETIC GYNECOLOGY?

Platelet-rich plasma (PRP) promotes the natural healing process through trombocytes and also by delivering growth factors to the interested treatment site, so it is used in many medical fields, such as plastic surgery, dentistry, musculoskeletal, ENT, spinal and gynecology.

But when did this PRP first appear? It was, of course, in hematology in 1970, used to treat thrombocytopenia patients [19]. Ten years later, it was introduced in maxilofacial surgery, having cellular proliferation proprieties, and then in sports medicine. The use of PRP in gynecology has gradually emerged, along with other medical fields such as dermatology.

The largest review of studies that concerns the use of PRP in gynecology includes studies on safety and efficacy in this field, conducted between 2000 and 2017. Therefore, PRP has been used in this field for over 20 years [20]. In the United States, it is estimated to be used in obstetrics and gynecology specifically in more than 100,000 cases annually [21]. PRP is used in Aesthetic Gynecology, including vaginal genito-urinary syndrome (GSM), female sexual dysfunction (O-Shot, G-Shot therapy) [22,23] and lichen sclerosus treatment [24,25], but also may be added to all genital surgery, in order to lower rates of wound infection, necrosis and wound dehiscence and shorter recovery time in vulvar reconstructive surgery and pelvic floor reconstructive procedures (with or without meshes) [26,27].

WHEN DID THE TREATMENT WITH LASER START BEING USED IN AESTHETIC GYNECOLOGY?

The laser concept was developed by Einstein in 1917, and it is an acronym for "light amplification by the stimulated emission of radiation" [28]. It took 40 years to finalize this concept, and the first laser was introduced in 1960 by Theodore Maiman and used a ruby as the active medium [29]. One year later, in 1961, the CO_2 laser was developed [30].

In gliterature from January 2000literature from January 2000ynecology, the CO_2 laser was first used in 1973 for treatment of cervical erosions, and later for treatment of cervical intraepithelial neoplasia and for microsurgery of the fallopian tube and become a popular instrument in laparoscopy, especially in the area of infertility [31–33].

Many advancements in laser technology have been made, and several other types of lasers started to be available from the early 1980s, including the neodymium:yttrium-aluminum-garnet (Nd:YAG), potassium-titanyl-phosphate (KTP), and argon, but the CO_2 laser remains the most versatile and safe because of limited depth penetration (0.1–0.5 mm) and lateral thermal damage (0.5 mm). During the early 1990s, alternative and less expensive technology was developed (unipolar instruments and loop electrical excision), the high costs led to a decrease in its use [31].

For vaginal rejuvenation, energy-based devices are a new trend gaining more and more confidence. By application of thermal or nonthermal energy to the various layers of the vaginal tissue, this device stimulates collagen regeneration, the contracture of elastin fibres, the neovascularization and also vaginal lubrication [34].

In menopause vulvovaginal atrophy, the CO_2 fractional laser has been intensively studied, both by clinical and histopathology trials, randomized, compared to placebo and to estriol, in order to evaluate efficacy and safety [35]. It was shown to improve in a safe way: dyspareunia, dryness, lubrication, desire, dysuria, vaginal flora, imperiosity, laxity, lichen sclerousus in patients in menopause and even in patients after cancer vaginal radiotherapy or systemic hormonal chemotheraphy [36–47]. Similar studies exist for the Er:YAG LASER and Nd:YAG [48].

However, the US Food and Drug Administration (FDA) approved only the CO_2 laser in 2010 for Gynecology use, but it is in debate for vaginal rejuvenation, and the Er:YAG LASER and Nd:YAG in 2011 and 2014 were licensed for "dermatologic uses: coagulation, vaporization, ablation, or cutting of skin in dermatology and plastic/aesthetic surgery". Even if there exists a large number of studies, the FDA states there is a need for larger and more robust data in order to recommend the laser for vulva-vaginal rejuvenation [49–51].

WHEN DID TREATMENT WITH RADIOFREQUENCY ABLATION (RFA) START BEING USED IN AESTHETIC GYNECOLOGY?

The basic technique of RFA was first described by D'Arsonval in 1891 [52]. It showed an increase in tissue temperature when an RF current passed through tissue [53]. Since then, only recently has the nonablative RF been developed as a noninvasive treatment in vaginal rejuvenation.

In 2002 and 2003, Fulmer et al. and Dmochowski et al. evaluated the safety and efficacy of a transvaginal RF applicator as a new treatment modality for genuine stress urinary incontinence, by delivering RF energy to the endopelvic fascia. They concluded that this procedure has "good efficacy and excellent safety at 1-year follow-up" [54,55].

In 2019, Dillon et al. studied the transurethral approach with RF for stress urinary incontinence (SUI). The data suggested that RF treatment of SUI has promising efficacy, while posing a minimal risk of adverse events [56]. In 2010, Millheiser et al. showed in their study subjective improvements after RF in vaginal tightness, sexual function and decreased dyspareunia [57]. Since then many studies have shown similar results, confirming the initial findings.

WHEN DID THE TREATMENT WITH FAT GRAFTING START BEING USED IN AESTHETIC GYNECOLOGY?

The first "fat grafting" procedure was described in 1893, by a German Plastic Surgeon, Gustav Neuber, that used fat tissue transferred from the arm to the orbital (eye) region to correct scars formed from osteomyelitis. In 1895, Dr. Viktor Czerny had the idea to transfer a lipoma to the breast, in order to establish symmetry after a unilateral partial mastectomy [58].

In the 1990s, a New York City Plastic Surgeon, Dr. Sydney Coleman, began publishing papers describing standardized techniques for fat extraction, processing, and injection. The procedure's popularity has increased, and even though usually fat grafting is associated with buttocks or breast augmentation, it has gained increased interest amongst ob-gyns specialized in the aesthetic and reconstructive female genitalia, due to its efficacy, safety, long-lasting results and reliability.

The American Society of Plastic Surgeons (2017) noted that fat grafting had seen an increase of 10% in 2017. In Aesthetic Gynecology, fat grafting started to be used for sexual dysfunction, vaginal laxity, retractile episiotomy scar or labia majora augmentation [59].

WHEN DID THE TREATMENT WITH BOTULINUM TOXIN START BEING USED IN AESTHETIC GYNECOLOGY?

Botulinum toxin was discovered in 1897; in 1946, it was produced in a purified form and studied, and the FDA approved the toxin for treatment of strabismus, blepharospasm, and hemifacial spasm (HFS) in 1989. As it inhibits the release of acetylcholine from the nerve endings, it is used in various treatments, including cervical dystonia, hyperactive bladder, sialorrhea, hyperhidrosis, migraine, and spasticity [60].

In gynecology, botulinum toxin A (BoNT-A) is used to treat refractory myofascial pelvic pain, vaginism, chronic pelvic pain, dyspareunia, vulvodynia, urinary incontinence and overactive bladder or sphincter dyssynergia [61].

The first case of vaginismus treated with BoNT-A was described in 1977, but the FDA approved the first study in 2010 on 31 patients, titled "Pilot Study Protocol BTX-PV-01: Open Label, Single Center, Pilot Study of the Use of Botox Injections, Sensorcaine Injections and Progressive Dilation Under Anesthesia for the Treatment of Primary Vaginismus" [62].

Many studies followed, showing efficacy and safety in vaginismus treatment, but there were case studies even from 2004 for vulvodynia treatment (20–40 U of botulinum toxin A were used in each injection in the vestibule, levator ani muscle or the perineal body, with a reinjection after 2 weeks if the symptoms did not fully disappear; effects were lasting at 24 months follow-up) [63,64].

Botulinum toxin has been demonstrated to treat vulvar vestibulitis from 2006 (100 U botulinum toxin A significantly reduced pain 3 and 6 months after injections without side effects) [65,66].

And from 2005 studies showed botulinum toxin reduces pelvic floor hypertonia more than placebo, so it could be used in women with refractory chronic pain (100 to 300 units injected intralevator) [67].

Even if botulinum toxin has long been used for different voiding disfunctions, onabotulinumtoxin A (onaBoNT-A) is receiving regulatory approval as a second-line treatment for detrusor overactivity NDO at a dose of 200 U and for overactive bladder OAB at a dose of 100 U) [68]. FDA approval for its use as a treatment for urinary incontinence only occurred in 2011 [69].

Interestingly, there have been studies in urogynecology since 1990: for example, a double-blind study shows treatment of detrusor-sphincter dyssynergia with botulinum A toxin [70] and the efficacy in the treatment of the neurogenic bladder (endoscopic injection of 100 units of botulinum A toxin) [71].

The FDA licensed botulinum toxin in urinary incontinence after the results of two large, placebo-controlled phase III studies: "OnabotulinumtoxinA 100 U significantly improves all idiopathic overactive bladder symptoms and quality of life in patients with overactive bladder and urinary incontinence: a randomised, double-blind, placebo-controlled trial" and "OnabotulinumtoxinA for the treatment of patients with overactive bladder and urinary incontinence: results of a phase 3, randomized, placebo controlled trial" [72,73].

Sievert pooled the studies, giving a sample size of 1105 patients, showing robust results [68,74].

They included patients with over three UI episodes in three days, over 8 micturitions per day and were randomized to 100 U onaBoNT-A (n = 557) and placebo (n = 548). The study showed a significant improvement of the urinary urgency incontinence (UUI) episodes per day in the treatment group compared to placebo (−2.80 *vs.* −0.95 episodes/day; $P < 0.001$). After 3 months, full continence was achieved in 27.1% of onaBoNT-A group *vs.* 8.4% in the placebo group ($P < 0.001$). Interestingly, the median time for re-treatment was 24 weeks for onaBoNT-A compared to 12 weeks in placebo group.

WHEN DID THE TREATMENT WITH HIFU START BEING USED IN AESTHETIC GYNECOLOGY?

The first investigations of HIFU (high-intensity focused ultrasound) for non-invasive ablation were reported by Lynn et al. in the early 1940s. Then, in the 1950s and 1960s it was used in clinical treatments of neurological disorders, then in accurate ablation of brain tumours [75].

In 1994, the first commercial HIFU machine was launched in Europe after receiving CE approval for benign prostatic hyperplasia (BPH), and now HIFU treatment for prostate cancer is currently approved in Europe, Canada, South Korea, Australia, and elsewhere. HIFU is used nowadays for treatment of tumours of the the brain, thyroid, liver, kidney, pancreas, breast, uterus, prostate, and bone.

In gynecology, treatment for symptomatic uterine fibroids became the first approved application of HIFU by the FDA in October 2004, and it has been used recently for placenta accreta (studies from 2015), adenomyosis and endometriosis as well, with good 2020 studies results [76,77].

In Aesthetic Gynecology, HIFU started being used recently, with good study results mostly after 2017. It was shown that intravaginal HIFU therapy results in vaginal tightening [78], urinary incontinence improvement [79], and atrophy and genito-urinary syndrome treatment [80,81].

WHEN DID TREATMENT WITH HIFEM START BEING USED IN AESTHETIC GYNECOLOGY?

High-intensity focused electromagnetic (HIFEM) technology is a novel approach for non-invasive targeting of pelvic floor muscles (PFM), in the treatment of urinary incontinence and vaginal laxity. HIFEM technology triggers intense PFM contractions by depolarizing motoneurons and inducing electric currents in the pelvic floor area. Urogynecology international societies highlight that non-invasive procedures addressing the PFM should be the first treatment option prior to any surgical intervention, and recent studies show that HIFEM technology is significantly more effective than electrical stimulation in treatment of pelvic PFM in postpartum women.

For example, a study published in 2020 on a total of 95 patients compared two intervention groups treated with HIFEM (G1) procedure and electrical stimulation (G2), along with the control group (G3). They measured the functionality objectively of the PFM by surface electromyography measurements (maximal voluntary contraction [MVC]; mean MVC; muscle activity at rest; endurance of contraction) and also subjectively, by patient's perception with the Pelvic Floor Impact Questionnaire–Short Form 7 (PFIQ-7) standardized questionnaire. The results show that women of age 18–45 years, who had vaginal delivery, have better results using HIFEM, as all their parameters significantly increased ($P < .001$) and moved toward the values of the healthy population [82].

Another study in 2019 included 75 women with symptoms of stress, urge or mixed urinary incontinence. Patients received 6 HIFEM treatments (2 per week) with a duration of 28 minutes. Outcomes were evaluated after the 6 sessions and at the 3-month follow-up; 61 out of 75 patients (81.33%) reported a significant reduction of their symptoms using HIFEM treatment [83].

WHEN DID TREATMENT WITH STEM CELLS START BEING USED IN AESTHETIC GYNECOLOGY?

Stem cells are getting more and more attention due to modern technology making them more available to collect and use, but they were discovered in 1961 by two Canadians, biophysicist James Till and cellular biologist Ernest McCulloch [84]. The first stem cell research began in 1970, along with the discovery of mouse embryonic stem cells (ESCs). In later 1998, human embryonic stem cells were described [85,86].

Stem cells have been categorized into: ESCs, stem cells derived from placenta or amniotic fluid (AFPS), induced pluripotent stem cells (IPSC), and adult stem cells (ASC) [85–88].

In order to correct insufficiencies in the pelvic floor, vulva-vaginal area, urogenital tract, and repair after local cancer treatment, several studies have focused on the use of regenerative medicine. Stem cells improve tissue repair by a multilineage differentiation and self-renewal, while having a therapeutic effect also via the secretion of bioactive factors with antiapoptotic, antiscarring, neovascularization, and immunomodulatory effects on the tissues, and this way can direct innate stem and progenitor cells to the area of injury [89].

Mesenchymal, muscle-derived and adipose-derived stem cells used in local injections in animal models showed successful results of mechanical, nerve, or external urethral sphincter injury in stress urinary incontinence or anal incontinence [89,90].

Nevertheless, for bladder overactivity, direct injection of mesenchymal and adipose-derived stem cells into the bladder in animal models has demonstrated efficacy. In addition, clinical trials, most published after 2012 in both male and female patients, using stem cells for the treatment of stress urinary incontinence, sexual disfunction, atrophy, dyspareunia, and erectile problems have also showed promising functional results with minimal adverse effects [89,91–93].

Even though the technology is yet to be further investigated and there are limited patient data and clinical trials to support this approach and there is yet no FDA approval on stem cells being used in the Regenerative Gynecology area, stem cell therapies seem to be a great discovery for urinary and sexual disfunctions and vaginal reconstruction.

WHEN DID THE TREATMENT WITH AMNIOTIC FLUID START BEING USED IN AESTHETIC GYNECOLOGY?

Placenta and amniotic fluid are intensively studied, both for their regenerative properties and for being a source of stem cells (AFPSs). AFPSs are a new class of stem cells with properties intermediate to those of ESCs and ASCs [94]. They represent a heterogeneous stem cell population derived from the amniotic fluid and placental membrane and possess extensive self-renewal capacity and also can be induced to differentiate into cells of all three germ cell layers, including cells of adipogenic, osteogenic, myogenic, endothelial, neural, and hepatic lineages.

AFPSs are currently being investigated for a variety of applications, including modulating the immune response, treating acute tubular necrosis, and regenerating cardiac valves [95–97] and also in treating urological and gynecological disfunctions [89,98].

Also, in the animal model, injected intravenously, they have been shown to improve cognitive and physical functions of naturally ageing rats and also extending life span [99].

As gynecologists we must be aware of this potential of the amniotic fluid and placenta, and as Aesthetic Gynecology specialists that have a great focus on regenerative medicine, we must have an idea about amniotic stem cells, as for their safety, non-tumorigenicity and a lack of ethical concerns, easy accessibility and non-invasive application procedure, and their major advantages compared with embryonic stem cells (ESCs) and induced pluripotent stem cells (iPSCs). Human amniotic epithelial stem cells (hAESCs) are even been used in clinical trials related to the global coronavirus disease 2019 (COVID-19) pandemic (Phase 1 trial (ACTRN12620000676910 p) efficacy in respiratory failure and multiorgan complications, by Australian New Zealand Clinical Trials Registry (ANZCTR) [100].

Nevertheless, amniotic fluid therapies do not consist only of stem cells focus. Amniotic fluid itself has antibacterial and proinflammatory properties, and also has been used in preclinical and clinical trials for its anti-fibrotic and anti-inflammatory cytokines, immune modulators, growth factors, and matrix protein composition and action [101].

There are also many clinical trials utilizing the amniotic membrane, amniotic fluid, amnion-derived cellular cytokine solution (ACCS), and amniotic membrane extract eye drop (AMEED) as biological interventions for therapies in ophthalmology, orthopedics, pneumology, aesthetics and urogynecology [102,103].

Even if the procedure to take amniotic fluid during delivery is not complicated, in order to be able to use it you need special technology for sterilizing the product without damaging it; hence, companies produce sterile and safe amniotic fluid that can be used for local injections at the site needed and that has regenerative mechanisms. Since 2020, there have been clinical trials in progress to address the efficacy of these products in Aesthetic Gynecology.

CONCLUSIONS

Aesthetic Gynecology can be the solution for improving the quality of life for so many patients, but the art of this specialization and the goal towards which we should go is that doctors performing it must have combined knowledge in gynecology, urogynecology, sexology, psychology, lasers and regenerative medicine.

REFERENCES

1. Rodriguez SB. Female circumcision and clitoridectomy In the United States: a history of a medical treatment. *Boydell Brewer*. Rochester, NY, USA; Woodbridge, Suffolk, UK.
2. Rodriguez SB. James Burt's "love surgery". Female sexuality and consent in public discourse. *Arch Sex Behav*. 2013; 42(3): 43–51.
3. Burt JC, Burt J. *Surgery of Love*. Carlton Press, 1975, New York.
4. Honoré LH, O'Hara KE. Benign enlargement of the labia minora: report of two cases. *Eur J Obstet Gynecol Reprod Biol*. 1978; 8(2): 61–64.
5. Hodgkinson DJ, Hait G. Aesthetic vaginal labioplasty. *Plast Reconstr Surg*. 1984 Sep; 74(3): 414–416.
6. Schick VR, Calabrese SK, Rima BN, Zucker AN. Genital appearance dissatisfaction: implications for women's genital image self-consciousness, sexual esteem, sexual satisfaction, and sexual risk. *Psychol Women Quarter*. 2010; 34(3): 394–404.
7. Fredrickson BL, Roberts TA. Objectification theory: toward understanding women's lived experiences and mental health risks. *Psychol Women Quarter*. 1997; 21(2): 173–206
8. Sharp G, Tiggemann M, Mattiske J. Factors that influence the decision to undergo labiaplasty: media, relationships, and psychological well-being. *Aesthet Surg J*. 2016; 36(4): 469–478.
9. Fredrickson BL, Noll SM. A mediational model linking self-objectification, body shame, and disordered eating. *Psychol Women Quarter*. 1998; 22: 623–636.
10. Henning SL, Syzmanski DM. The role of self-objectification in women's depression: a test of objectification theory. *Sex Roles*. 2007; 56: 45–53.
11. Pruzinsky T, Cash TF. *Body Image: A Handbook Of Theory, Research, and Clinical Practice*. New York, NY: The Guildford Press, 2002.
12. McCabe Davison TE. Relationship between men's and women's body image and their psychological, social and sexual functioning. *Sex Roles*. 2005; (7/8): 463–475.
13. Moore RD, Miklos JR. Vaginal rejuvenation and cosmetic vaginal surgery. In; Cardozo L, Staskin D, eds, *Textbook of Female Urology and Urogynecology* (Third Edition). London: Informa Healthcare, 2010, 1056–1074.
14. Barbara G, Facchin F, Buggio L, et al. Vaginal rejuvenation: current perspectives. *Int J Women's Health*. 2017; 9: 513–519.
15. The American Society for Aesthetic Plastic Surgery, Cosmetic Surgery National Data Bank Statistics. ASAPS, New York, 2017, available at: https://cdn.theaestheticsociety.org/media/statistics/2017-TheAestheticSocietyStatistics.pdf.

16. Güneş A, Alinsod RM. A mini-review of aesthetic gynecology and leading gynecology associations' approaches to this issue. *Turk J Obstet Gynecol.* 2018; 15(2): 105–111.
17. Desai SA, Kroumpouzos G, Sadick N. Vaginal rejuvenation: from scalpel to wands. *Int J Womens Dermatol.* 2019; 5(2):79–84.
18. Goodman MP. Female cosmetic genital surgery. *Obstet Gynecol.* 2009 Jan; 113(1): 154–159.
19. Alves R, Grimalt R. A review of platelet-rich plasma: history, biology, mechanism of action, and classification. *Skin Appendage Disord.* 2018; 4: 18–24.
20. Dawood AS, Salem HA. Current clinical applications of platelet-rich plasma in various gynecological disorders. An appraisal of theory and practice. *Clin Exp Reprod Med.* 2018; 29; 45(2): 67–74.
21. Stammers AH, Trowbridge CT, Marko M, et al. Autologous platelet gel: fad of savoir? Do we really know? *J ExtraCorporeal Technol.* 2009; 41: P25–P30.
22. Jain A, Bedi RK, Mittal K. Platelet-rich plasma therapy: a novel application in regenerative medicine. *Asian J Transfus Sci.* 2015; 9(2): 113–114.
23. Runels C, Melnick H, Debourbon E, Roy L. A pilot study of the effect of localized injections of autologous platelet rich plasma (PRP) for the treatment of female sexual dysfunction. *J Womens Health Care.* 2014; 3: 169.
24. Casabona F, Priano V, Vallerino V, et al. New surgical approach to lichen sclerosus of the vulva: the role of adipose-derived mesenchymal cells and platelet-rich plasma in tissue regeneration. *Plast Reconstr Surg.* 2010; 126(4): 210E–211E.
25. Behnia-Willison F, Pour NR, Mohamadi B, et al. Use of Platelet-rich plasma for vulvovaginal autoimmune conditions like Lichen sclerosus. *Plast Reconstr Surg Glob Open.* 2016; 4(11): E1124.
26. Medel S, Alarab M, Kufaishi H, et al. Attachment of primary vaginal fibroblasts to absorbable and non-absorbable implant materials coated with platelet-rich plasma: potential application in pelvic organ prolapse surgery. *Female Pelvic Med Reconstr Surg.* 2015; 21: 190–197.
27. Gorlero F, Glorio M, Lorenzi P, et al. New approach in vaginal prolapse repair: mini-invasive surgery associated with application of platelet-rich fibrin. *Int Urogynecol J.* 2012; 23(6): 715–722.
28. Einstein A. Zur Quantentheorie der Strahlung. *Physikalische Zeitschrift.* 1917; 18: 121.
29. Maiman TH. Stimulated optical radiation in ruby. *Nature.* 1960; 187: 493.
30. Patel CKN. Continuous wavelength action on vibrational rotational transitions of CO_2. *Physical Rev.* 1964; 136: 1187.
31. DeLeon F, Baggish M. Lasers in dermatology, *Glob Libr. Women's Med.* 2008. 10.3843/GLOWM.10023.
32. Kaplan I, Goldman J, Ger R. The treatment of erosions of the uterine cervix by means of the CO_2 laser. *Obstet Gynecol.* 1973; 41: 795.
33. Bellina JH. Gynecology and the laser. *Contemp Obstet Gynecol.* 1974; 4: 24.
34. Karcher C, Sadick N. Vaginal rejuvenation using energy-based devices. *Int J Women's Dermatol.* 2016; 2(3): 85.
35. Mihai D. The efficacy of fractional microablative CO_2 laser for the treatment of menopausal vulvovaginal atrophy – systematic review. *Maturitas.* 2019; 124: 132–133.
36. Zerbinati N. Microscopic and ultrastructural modifications of postmenopausal atrophic vaginal mucosa after fractional carbon dioxide. *Lasers Med Sci.* 2015; 30(1): 429–436.
37. Salvatore S. Sexual function after fractional microablative CO_2 laser in women with vulvovaginal atrophy. *Climacteric.* 2015; 18(2): 219–225.
38. Pieralli A. Fractional CO_2 laser for vulvovaginal atrophy (VVA) dyspareunia relief in breast cancer survivors. *Arch Gynecol Obstetrics.* 2016 Oct; 294(4): 841–846.
39. Perino A. Is vaginal fractional CO_2 laser treatment effective in improving overactive bladder symptoms in post-menopausal patients? Preliminary results. *Eur Rev Med Pharmacol Sci.* 2016; 20(12): 2491–2497.
40. Athanasiou S, et al. The effect of microablative fractional CO_2 laser on vaginal flora of postmenopausal women. *Climacteric.* 2016; 19(5): 512–518.
41. Pitsouni E, et al, Microablative fractional CO_2 laser therapy and the genitourinary syndrome of menopause: an observational study. *Maturitas.* 2016; 26(3): 248–255
42. Sokol ER. An assessment of the safety and efficacy of a fractional CO_2 laser system for the treatment of vulvovaginal atrophy. *Menopause.* 2016; 23(10): 1102–1107.
43. Pagano T. Fractional microablative CO_2 laser for vulvovaginal atrophy in women treated with chemotherapy and/or hormonal therapy for breast cancer: a retrospective study. *Menopause.* 2016; 25(6): 657–662.
44. Baggish SM. Fractional CO_2 laser treatment of the vestibule for patients with vestibulodynia and vulvar lichen sclerosus. *J Gynecologic Surg.* 2016; 32(6): 309–317.
45. Sokol ER, Karram M. Use of a novel fractional CO_2 laser for the treatment of genitourinary syndrome of menopause: 1-year outcomes. *Menopause.* 2017; 24(7): 810–814.
46. Siliquini GP. Fractional CO_2 laser therapy: a new challenge for vulvovaginal atrophy in postmenopausal women. *Climacteric.* 2017; 20(4): 379–384.
47. González Isaza P, et al. Long-term effect of thermo-ablative fractional CO_2 laser treatment as a novel approach to urinary incontinence management in women with genitourinary syndrome of menopause. *Int Urogynecol J.* 2017; 29(2): 211–215.
48. Mitsuyuki M, Štok U, Hreljac I, et al. Treating vaginal laxity using nonablative Er:YAG laser: a retrospective case series of patients from 2.5 years of clinical practice. *Sex Med.* 2020; 8(2): 265–273.
49. 510(K) Notification, DEKA SmartXide2 Laser, available at: https://www.accessdata.fda.gov/CDRH510K/K133895.pdf.
50. 510(K) Notification, Apex Er:YAG/IPL, available at: https://www.accessdata.fda.gov/cdrh_docs/pdf13/k133254.pdf.
51. 510(K) Notification, RevLite 0-Switched Nd:YAG Laser, available at: https://www.accessdata.fda.gov/cdrh_docs/pdf13/k133254.pdf.
52. D'Arsonval MA. Action physiologique des courants alternatifs. *C R Soc Biol.* 1891; 43: 283–286.
53. Lee BB, Yu SP. Radiofrequency ablation of uterine fibroids: a review. *Curr Obstet Gynecol Rep.* 2016; 5(4): 318–324.
54. Dmochowski RR, Avon M, Ross J, et al. Transvaginal radio frequency treatment of the endopelvic fascia: a prospective evaluation for the treatment of genuine stress urinary incontinence. *J Urol.* 2003; 169(3): 1028–1032.

55. Fulmer BR, Sakamoto K, Turk TM, et al. Acute and long-term outcomes of radio frequency bladder neck suspension. *J Urol.* 2002; 167(1): 141–145.
56. Dillon B, Dmochowski R. Radiofrequency for the treatment of stress urinary incontinence in women. *Current Urol Reports.* 2009; 10: 369–374.
57. Millheiser L, Pauls R, Herbst S et al. Radiofrequency treatment of vaginal laxity after vaginal delivery: non-surgical vaginal tightening. *J Sexual Med.* 2010: 3088–3095.
58. Zielins ER, Brett EA, Longaker MT, Wan DC. Autologous fat grafting: the science behind the surgery. *Aesthet Surg J.* 2016; 36(4): 488–496.
59. Aguilar P, Hersant B, SidAhmed-Mezi M, et al. Novel technique of vulvo-vaginal rejuvenation by lipofilling and injection of combined platelet-rich-plasma and hyaluronic acid: a case-report. *Springerplus.* 2016; 26. 5(1):1184.
60. Jabbari B. History of botulinum toxin treatment in movement disorders. *Tremor Other Hyperkinet Mov.* 2016; 6: 394.
61. Moga MA, Dimienescu OG, Bălan A, et al. Therapeutic approaches of botulinum toxin in gynecology. *Toxins.* 2018; 10(4): 169.
62. Pacik PT, Geletta S. Vaginismus treatment: clinical trials follow up 241 patients. *Sex Med.* 2017; 5(2): e114–e123.
63. Gunter J, Brewer A, Tawfik O. Botulinum toxin A for vulvodynia: a case report. *J Pain.* 2004; 5(4): 238–240.
64. Yoon H, Chung WS, Shim BS. Botulinum toxin A for the management of vulvodynia. *Int J Impot Res.* 2007; 18, 19(1): 84–87.
65. Bertolasi L, Frasson E, Cappelletti JY, et al. Botulinum neurotoxin type A injections for vaginismus secondary to vulvar vestibulitis syndrome. *Obstet Gynecol.* 2009; 114(5): 1008–1016.
66. Pelletier F, Parratte B, Penz S, et al. Efficacy of high doses of botulinum toxin A for treating provoked vestibulodynia. *Br J Dermatol.* 2011; 164(3): 617–622.
67. Adelowo A, Hacker MR, Shapiro A, et al. Botulinum toxin type A (BOTOX) for refractory myofascial pelvic pain. *Female Pelvic Med Reconstr Surg.* 2013; 19(5): 288–292.
68. Eldred-Evans D, Dasgupta P. Use of botulinum toxin for voiding dysfunction. *Transl Androl Urol.* 2017; 6(2): 234–251.
69. Linsenmeyer TA. Use of botulinum toxin in individuals with neurogenic detrusor overactivity: state of the art review. *J Spinal Cord Med.* 2013; 36(5): 402–419.
70. Dykstra DD, Sidi AA. Treatment of detrusor-sphincter dyssynergia with botulinum A toxin: a double-blind study. *Arch Phys Med Rehabil.* 1990; 71(1): 24–26.
71. Schurch B, Hauri D, Largo M, et al. Effets de la Toxine Botulinique A sur le sphincter strié périurétral des vessies neurogènes. Etude préliminaire [Effects of botulinum A toxin on the periurethral striated sphincter of the neurogenic bladder. Preliminary study]. *J Urol.* 1990; 96: 375–380.
72. Chapple C, Sievert KD, MacDiarmid S, et al. OnabotulinumtoxinA 100 U significantly improves all idiopathic overactive bladder symptoms and quality of life in patients with overactive bladder and urinary incontinence: a randomised, double-blind, placebo-controlled trial. *Eur Urol.* 2013; 64(2): 249–256.
73. Nitti VW, Dmochowski R, Herschorn S, et al. EMBARK study group. OnabotulinumtoxinA for the treatment of patients with overactive bladder and urinary incontinence: results of a phase 3, randomized, placebo controlled trial. *J Urol.* 2013; 189(6): 2186–2193.
74. Sievert KD, Chapple C, Herschorn S, et al. OnabotulinumtoxinA 100U provides significant improvements in overactive bladder symptoms in patients with urinary incontinence regardless of the number of anticholinergic therapies used or reason for inadequate management of overactive bladder. *Int J Clin Pract.* 2014; 68(10): 1246–1256.
75. Duc NM, Keserci B. Emerging clinical applications of high-intensity focused ultrasound. *Diagn Interv Radiol.* 2019; 25(5): 398–409.
76. Zhang X, Duan H. One-time high-intensity focused ultrasound ablation of abdominal wall endometriosis with concurrent uterine fibroids or adenomyosis: two cases and literature review. *Quant Imaging Med Surg.* 2020; 10(2): 511–517.
77. Philip CA, Warembourg S, Dairien M, et al. Transrectal high-intensity focused ultrasound (HIFU) for management of rectosigmoid deep infiltrating endometriosis: results of phase-I clinical trial. *Ultrasound Obstet Gynecol.* 2020; 56(3): 431–442.
78. Sekiguchi Y, Nakamura R, Ninomiya N, et al. Safety and efficacy of high intensity focused ultrasound (HIFU) treatment for vagina ultra vera – preliminary results, *J Sexual Medicine.* 2017; 14(6): Suppl 5, e353.
79. de la Torre S. Effectiveness of a novel technology on women's urogenital health and sexual function. *J Sexual Medicine.* 2017; 14(6), Suppl 5, e353.
80. Jorge Alberto E. Management of vaginal atrophy, vaginal hyperlaxity and stress urinary incontinence with intravaginal high-intensity focused ultrasound (HIFU). *Int J Obstetrics and Gynaecology Res. IJOGR.* 2019; 6(2): 735–765.
81. Kolczewski P, Kozłowski M, Cymbaluk-Płoska A. Micro-focused ultrasound therapy in patients with urogenital atrophy and vaginal laxity. *J Clin Med.* 2022; 11(23): 6980.
82. Elena S, Dragana Z, Ramina S, et al. Electromyographic evaluation of the pelvic muscles activity after high-intensity focused electromagnetic procedure and electrical stimulation in women with pelvic floor dysfunction. *Sex Med.* 2020; 282–289.
83. Samuels JB, Pezzella A, Berenholz J, et al. Safety and efficacy of a non-invasive high-intensity focused electromagnetic field (HIFEM) device for treatment of urinary incontinence and enhancement of quality of life. *Lasers Surg Med.* 2019; 51(9): 760–766.
84. Weissman ILH. The road ended up at stem cells. *Immunol Rev.* 2002; 185: 159–174.
85. Martin G. Isolation of a pluripotent cell line from early mouse embryos cultured in medium conditioned by teratocarcinoma stem cells. *Proc Natl Acad USA.* 1981; 78: 7634–7638.
86. Thomson J, Itskovitz-Eldor J, Shapiro S, et al. Embryonic stem cell lines derived from human blastocysts. *Science.* 1998; 282: 1145–1147.
87. Vaegler M, Lenis, Daum L, et al. Stem cell therapy for voiding and erectile dysfunction. *Nat Rev Urol.* 2012; 9: 435–447.
88. Kim J, Lee S, Song Y, Lee H. Stem cell therapy in bladder dysfunction: where are we? And where do we have to go? *Biomed Res Int.* 2013: 930713.

89. Tran C, Damaser MS. The potential role of stem cells in the treatment of urinary incontinence. *Ther Adv Urol.* 2015; 7(1): 22–40.
90. Gräs S, Tolstrup CK, Lose G. Regenerative medicine provides alternative strategies for the treatment of anal incontinence. *Int Urogynecol.* 2017; 28(3): 341–350.
91. Lin G, Wang G, Banie L, et al. Treatment of stress urinary incontinence with adipose tissue-derived stem cells. *Cytotherapy.* 2010; 12(1): 88–95.
92. Casarotti GA, Chiodera P, Tremolada C. Menopause: new frontiers in the treatment of urogenital atrophy. *Eur Rev Med Pharmacol Sci.* 2018; 22(2): 567–574.
93. Stangel-Wojcikiewicz K, Jarocha D, Piwowar M, et al. Autologous muscle-derived cells for the treatment of female stress urinary incontinence: a 2-year follow-up of a Polish investigation. *Neurourol Urodyn.* 2014; 33(3): 324–330.
94. T Anker P, Scherjon S, Kleijburg-Van Der Keur C, et al. Amniotic fluid as a novel source of mesenchymal stem cells for therapeutic transplantation. *Blood.* 2003; 102: 1548–1549.
95. Perin L, Sedrakyan S, Giuliani S, et al. Protective effect of human amniotic fluid stem cells in an immunodeficient mouse model of acute tubular necrosis. *PLoS One.* 2010; 5: e9357.
96. Askari A, Unzek S, Popovic Z, Goldman C, Forudi F, Kiedrowski M, et al. Effect of stromal-cell-derived factor 1 on stem-cell homing and tissue regeneration in ischaemic cardiomyopathy. *Lancet.* 2003; 362: 697–703.
97. Moorefield E, Mckee E, Solchaga L, et al. Cloned, CD117 selected human amniotic fluid stem cells are capable of modulating the immune response. *PLoS One.* 2011; 6: e26535.
98. Weber B, Emmert M, Behr L, et al. Prenatally engineered autologous amniotic fluid stem cell-based heart valves in the fetal circulation. *Biomaterials.* 2012; 33: 4031–4043.
99. Liang CC, Shaw SWS, Ko YS. Effect of amniotic fluid stem cell transplantation on the recovery of bladder dysfunction in spinal cord-injured rats. *Sci Rep.* 2020; 10: 10030.
100. Kim D, Kyung J, Park D, et al. Health span-extending activity of human amniotic membrane- and adipose tissue-derived stem cells in F344 rats. *Stem Cells Transl Med.* 2015; 4(10): 1144–1154.
101. Qiu C, Ge Z, Cui W, et al. Human amniotic epithelial stem cells: a promising seed cell for clinical applications. *Int J Mol Sci.* 2020; 21(20): 7730.
102. Rennie K, Gruslin A, Hengstschläger M, Pei D, Cai J, Nikaido T, Bani-Yaghoub M. Applications of amniotic membrane and fluid in stem cell biology and regenerative medicine. *Stem Cells Int.* 2012; 2012: 721538. doi: 10.1155/2012/721538.
103. Murri MS, Moshirfar M, Birdsong OC, et al. Amniotic membrane extract and eye drops: a review of literature and clinical application. *Clin Ophthalmol.* 2018; 12: 1105–1112.

2 Anatomical Aspects

Dawid Serafin

The object of this chapter is a detailed description of the practical anatomy of the female reproductive system in the context of Aesthetic Gynecology therapy and reconstruction. This knowledge is crucial to choosing the proper treatment while taking into consideration the patient's safety.

The female reproductive organs can be divided into internal and external organs. The internal organs consist of the uterus, ovaries, fallopian tubes, and vagina. The external organs, comprising the vulva (Latin *pudendum femininum*), consist of:

- Mons pubis
- Labia majora
- Clitoris
- Labia minora
- Vaginal opening

VAGINA

Part of the female birthing canal, the vagina is a myomembranous canal, extremely elastic and flexible, from 5 to 14 cm long (usually 6 to 8 cm), which connects the uterus to the vestibule of the vagina, which is part of the vulva. The narrowest inferior part widens gradually. Its central part is 2 to 3 cm wide. The bladder is located anteriorly to the vagina, and both ureters run between the bladder and the vagina. The urethra connected to the anterior vaginal wall with the urethrovaginal septum, which fills the urethrovaginal space (spatium urethrovaginale), is located inferiorly to the vagina. This area is often treated with energy transmission methods, such as laser, high-intensity focused ultrasound (HIFU), or radiofrequency, due to stress urinary incontinence [1–3].

Posteriorly, the superior part of the vagina (1 to 2 cm) is covered with the peritoneum, which extends onto the rectal ampulla, forming the fundus of the rectouterine pouch, which is usually a crevicular space. This area is treated in cases of vaginal dryness, also using the aforementioned methods. Indications for this treatment are vaginal atrophy or the necessity to narrow the lumen of the vagina due to loosening of the vaginal introitus, and rectocele [4].

The superior part of the vagina includes the vaginal part of the cervix. In virgins, this inferior end is closed off by the hymen, which is torn during the first sexual intercourse or spontaneously due to the use of tampons, which results in the presence of hymenal caruncles (carunculae hymenales). This area is often subject to post-partum plastic surgery [5].

The vaginal wall has three layers, which consists of an external membrane consisting of continuous tissue; a muscularis layer consisting of smooth muscle and continuous tissue; and a mucous membrane, which smoothly transforms from muscularis and includes two layers (the lamina propria and epithelium).

In some women, the anterior wall contains a sensitive sensory area with richer innervation. This area was described in 1950 by Grafenberg, who called it the G-spot [6], and in 2012 it received a histopathological description by Ostrzeński [7]. This area is often treated with platelet-rich plasma or hyaluronic acid to increase sensitivity or accessibility for the partner during intercourse [8].

Vascularization

- The vaginal artery – the descending branch of the uterine artery (or the direct branch of the internal iliac artery reaching the lateral margin of the vagina)
- Branches of the inferior vesical artery
- Branches of the middle rectal artery
- Branches of the internal pudendal artery

An azygos artery of the vagina can form on its posterior wall (arteria azygos vaginae).

Innervation

Fibres transmitting sensation as well as anatomical fibres emerge from the pelvic plexus. From there, nerves go out to the muscularis and mucous membrane. The anterior portion of the vagina where the G spot is located is innervated with branches of the pudendal nerve.

MONS PUBIS

The mons pubis is a cutaneous mound covered with pubic hair, whose shape depends on the presence of adipose tissue located above the pubic symphysis. Inferiorly it borders with the upper ridge of the labia majora. In the case of excessive adipose tissue, reduction procedures, like injection lipolysis or liposuction, can be performed. In the

DOI: 10.1201/9780429353079-2

case of deficiencies, a common procedure is autologous fat transfer or hyaluronic acid injections [9].

LABIA MAJORA

The labia majora is a paired organ. These structures border superiorly with the mons pubis. The upper part of both labia descends centrally into the anterior commissure of the labia majora. Clitoral hood (prepuce) hypertrophy is often accompanied by the separation of this commissure, which should also be corrected in the case of clitoral hood reduction. The lower part of the labia forms the posterior commissure of the labia majora. Both labia are medially separated from the central structures by the pudendal cleft, and the lateral margin of the labium is also the margin of the vulva. The skin of the labia can be divided into the pilose outer part and the hairless inner part, which adheres to the labia minora and the clitoral prepuce. The labium majora resembles the anterior abdominal wall.

The volume, shape, and size of the labia are defined by the presence of the adipose sac with variable adipose tissue content. The adipose tissue has a rich venous plexus. During pregnancy these veins often become distended, causing labia majora varices due to the increased venous pressure generated by the expanding uterus. The subdermal layer of the mons pubis and labia majora consists of a superficial adipose layer described by Ostrański [7], which is similar to the Camper fascia and is connected to it, and of a deeper membranous layer, called the Colles fascia, which corresponds to the Scarpa fascia in the abdominal wall. The Colles fascia is attached to the ischiotibial branch inferiorly and the urogenital diaphragm posteriorly; it does not have an anterior insertion. This can be of clinical significance, since hematomas and infections cannot expand into the thigh area, but they can reach the anterior abdominal wall. The adipose sac is used in a procedure called the Martius labial fat pad graft. In the case of fat atrophy or lack of adipose tissue in slim patients, procedures with autologous fatty tissue or hyaluronic acid are often performed [10]. In cases of increased labia majora volume, a commonly performed procedure is labia majora reduction using a simple incision or the presented Double Hockey Stick Technique (Figs. 2.1 and 2.2) [11].

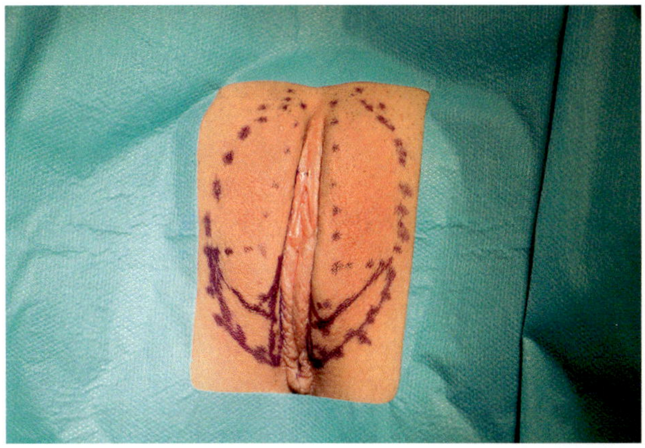

FIGURE 2.1 Labia majora plasty (Double Hockey Stick Technique) – marking lines.

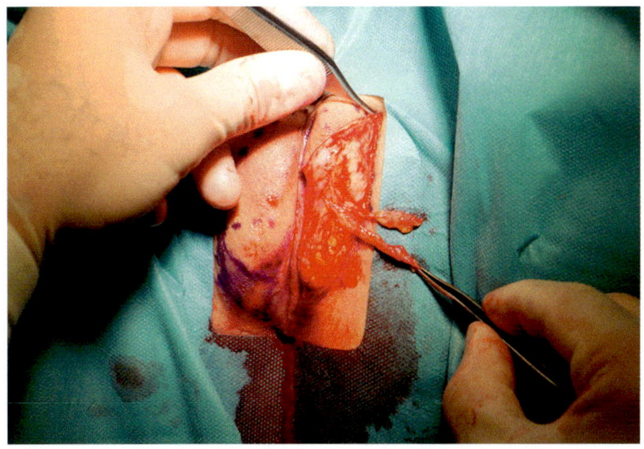

FIGURE 2.2 Labia majora plasty (Double Hockey Stick Technique) – tissue reduction.

CLITORIS

The clitoris is homologous with the male penis; similarly to the penis it consists of the glans and corpus cavernosum. The paired corpora cavernosa (*corpora cavernosa clitoridis*), which begin as the crura of the clitoris (*crura clitoridis*), are attached to the inferior rami of the pubic bones. They merge forming the body of the clitoris (*corpus clitoridis*) in the centre, which consists of the ascending and descending part, the latter ending with the glans, which is covered with the clitoral prepuce. Superiorly, the prepuce is separated from the mons pubic by the anterior labial commissure and laterally by the labia majora. The clitoral glans changes into the frenulum of the clitoris, which then branches out forming the initial part of the right and left labium.

The prepuce is often involved in labia minora hypertrophy, which requires a complex approach to labia minora reduction procedures (Fig. 2.3). A common problem is significant prepuce elongation, which is often accompanied by hypertrophy.

As a result, the prepuce covers the whole glans, which in turn can lead to weakened sexual stimulation during clitoral excitement. In this case the reduction is performed by decreasing the width and length, and changing the shape of the clitoral prepuce, while remembering to correct the anterior labial commissure if it separated. A common result of improperly planned labiominorrhaphy with omission of clitoral foreskin hypertrophy reduction is the penile effect (Fig. 2.4).

In the case of severe clitoral foreskin hypertrophy, the lateral folds can result in incorrect assessment of the anatomy, particularly identification of the proper margins of the labia minora.

(a) (b)

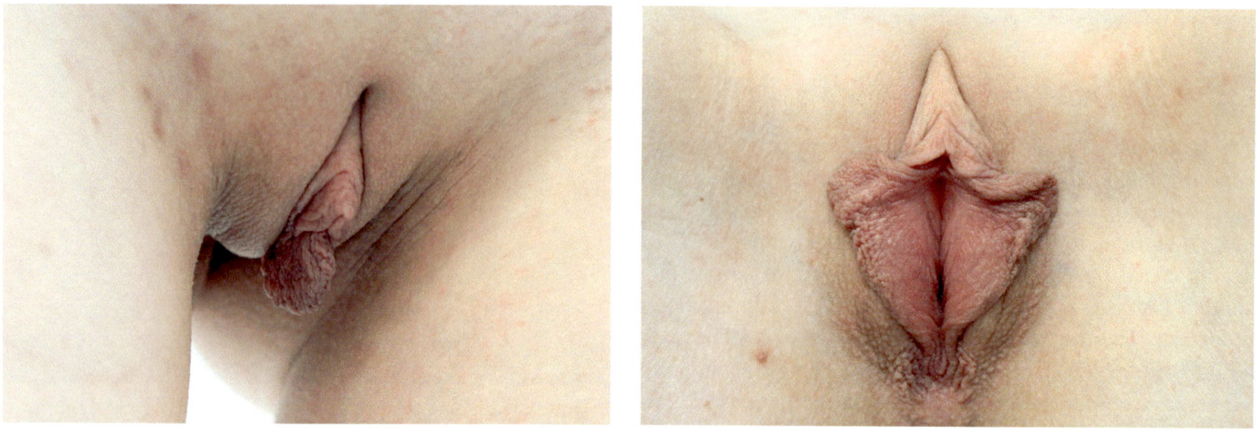

FIGURE 2.3 Clitoral prepuce hypertrophy: (a) Vulva in standing position – side view, (b) Vulva in lying position – front view.

(a) (b)

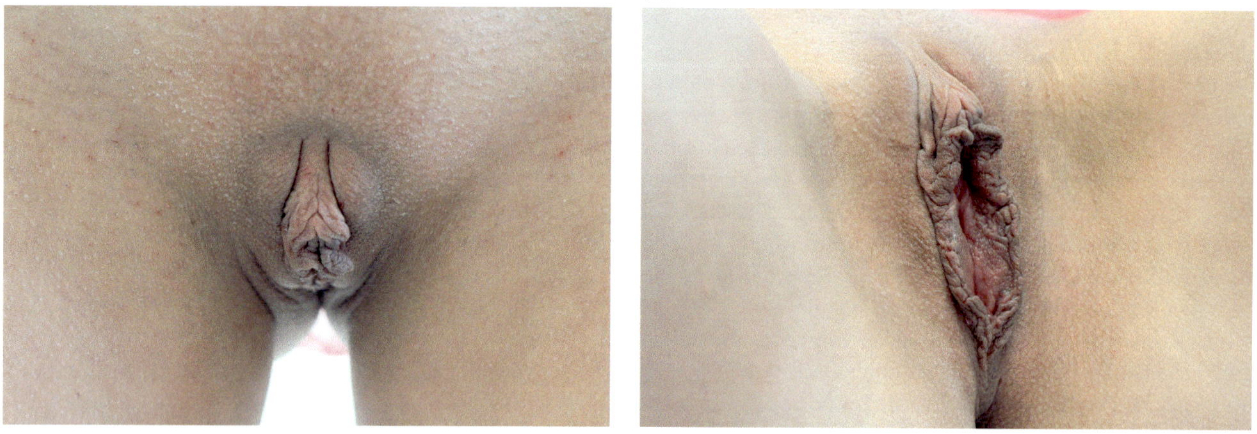

FIGURE 2.4 Penile effect after labiaplasty (Trim technique): (a) Vulva in standing position – front view, (b) Vulva in lying position – side view.

LABIA MINORA

The labia minora is a paired organ, located bilaterally between the labia majora. In the centre, they close off the area called the vestibule of the vagina. Superiorly, the ridges of both labia come down across the middle line forming the frenulum of the clitoris. The lower part of the labia minora extends downward forming the frenulum of the labia minora. The labia minora are covered by hairless skin, both externally and internally, divided by tissue homologous to the structure of the corpus spongiosum. The labia minora are very often afflicted with congenital shape, size, and thickness deformations. Labia minora hypertrophy can cause the skin structure to change, which is often associated with darkening of the labia (Fig. 2.5). This kind of hypertrophy is often an indication for labia reduction. This procedure has been performed for many years, and there are many techniques depending on the shape, size and type of hypertrophy. The types of labia hypertrophy have not been classified such as to mandate choosing a specific surgical technique. The current classification takes into consideration the size and characteristics of the hypertrophy, but the choice of the

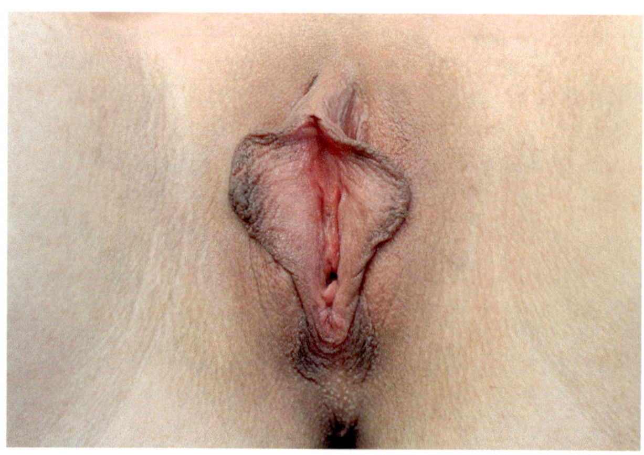

FIGURE 2.5 Labia minora hypertrophy.

surgical technique depends on the skills and experience of the surgeon.

Vaginal Opening (Introitus, Vestibule)

This central orifice is partially closed off by the hymen. Anatomically, this area is limited superiorly at the frenulum of the clitoris, laterally by the labia majora, and inferiorly by the frenulum of the labia minora. From the top, it consists of the urethra and the vaginal introitus beneath located in the midline. The vestibule of the vagina is also an essential area for minimally invasive procedures, since it may require e.g., platelet-rich plasma injections used in treating dysfunctions consisting in a weakened ability to experience sexual satisfaction during intercourse or masturbation [12].

Vascularization

Blood to the external genitalia is supplied by arteries forming many anastomoses. The internal pudendal artery, which is the main branch supplying blood to the external genitalia, is a branch of the internal iliac artery and branches out into:

- The inferior rectal artery descending into the rectal canal
- The perineal artery supplying the superficial transverse muscles of the perineum
- The posterior arterial branches supplying the labia
- The artery supplying the bulb of the vaginal vestibule
- The dorsal artery of the clitoris
- The deep artery of the clitoris supplying the corpora cavernosa of the clitoris

The external iliac artery extending into the external pudendal artery branches out into:

- The anterior labial artery

The femoral artery is an extension of the external iliac artery, which branches out into:

- The external pudendal artery additionally supplying the labia majora

Innervation

The innervation of the vaginal vestibule stems mostly from the pudendal nerve. It is a mixed nerve, which extends from the abdominal branches of the S2, S3, S4 spinal nerves and the intermediomedial nucleus.

The muscle branches innervating the muscles in the pelvis, the cutaneous nerves innervating the skin of the vulva, except for the mons pubis and the anterior part of the labia majora, which is additionally innervated with the anterior labial nerves extending from the ilioinguinal nerve, the perineal branches of the posterior cutaneous femoral nerve, and the genital branch of the genitofemoral nerve (*ramus genitalis nervi genitofemoralis*) extending from the lumbar plexus.

Labia Minora Classification

Until now, the sole classification of external female genitalia abnormalities included only hypertrophy of the labia minora.

The first attempt to create a classification system was made by Felicio in 1992 [13]. This classification included four size variations, where the width of the labia was assessed from 2 to 6 cm:

1. Up to 2 cm
2. 2–4 cm
3. 4–6 cm
4. Over 6 cm

This did not exhaust all the possibilities in the case of labia reduction.

In 2011, Cuhna presented a classification that assessed the characteristics of the hypertrophy instead of its size [14], which consisted of three grades of excess skin:

1. In the posterior/inferior region adjacent to the vaginal introitus
2. Extending laterosuperiorly to the clitoris
3. In the entire region, including the clitoral prepuce

This was the first classification to include the clitoral prepuce.

The widest classification, presented by Gonzalez in 2015, describes both the length of the labium from the base, the presence of clitoral prepuce hypertrophy, and symmetry [15]. This classification allows the clinician to organize medical documentation in a systemic way and is also helpful at the initial stage of reduction procedures, since it helps select which technique should be used for the specific type of hypertrophy based on its classification.

Grade of hypertrophy		***By location***	***By symmetry***
1	Up to 2 cm	A: Anterior	Symmetrical
2	2–4 cm	B: Central	Asymmetrical
3	4–6 cm	C: Generalized	
4	Over 6 cm		

Type-based hypertrophy classification is certainly a helpful tool in planning surgical procedures and preparing proper documentation, both pre-operatively and post-operatively. At the same time, it is this author's opinion that the extent of the procedure and the selected surgical technique should not be based solely on a classification system. The decision should be made after consulting with the patient and receiving a full set of information concerning postoperative expectations, and should be based on the preoperative examination in order to fulfil aesthetic and functional expectations while maintaining the maximum safety of the patient.

REFERENCES

1. Alsulihem A, Corcos J. The use of vaginal lasers in the treatment of urinary incontinence and overactive bladder, systematic review. *Int Urogynecol J.* 2021 Mar;32(3):553–572.
2. Ogrinc UB. Senčar S. Lenasi H. Novel minimally invasive laser treatment of urinary incontinence in women. *Lasers Surg Med.* 2015 Nov;47(9):689–697.
3. Liu D. Transurethral high-intensity ultrasound for treatment of stress urinary incontinence (SUI): Simulation studies with patient-specific models. *Int J Hyperthermia.* 2018 Dec;34(8):1236–1247.
4. Samuels JB, Garcia MA. Treatment to external labia and vaginal canal with CO_2 laser for symptoms of vulvovaginal atrophy in postmenopausal women. *Aesthet Surg J.* 2019 Jan 1;39(1):83–93.
5. Meekins AR, Siddiqui NY. Diagnosis and management of postpartum pelvic floor disorders. *Obstet Gynecol Clin North Am.* 2020 Sep;47(3):477–486.
6. Grafenberg E. The role of urethra in female orgasm. *Int J Sexol.*1950;3:145–148.
7. Ostrzenski A. G-spot anatomy: A new discovery. *J Sex Med.* 2012;9:1355–1359.
8. Wilkie G, Bartz D. Vaginal rejuvenation: A review of female genital cosmetic surgery. *Obstet Gynecol Surv.* 2018 May;73(5):287–292.
9. Hexsel D, dal'Forno T, Caspary P, et al. Soft-tissue augmentation with hyaluronic acid filler for labia majora and mons pubis. *Dermatologic Surg.* 2016;42(7):911–914.
10. Zerbinati N, Haddad RG, Bader A, et al. A new hyaluronic acid polymer in the augmentation and restoration of labia majora. *J Biol Regul Homeost Agents.* 2017;31(2 Suppl. 2):153–161.
11. Serafin W. Master individual course 'perfect labiaplasty', at www.papag.pl.
12. Sukgen G, Kaya AE, Karagun E, et al. Platelet-rich plasma administration to the lower anterior vaginal wall to improve female sexuality satisfaction. *Turk J Obstet Gynecol.* 2019;16(4):228–234.
13. Felicio Y. Chirurgie intime. *Rev Chir Esth Lang Franc.* 1992;27(67):37–43.
14. Cunha FI, Silva LM, Costa LA, et al. Ninfoplasatia: Classificação e refinamentos técnicos. *Rev Bras Cir Plást.* 2011;26(3):507–511.
15. González PI. Classification of hypertrophy of labia minora: Consideration of a multiple component approach. *Surg Technol Int.* 2015;27:191–194.

3 Labiaplasty

Wedge Technique

Dawid Serafin

Labia minora hypertrophy is the most common external genitalia defect reported by patients seeking surgical treatment. As early as 1976, Radman presented a simple amputation technique of the labia minora [1]. Unfortunately, if we use this technique while omitting the clitoral prepuce hypertrophy, we could end up with a protruding clitoral hood, also called a micropenis or the penile effect (Fig. 3.1).

In addition, amputating the margins of the labia and replacing them with newly formed scars increases the risk of hypersensitivity and pain during sexual intercourse.

Laufer's 1995 paper proposed a new insight into reduction techniques [2]. Just 3 years later, in 1998, Alter presented his new technique: a central wedge resection of a fragment of the labium minus [3]. The most important difference between this technique and amputation was to preserve the natural margin of the labia minora, which resulted in a more natural post-surgical appearance. It also minimized the risk of functional impairments, which would result from the longitudinal scar replacing the natural margin of the labia.

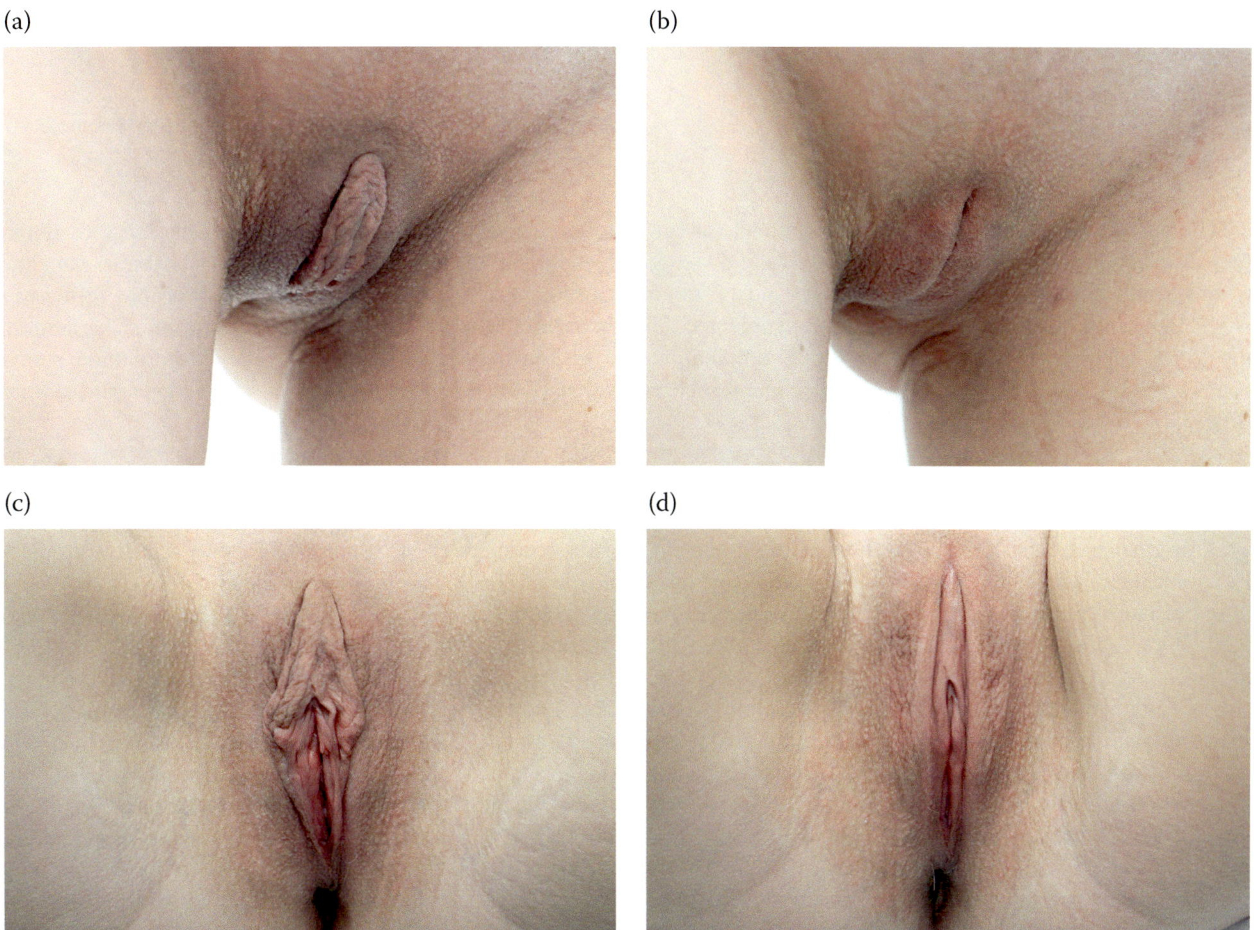

FIGURE 3.1 Micropenis effect after labiaplasty. (a) View in standing position before reconstruction. (b) View in standing position after reconstruction. (c) View in gynecological chair before reconstruction. (d) View in gynecological chair after reconstruction.

DOI: 10.1201/9780429353079-3

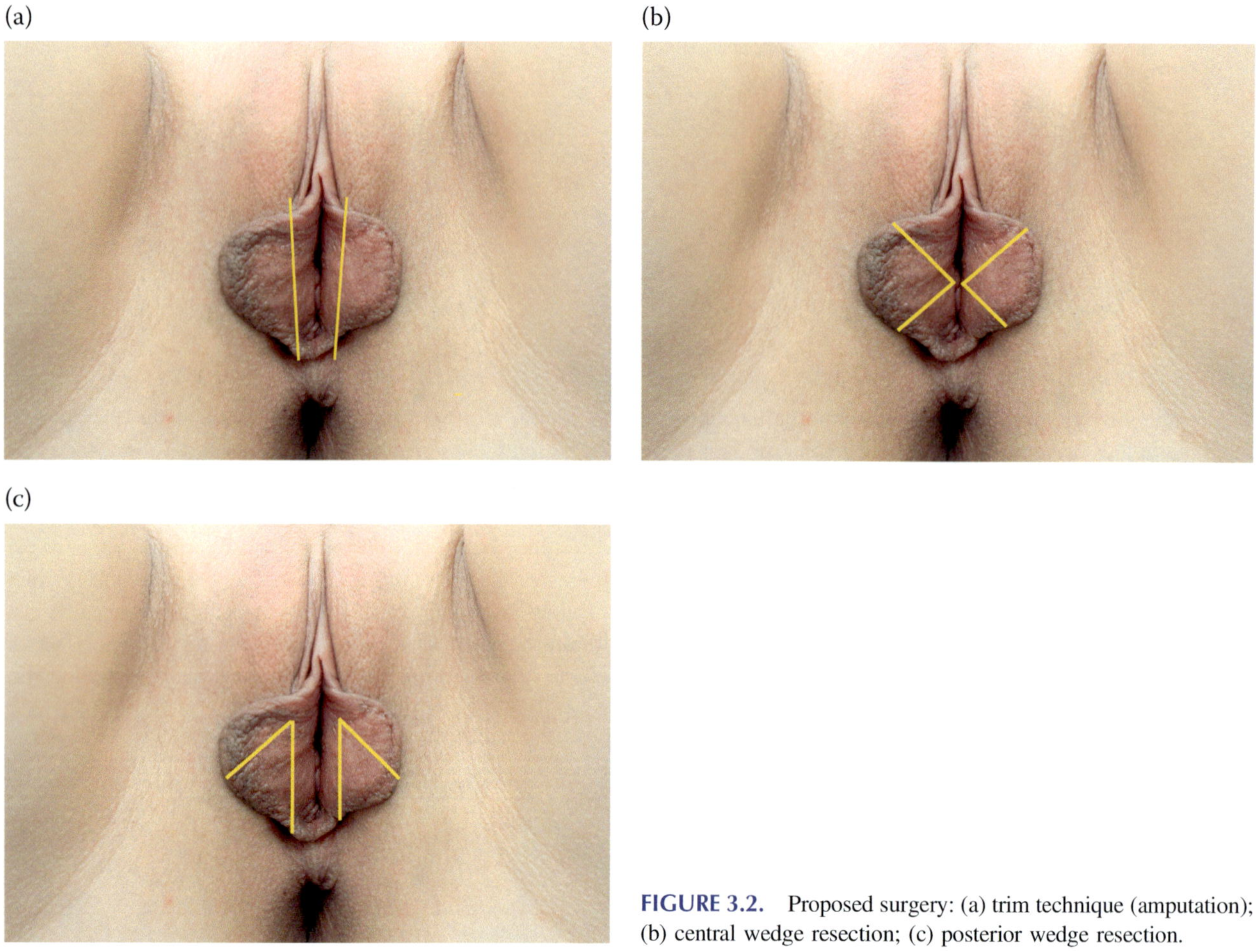

FIGURE 3.2. Proposed surgery: (a) trim technique (amputation); (b) central wedge resection; (c) posterior wedge resection.

The central wedge technique became a model for further modifications, which consisted in moving the wedge to the front or to the back, called anterior and posterior wedge resection, respectively. According to surgeons, the most commonly used techniques are simple amputation, central wedge resection, and posterior wedge resection (Fig. 3.2).

CENTRAL WEDGE RESECTION

This surgical technique can be performed under general, field block, or local anesthesia. It consists in resecting a triangle-shaped piece of tissue, with the top pointed at the base of the labia. The incision is perpendicular and made through all layers of the labia. Next, the surgeon places single sutures. In this case, a continuous suture would increase the risk of pulling in the tissue and permanently deforming the labium at the suture site. This technique is a relatively simple procedure, provided a few rules are followed. When choosing this surgical technique, it is important to remember that the outer surface of the labium should have a homogeneous colour and structure. The resected triangle should be equilateral in order to avoid the risk of the upper and lower stump of the labium not matching. The resection angle should exceed 60 degrees. A wider wedge increases the risk of disturbed healing due to excessive stress in both stumps. The most common reasons for dissatisfaction in patients who underwent the central wedge procedure stem from a visible difference between the sutured upper and lower stump of the labium, a visible transverse scar and a relatively common dehiscence of the labium at the incision site, which could require a secondary intervention (Fig. 3.3).

POSTERIOR WEDGE RESECTION

This technique is the most commonly chosen surgical technique for labia minora reductions due to its beneficial aesthetic effect and well-preserved function of the labia. The posterior wedge resection technique allows the surgeon to simultaneously perform a clitoral prepuce correction. During the surgery, the resected piece of tissue in the shape of a wedge is placed at the base, as shown in the picture. The superior, free margin of the labium should have the same length as the incision at the base. A straight incision is also performed transversely to the labium, through all its layers. In the case of clitoral prepuce reduction, a lateral incision is performed in the interlabial sulcus, above the clitoral glans, towards the anterior commissure of the labia majora. After preparing the tissue, layer suturing is performed. A properly performed suture should result in a scar hidden in the interlabial sulcus. It

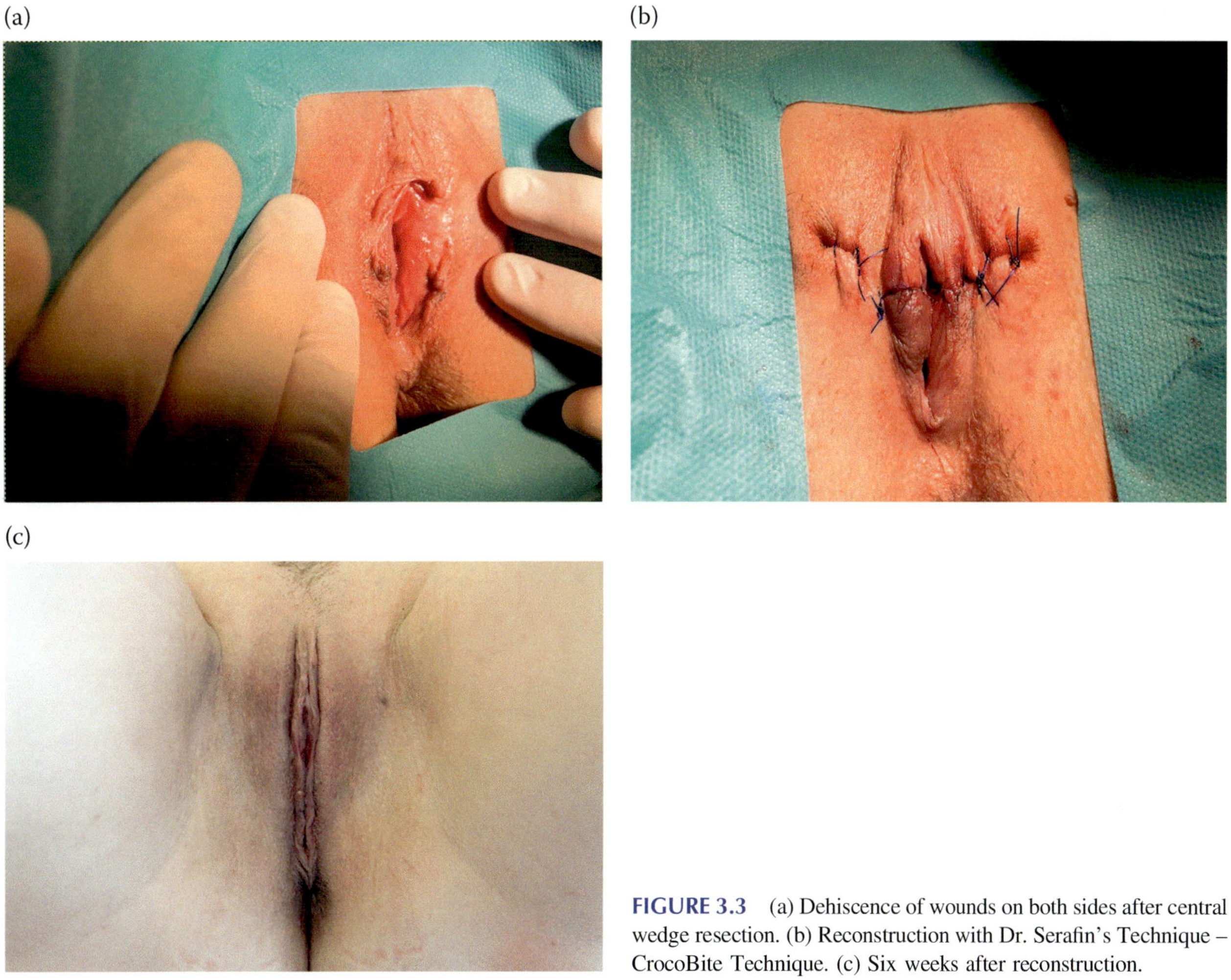

FIGURE 3.3 (a) Dehiscence of wounds on both sides after central wedge resection. (b) Reconstruction with Dr. Serafin's Technique – CrocoBite Technique. (c) Six weeks after reconstruction.

should be noted that this surgical technique comes with the largest destruction of natural vascularity, since the central artery of the labium minus and the two smaller posterior arteries are being cut, which results in heavy intra-operative bleeding. Excessive coagulation of large vessels can lead to vast necrotic areas, which prevents correct healing and can disrupt proper fusion of the tissue by

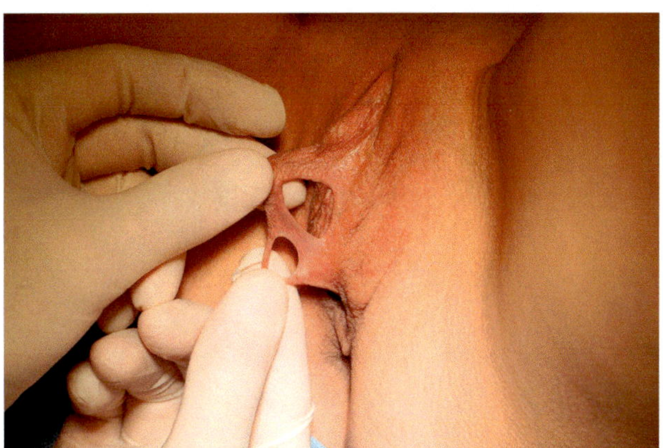

FIGURE 3.4 Labium minor after plastic surgery – Complications due to excessive coagulation.

forming visible holes in the labium (Fig. 3.4). Due to its aggressive nature, this technique is burdened with the highest complication rate (23%) amongst the presented techniques. This is a result of disrupting the vascularity of the leftover middle fold of the labium in the case of excessive reduction, which leads to necrosis of the distal labial stump. The most common cause of secondary interventions post-labial reduction is dehiscence of post-operative wounds (Fig. 3.5). This occurs due to excessive stress in the fold sutured to the basis of the amputated part of the labium in order to match the sutured sides symmetrically.

A rapid development in aesthetic gynecology allowed surgeons to fine-tune current surgical methods and create further modifications of the existent techniques. As a result, Gress presented his technique in 2013 [4], which is a hybrid posterior wedge resection with a partial amputation of the lower portion of the labia minora and a simultaneous correction of the clitoral prepuce. In 2014, Ostrzeński presented the fenestration technique, which allowed for an aesthetic correction of the labia minora and clitoral prepuce hypertrophy [5]. In 2017, during the 2nd European Society of Aesthetic Gynecology, the present author presented the new de-wedge surgical technique [6]

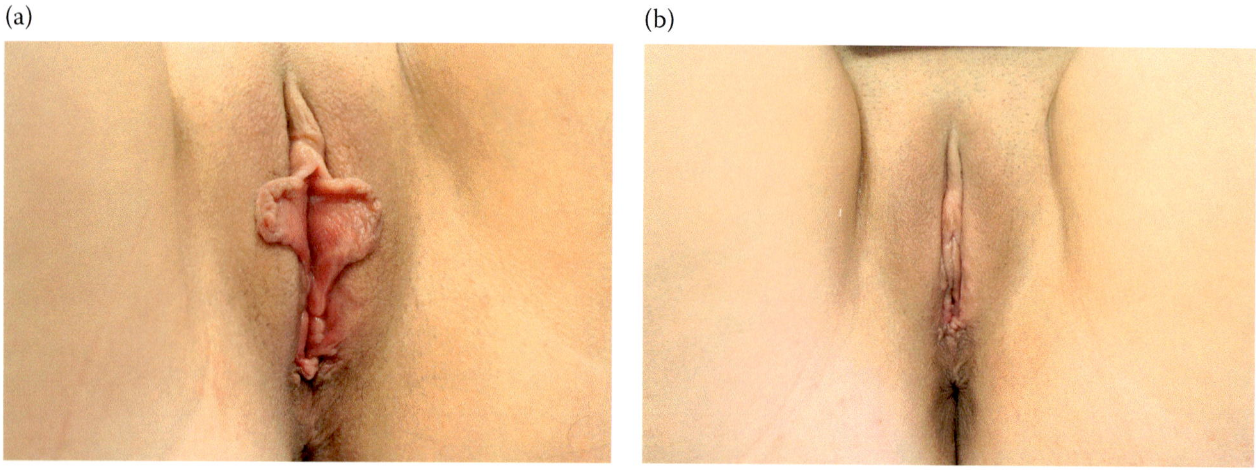

FIGURE 3.5 (a) Dehiscence of the wound after labiaplasty (posterior wedge resection) before reconstruction; (b) after reconstruction.

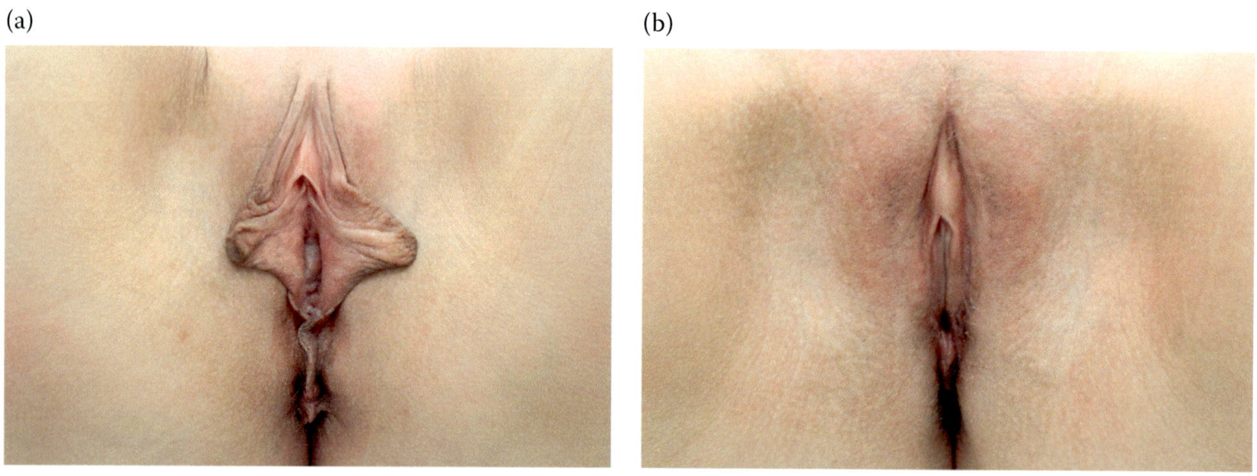

FIGURE 3.6 (a) Before labiaplasty (de-wedge technique); (b) 6 weeks after surgery.

(Fig. 3.6). It introduced an additional delamination of the marginal labial fold using a fish-hook incision. This reduction technique, which preserves a larger amount of the corpus spongiosum, enables an almost complete elimination of complications, such as necrosis at the top of labia and wound dehiscence.

REFERENCES

1. Radman HM. Hypertrophy of the labia minora. *Obstet Gynecol*. 1976 Jul; 48(1 Suppl): 78S–79S.
2. Laufer MR, Galvin WJ. Labia hypertrophy: A new surgical approach. *Adolesc Pediatr Gynecol*. 1995; 8: 39–41.
3. Alter GJ. A new technique for aesthetic labia minora reduction. *Ann Plast Surg*. 1998; 40(3): 287–290.
4. Gress S. Composite reduction labiaplasty. *Aesthet Plast Surg*. 2013; 37(4): 674–683.
5. Ostrzenski A. Fenestration labioreduction of the labium minus: A new surgical intervention concept. *ISRN Obstetr Gynecol*. 2014; 10.1155/2014/671068.
6. Serafin D. The de-wedge laser-based labiaplasty technique: Extended posterior wedge resection with de-epithelialization. *Gynecol Obstet*. 2018; 8. 10.4172/2161-0932-C3-029.

4 Curvilinear Technique

Alexander Bader

INTRODUCTION

To perform this technique, the surgeon will need to recognize that this is the indicated technique for the specific shape. Also, the surgeon must have skills on what and from where the excision will be done but also be able to use a precise cutting tool. Generally, curved linear excision provides patients with any degree of cosmetic appearance they desire but does not maintain the appearance of the dark and irregular edges. The more radical reductions are not possible with wedge techniques [1]. One of the most popular tools is the cutting laser. Surgeons can use radiofrequency (RF) fine needle, common electrocautery sharp tip, plasma cut, microplasma or just using the traditional cold surgical knife or scissors. The absolute fact is that surgeons must be able to use the tool that they are familiar with and know how to use it the best way. The precision of the cut differs between the devices. Some surgeons prefer to use more than one cutting device at the same surgery but for different purposes. The curvilinear technique seems to show better outcomes with a combination of RF and common electrocautery sharp tip/laser – RF to perform the incision and electrocautery sharp tip/laser to perform the excision and reach an excellent coagulation. Emerging evidence supports the increased safety, precision, functional, and aesthetics of RF labia minora labiaplasty, compared with other minora reduction procedures, performed by a properly trained and experienced practitioner [2].

The art of using the electrosurgery goes beyond that. Skilled surgeons are able to use the thermal heat released from the electrocautery tip or the laser head to sculpt the edges and modify the final shape of the labia. Variation of the wound closure also involves several techniques, tips, and tricks over each technique. The challenge is how to perform tissue closures by achieving great and symmetrical approximation but maintaining minimal tension, allowing for better blood flow and therefore less scaring.

CONSULTATION AND EVALUATION

This is one of the most important steps during the patient's journey of having labiaplasty. The patient needs to understand and take an active role when making the decision about undergoing any type of labiaplasty and equally choosing the curvilinear technique. The consultation must take place face to face with the prospective candidate. During the consultation, the surgeon needs to be able to demonstrate the way the procedure will be performed. After taking all the patient's records, the next step is the physical examination. This is a crucial point during the process as the patient is usually under stress, and she might not be able to cooperate as the surgeon needs. A relaxed environment is very important; staff acting as a chaperone has to be well trained and familiar with the process. The patient should be asked to change in privacy and lay on her back in a lithotomy position. The examiner must assure the candidate that the process is fast and has the objective to understand what she wants to achieve and what the surgeon can offer. The patient should be advised to hold a mirror so both the surgeon and she can discuss more in detail. The patient will be requested to show and point to what she doesn't like. Initially the examiner should unfold the labia and discuss the details with the patient while she is holding and looking at the mirror (Fig. 4.1). The examiner can refold the labia and bring them together showing the different

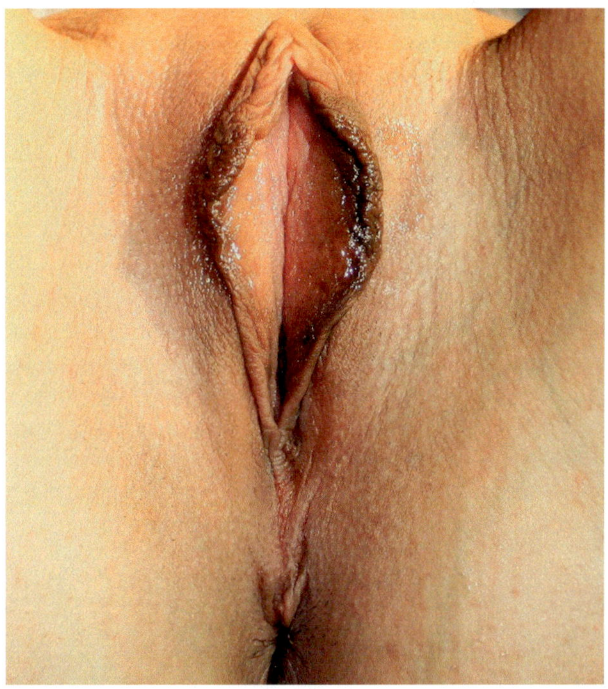

FIGURE 4.1 Labia minora examination in lithotomy, with unfolded labia.

DOI: 10.1201/9780429353079-4

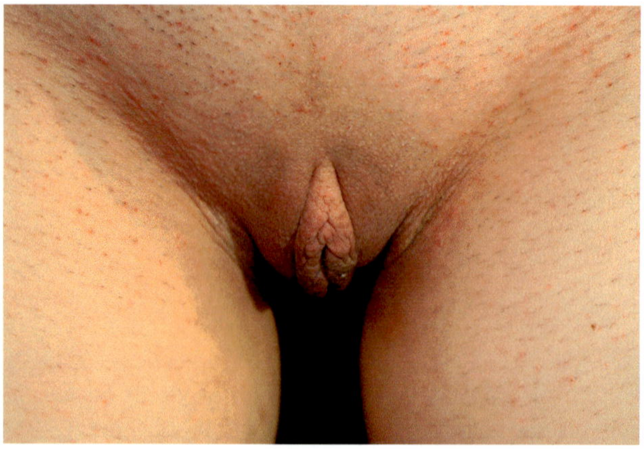

FIGURE 4.2 Examination in standing position.

length of both sides to the patient, and finally the examiner has the option to ask or suggest if the patient wishes to be examined in a standing position (Fig. 4.2). The following step is for the surgeon to show how much tissue will be removed. The most effective way is if the surgeon marks the area with a disposable medical skin marker. The surgeon must draw the entire labial tissue in a linear way but following the curves of the labia. The next step is to perform a "kissing" technique by stamping and attaching the marked labia on the unmarked one (Fig. 4.3). This way, the patient will be able to observe one of the surgeon's most important steps that will be done during the actual surgery. This action will show the patient herself where the cut will be done, show how much labial tissue will be preserved, but also confirm the surgeon's skills on how the symmetric results will be achieved. As mentioned, it is always recommended that the examination be completed with a standing position. This also allows both sides to understand how far the reduction can go. After the physical examination, the candidate shall attend a comprehensive discussion with the surgeon to go over all points and agree on what should be done in her case. Before and after photos need to be shown by the surgeon explaining the method and technique used to achieve the results. The session will end by answering questions and advising the steps forward. A cooling period should be honoured to allow some time for the patient to think and make a decision. Having a consultation and surgery on the same day is not recommended. Sometimes, the surgeon might provide a suggestion for the sake of reaching better results. This might combine labiaplasty with clitoral hood reduction or labia minora plasty with labia majora plasty combined, as prescribed by Miklos and Moore [3].

PRESURGICAL PREPARATION

The admission process should include a general health screen and pregnancy test. The patient has been advised to come with the area very well shaved. She also has been advised to bring with her a loose outfit so she feels comfortable going home after the surgery. The patient should sign an informed risks procedure consent form and a photography consent form and get prepared for photographs and marking the area. Photography should be taken before prepping the area, ideally both in lithotomy and in standing position captures. Prep the area with an antiseptic solution while the patient is comfortable in a lithotomy position.

TOOLS AND INSTRUMENTS

To perform the labiaplasty procedure, the surgeon must have prepared the surgery table. The standard set for minor surgeries includes needle holders, forceps, and scissors. The table should include:

- Monocryl 5/0
- Vicryl Rapid 5/0
- Diathermy attached to surgical pencil and Colorado dissection needle tip (Fig. 4.4)
- Radiofrequency cautery attached to rurgical pencil and RF Colorado tip (Fig. 4.5)
- Sterile skin marker

SURGICAL PERFORMANCE (STEP BY STEP)

Anaesthesia

- Local Anaesthesia

Thirty minutes before surgery, the patient places numbing cream (compounded topical anaesthetics of Benzocaine, Lidocaine, Tetracaine) directly on the labia and at the clitoral body. Local anaesthesia should be administrated directly to the labia; Marcaine 0.25% should be injected unmixed. The injections should be done under the marking lines using a 30 G needle. The area will appear slightly swollen, but it will still be possible to intervene. Sometimes it is necessary to reinforce the marking as this might otherwise disappear while injecting the local anaesthesia. It is highly recommended to anesthetize and operate directly on the same side; the other side should be done separately.

- I.V. sedation/general

This is a process usually performed by an anaesthetist, outside the scope of the current chapter.

Marking

Marking is one of the important skills the cosmetic surgeon must have. When it comes to the labia minora, marking is quite demanding, given the various shapes of the labia minora. The marking for simple and symmetrical labia minora starts medially and approximately 0.5–1 cm below the frenulum and extending down to the introitus. Usually, we need to stop marking when labial tissue

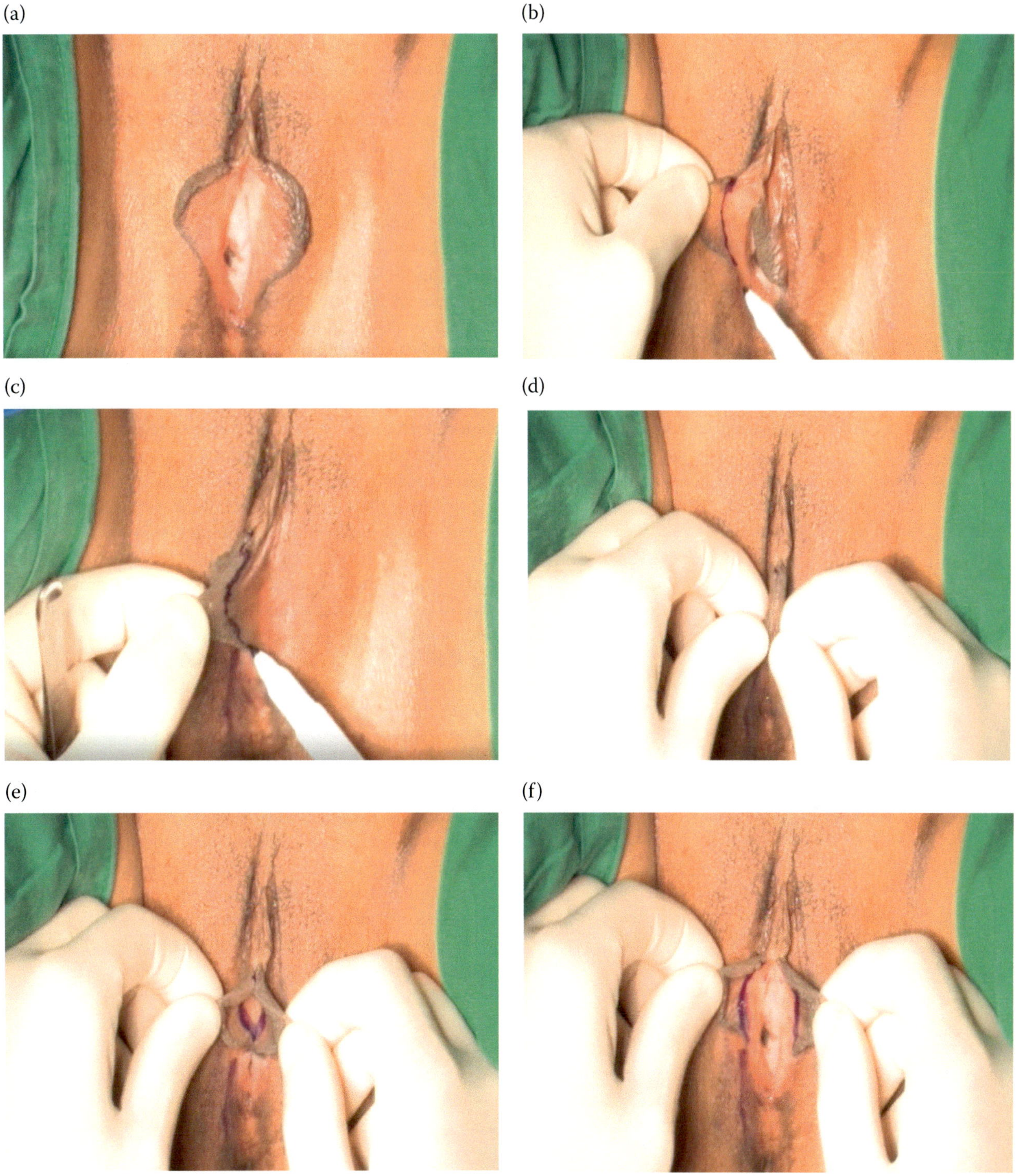

FIGURE 4.3 (a–f) Marking the labia starting slightly below the bifurcation, going linearly up to the lowest edge of the labia, from the outer part, and finishing with bringing both labia together to copy the marking from one side to the other one (the "Kissing" technique).

finishes at the introitus. Once one side has been fully marked, then we bring both labia together to allow copying the markings to the other labia with a perfect symmetry. Removal of slightly more medial minora while leaving a slightly wider lateral minora will result in a medially hidden surgical scar [2]. When the labia are asymmetric, we mark the shorter side first and copy it to the large side. This way we secure symmetry after the tissue excision and closure (Fig. 4.3).

Technique

Any atypical prepping and draping should be done. Photographs should be taken; the area should be marked out

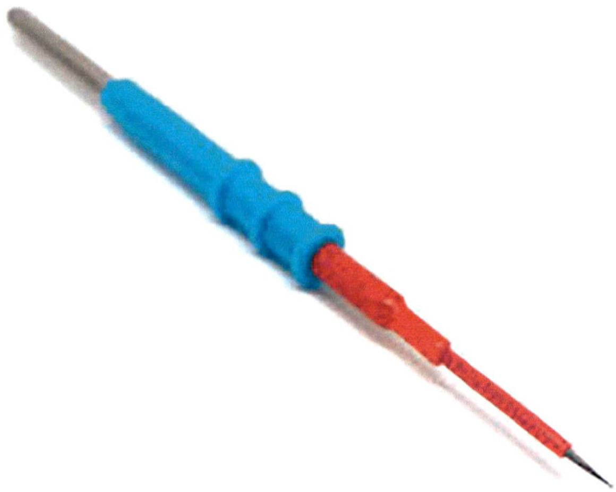

FIGURE 4.4 RF.

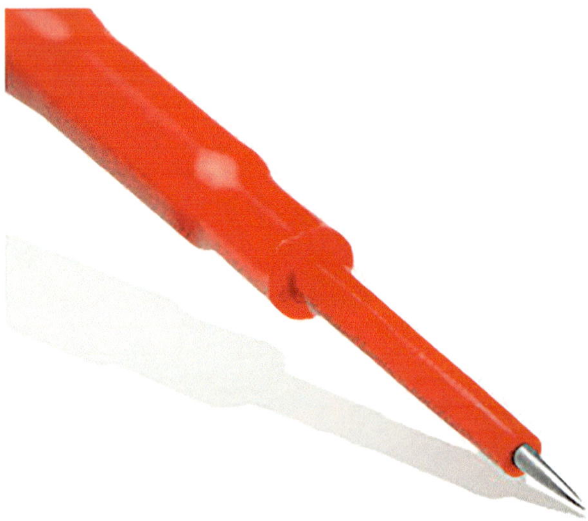

FIGURE 4.5 Cautery.

for surgery. If local anaesthesia is to be used, then approximately 5 mL of the anaesthetic is injected directly under the skin, specifically subcuticular under the markings; a 27–30 gauge needle is recommended. The best option is to inject the local anaesthetic just under the line of marking. It is recommended to start the infiltration from the lower part and go higher until reaching the bifurcation. It is always recommended to inject a small amount of anaesthesia at the frenulum as this part might become extremely painful and make the patient feel uncomfortable. Tissue can be substantially debulked by making an angled incisions toward the middle of the labia minora from the medial and lateral sides. This technique leaves a small "canal" that causes the edges of the minora to cling together as they fall medially toward it [4]. Tissue cutting will follow. The surgeons can use any tool they are familiar with. It is noticeable that fewer tissue disasters occur when using an RF fine tip (Fig. 4.4) and coagulating with a cautery Colorado tip (Fig. 4.5). Once haemostasis has been achieved, adjustments and refinements can be made by using the thermal heat of the cautery to even the edges or the thermal heat of the RF to slightly shrink the inner parts. RF does not carbonize the tissue, hence the safety of using it to shrink the inner parts.

Wound closure on such a soft tissue also requires high skill. The surgeon must be able to choose the correct and suitable tools and instruments on the surgical table. Labiaplasty does not require any complicated instrument, but using the correct ones plays a crucial part in the final outcome. Using absorbable Monocryl 5–0 seems to be the best option to close the deep layers of the surgical wound alongside the medial and superficial layers. Some surgeons prefer 5-0 Vicryl or Vicryl Rapid-type sutures. However, Monocryl has much less inflammatory reaction and therefore topical reaction in the surgical wound. My technique involves using Monocryl 5/0 running and unlocked on two layers, and I use Vicryl Rapid 5/0 just to approximate the edges superficially at the end of the procedure. The actual suturing technique starts with inserting the stitches subcutaneously and burying them at the low end of the surgical wound. Subsequently, perform the closure in a running unlocked technique at the deep layers to eliminate the dead space. Once you have reached the top of the surgical wound, one lock should be made; you then go back again with subdermal-to-subdermal closure (this also should be running and unlocked). Smooth and loose approximation is recommended to avoid strangulation and microvessel obstruction. You should perform a smooth, gentle massage on the labia, whenever possible, to spread the thread and avoid any shrinkage. Monocryl thread has the beauty of spreading easily when massaged. Once you reach the low end, you need to secure with the initial buried edge. In principle, Monocryl needs to be locked five times to be secure. (See Video 4.1: Curvilinear labiaplasty.)

Frequently, the hypertrophic labia minora are a continuation of hypertrophic excess skin at the lateral sides of the clitoral hood. In this case, it is indicated to perform a slightly modified procedure that includes the reduction of this excess skin on the same cut of the labia minora. Technically, in this case, the surgeon has to start the reduction from a higher level, basically at the lateral prepuce of the clitoral area. A superficial trim should be performed here, which gets thicker as we descend towards the bifurcation and the labia themselves. It is important to perform such a variation in the surgery when needed. Alternatively, the patient might end up with a hat-shaped excess skin overlapping the reduced labia minora. This can cause major distress to the patient when they realize it as it shows an extremely protruded shape that patients describe as a "mini penis". The surgical intervention is like the typical curvilinear technique. On many occasions, labia majora enhancement might be considered to balance the protrusion even after the surgery. The filling can be done either by injectable hyaluronic acid or by autologous fat transfer. Both options can be performed at the same time as the labiaplasty. (See Video 4.2: Extended linear labiaplasty.)

(a) (b)

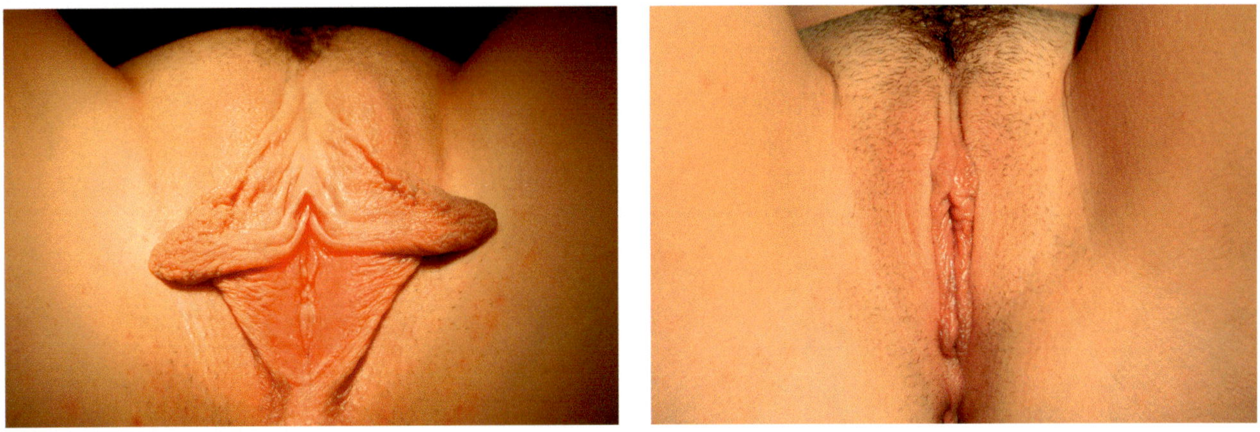

FIGURE 4.6 Case 1: (a) before and (b) after.

(a) (b)

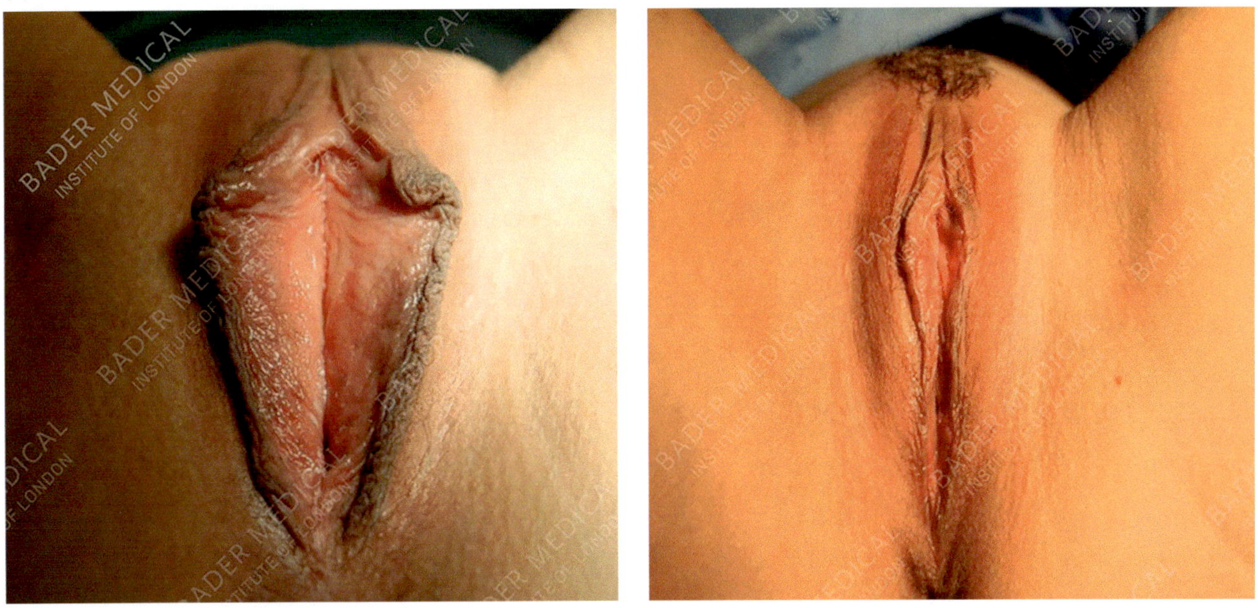

FIGURE 4.7 Case 2: (a) before and (b) after.

Postoperative Care

The patient is advised to avoid physical exercise, swimming, and sexual intercourse for 6–8 weeks. Cleaning and drying the area are mandatory as some patients are reluctant to clean the area. Washing with tap water without using any special products protects the sutures from early dissolve. Drying by tapping the area with a clean towel followed by using the hair dryer for a few minutes is very helpful. Medium temperature is recommended to achieve dryness. The patient is advised to leave the area free and not covered. Avoid touching the wound with nails or naked fingers. A course of oral antibiotics, NSAIDs, and topical antibiotic ointment (Fucidin Oint) should be prescribed. Estradiol cream can also be prescribed as it helps in the healing process. On a few occasions, we recommend applying zinc powder to speed the healing. Platelet-rich plasma (PRP) can also be used to improve the speed and quality of the healing. PRP can be applied immediately after the surgery and be repeated when the patient returns after 2 months for her third follow-up visit. Advise cessation of smoking before the surgery takes place; we need to make it clear to patients that their quality of healing might be affected. The standard post operative follow-up schedule is a visit 1 week after the surgery, a visit 1 month after the surgery, and one more visit 2 months after the surgery. This might be modified based on the progress of the healing and recovery. It is highly recommended to inform the patient that the final results might take up to 6 months to show and up to 2 years to be final. The process of healing differs between patients and depends on many factors.

(a) (b)

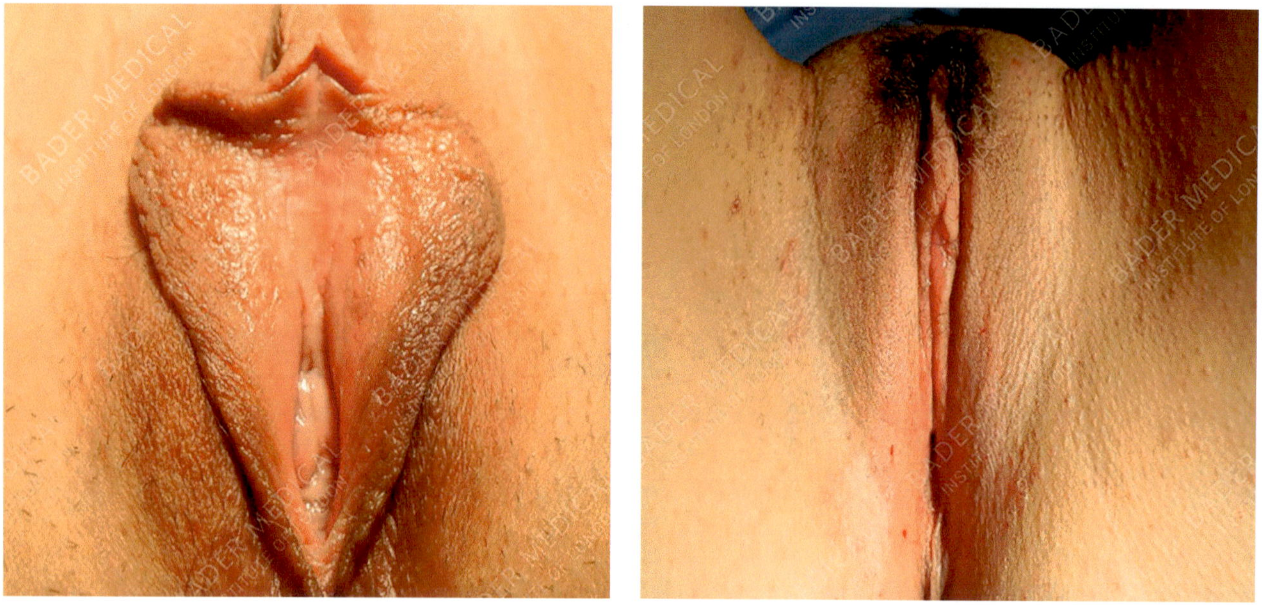

FIGURE 4.8 Case 3: (a) before and (b) after.

(a) (b)

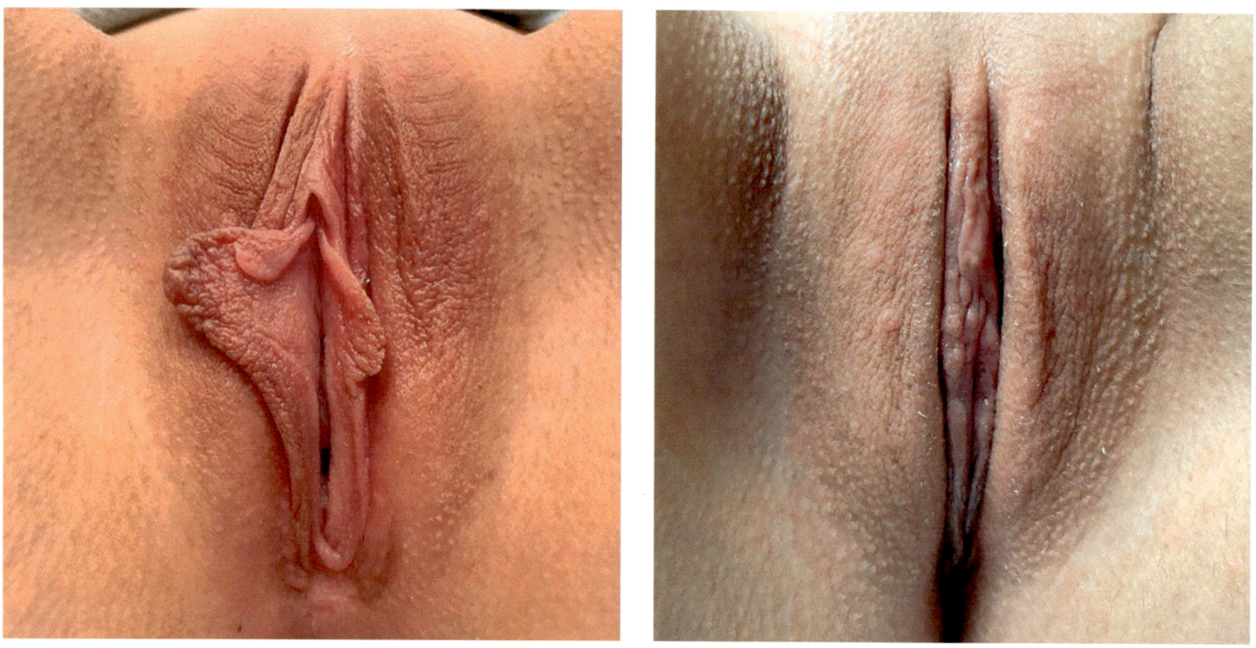

FIGURE 4.9 Case 4: (a) before and (b) after.

Complications

Adverse effects linked with labia minora reductions overall have been very low, ranging from 2.65% [1] to 4% [2,5] and 6% [6]. Complications associated with labiaplasties include postoperative infection [7], hematoma [7–9], infection, asymmetry, poor wound healing, premature suture absorption or breakage, under correction or overcorrection [8,10], urinary retention [8–10], skin retraction [11], late local pain, and transient dyspareunia [4]. Dyspareunia occurred primarily when the labial suturing involved the introitus [4]. In a case report, the wedge excision technique was associated with postoperative complications of bleeding and transient hypersensitivity for 4 to 6 weeks after surgery [5]. A running

(a) (b)

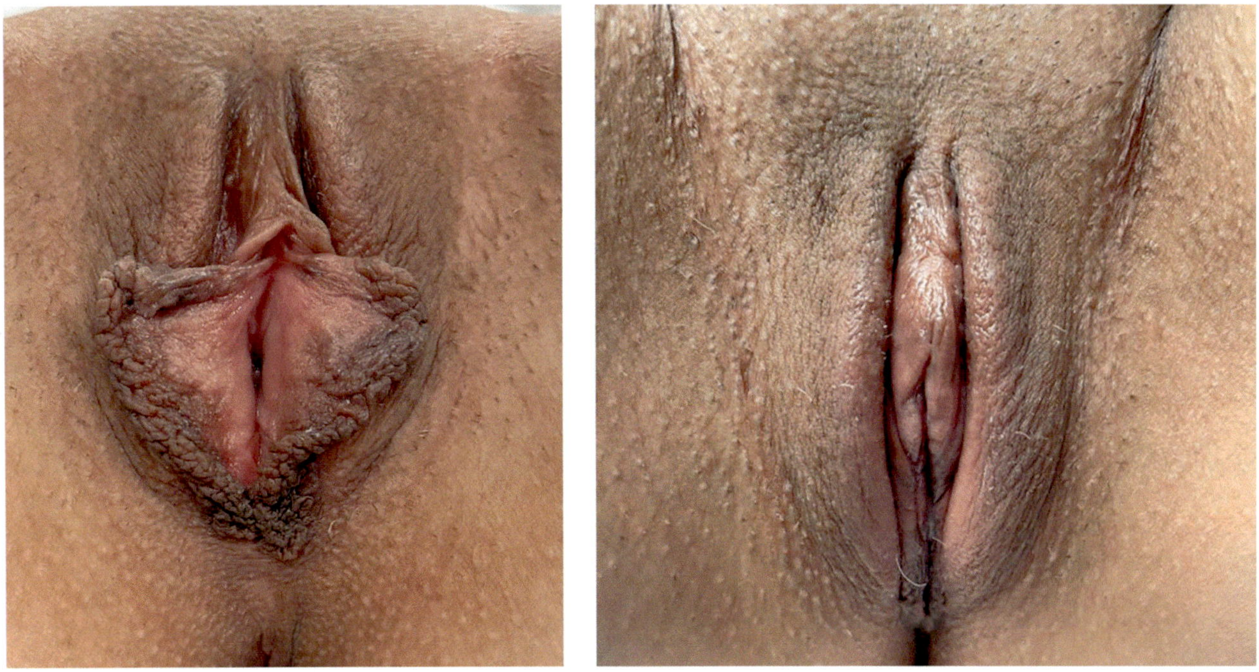

FIGURE 4.10 Case 5: (a) before and (b) after.

absorbable rather than buried suture can lead to scalloping along the free border of the labia minora [8,10]. There are few statistics on revision surgeries of labiaplasties, but overcorrection and under correction potentially can occur in any labia minora reduction procedure [11]. Studies of labia minora labiaplasties reveal high rates of overall satisfaction with cosmetic and functional results and psychosocial outcomes, including improved self-esteem [6,8,12,13].

Figures 4.6–4.10 illustrate clinical cases and results.

REFERENCES

1. Hamori CA, Banwell P, Alinsod R, eds. *Female Cosmetic Genital Surgery: Concepts, Classifications, and Techniques*. Thieme, New York, 2017.
2. Alter GJ. Aesthetic labia minora and clitoral hood reduction using extended central wedge resection. *Plast Reconstr Surg* 122:1780, 2008.
3. Miklos JR, Moore RD. Postoperative cosmetic expectations for patients considering labiaplasty surgery: Our experience with 550 patients. *Surg Technol Int* 21:170, 2011.
4. Alinsod R. Awake in-office Barbie labiaplasty. Awake in-office labia minora plasty, awake in-office labia majora plasty, awake in-office vaginoplasty, awake in-office labial revision, sutureless band release, awake In-office mesh excision, labia majora pelleve. Presented at the Congress of Aesthetic Gynaecology, Tuscon, AZ, 2011.
5. Trichot C, Thubert T, Faivre E, et al. Surgical reduction of hypertrophy of the labia minora. *Int J Gynaecol Obstet* 115:40, 2011.
6. Goodman MP, Placik OJ, Benson RH III, et al. A large multicenter outcome study of female genital plastic surgery. *J Sex Med* 7 (4Pt 1):1565, 2010.
7. Tepper OM, Wulkan M, Matarasso A. Labioplasty: Anatomy, etiology and new surgical approach. *Aesthet Surg* 31:511, 2011.
8. Davison SP, West JE, Baker CL, et al. Labiaplasty and labia minora reduction. *Medscape*. https://reference.staging.medscape.com/article/1372175-overview
9. Solanki NS, Tejero-Trujeque R, Stevens-King A, et al. Aesthetic and functional reduction of the labia minora using the Maas and Hage technique. *J Plast Reconstructive Surg* 63;1181, 2010.
10. Alinsod R. Review of vaginal rejuvenation: A new frontier in pelvic surgery. Presented at the Annual Meeting of National Society of the American Academy of Cosmetic Gynaecologists, Las Vegas, NV, Sep 2006.
11. Alter GJ. Labia minora reconstruction using clitoral hood flaps, wedge excisions and YV advancement flaps. *Plast Reconstr Surg* 127:2356, 2011.
12. Goodman MP. Female genital cosmetic and plastic surgery: A review. *J Sex Med* 8:1813, 2011.
13. Goodman MP. Female genital cosmetic and plastic surgery. *Obstet Gynecol* 113:154, 2009.

5 Hybrid Labiaplasty

Rafal Kuzlik

Hybrid labiaplasty means that different techniques are mixed to reduce the labia minora and clitoral hood simultaneously during one procedure. A similar idea of simultaneous labia and hood reduction procedure is described in Chapter 7 on deepitheliazation (the "one-cut technique"), but here I would like to present a true surgical hybrid – "Linear Z technique". It is a mix of two different techniques: curvilinear resection of labia minora (classic technique – "edge resection") and simultaneous clitoral hood reduction ("one-cut technique").

Alinsod described his hybrid labiaplasty method in his book, but in his view, "hybrid" means a type of look of the labia after the procedure. In his opinion, the hybrid look refers to a middle-road approach involving removing nearly all the labia minora and preservation of a small "peekaboo" (below or to the level of the labia majora) amount of tissue [1]. Of course, the idea of simultaneous procedures in labia minora and the clitoral hood protrusion is not new. Gress described his method as composite reduction labiaplasty [2]. However, his technique consists of two cut lines and two scars afterwards – one longitudinal (labia minora) and one transverse (clitoral hood) (Fig. 5.1). In my opinion, more than one scar is worse than one, and this question should be discussed with the patient.

Sometimes we have to make two incisions – one for labia minora excision and one for clitoral hood reduction.

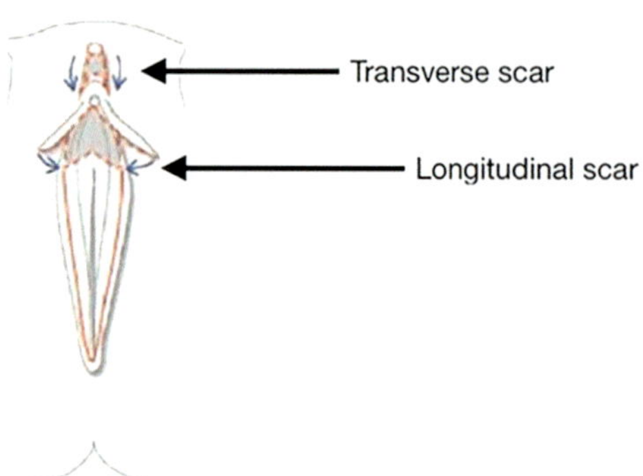

FIGURE 5.1 Gress technique of *composite reduction labiaplasty* (two perpendicular scars). (From Ref. [2], with permission, with annotations.)

In cases where the dark edges of the labia minora are unacceptable for the patient and there is protrusion of the clitoris and its hood, the double approach is obligated, and the surgeon needs to reduce two sides – first a hood reduction from the side and then a labia reduction from frontal access (Fig. 5.2). Although we have two cut lines, they are running longitudinally, and because the vulva is the longitudinal organ, scars will be almost invisible. In my opinion, any transverse scars should not be created on a longitudinal organ.

Another example of a transverse scar appears in central wedge excision of the labia minora, described by Gary Alter in 2008 [3]. In his technique, labia minora are reduced in their central part. The V shape of the skin and mucosa are excised without underlying subcutaneous tissues. Wounds on both sides are closed with interrupted stitches. This last fact is also, in my opinion, not to be accepted because after the stitches have dissolved small, multiple scars will remain. Of course, the transversal

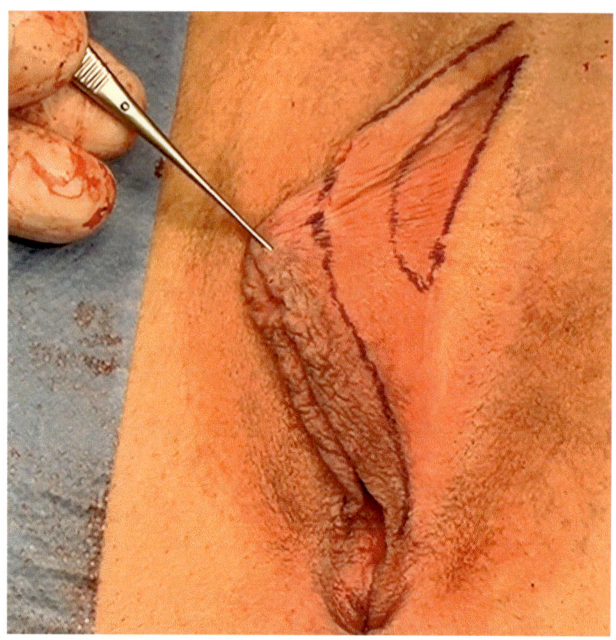

FIGURE 5.2 Labia minora and clitoral hood reduction with two longitudinal cut lines.

DOI: 10.1201/9780429353079-5

(a) (b)

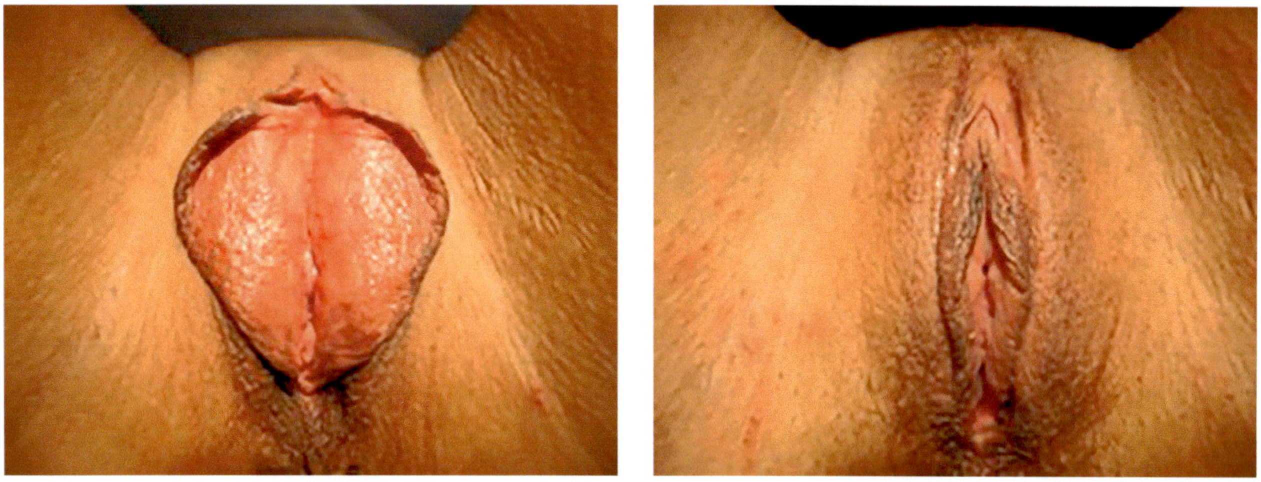

FIGURE 5.3 (a) Before and (b) after posterior wedge resection of labia minora with longitudinal running sutures.

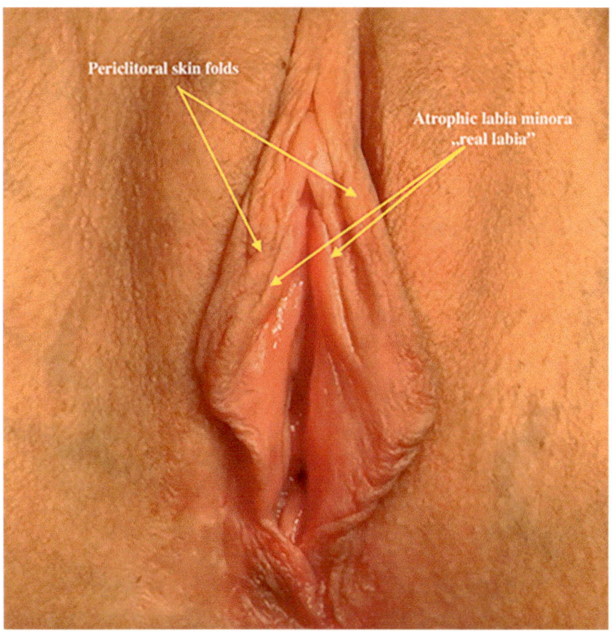

FIGURE 5.4 Overgrown labia minora are created by periclitoral skin folds.

wound is impossible close using running suture, which is why when I perform the wedge resection procedure, I always perform the posterior wedge, where cut lines are longitudinal and running sutures are obligatory (Fig. 5.3).

Everybody knows that a universal technique for every patient does not exist. One question appeared in my mind when I met a patient with overgrown labia minora and clitoral hood. To be honest, the "real" labia were very small, almost atrophic, but the periclitoral skin folds were so prominent that they created labia (Fig. 5.4). The labial structure is based on the fact that "real" labia have their roots; they grow out of the clitoral frenulum. In this case, the central mass and actual shape of the labia minora are the folds of the clitoral hood (periclitoral folds) running on both sides of the clitoris, optically and physically enlarging this area, creating a small penis in a standing position of the patient, which was very embarrassing for her. This kind of labia can be indicated by the one-cut technique, but this procedure could be challenging for a not-yet-experienced surgeon. This is why I created a new surgery method, more manageable than the one-cut technique and with a broader spectrum than ordinary edge resection.

The linear Z technique is dedicated primarily for beginners who want to make a simultaneous reduction of the labia minora and clitoral hood and want to avoid two scars, but the one-cut technique is too tricky for them. This new method was presented for the first time in 2019. Thanks to this procedure, the labia minora are reduced in their height, their shape, and the colour of the edges, and the clitoral hood is reduced in its height and shape, simultaneously.

INDICATIONS AND CONTRAINDICATIONS

The patient indicated for this hybrid method needs to have protrusion of labia minora and clitoral hood. Of course, the surgeon always needs to consider which method is the best to use, but if the "real labia" are atrophic and curvilinear

(a) (b)

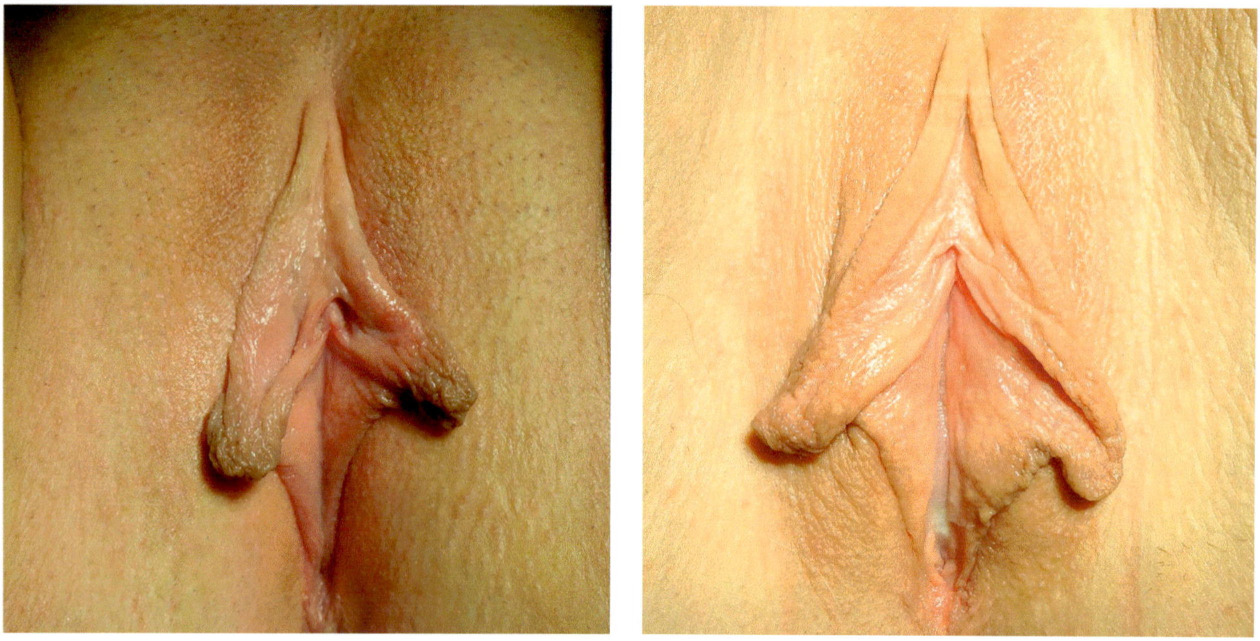

FIGURE 5.5 (a, b) Patient properly qualified for linear Z technique, with protruded labia minora and clitoral hood.

(a) (b)

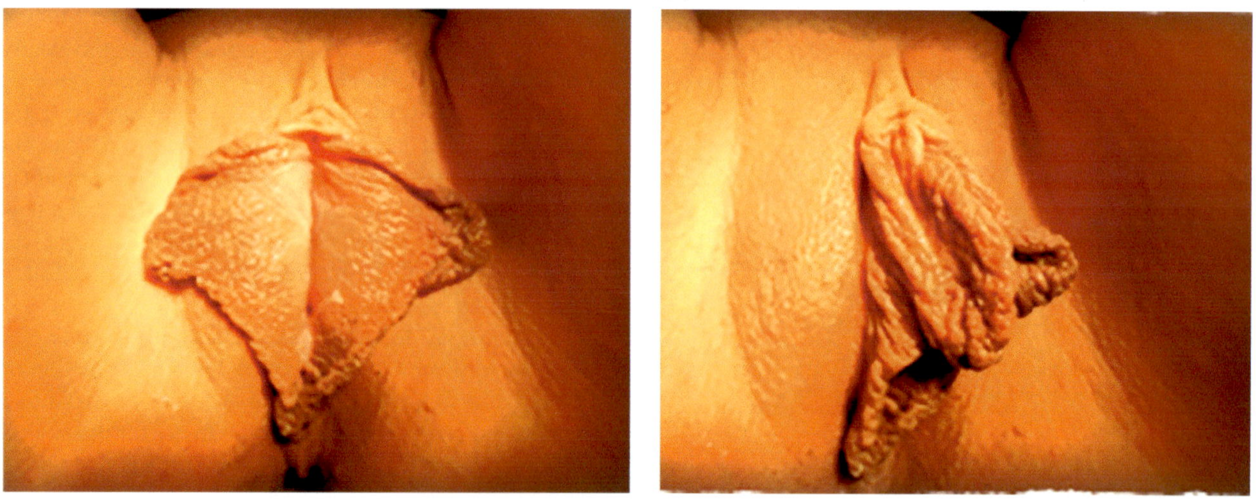

FIGURE 5.6 (a, b) Patient who would *not* qualify for linear Z technique with protruded labia minora without clitoral hood protrusion.

(a)

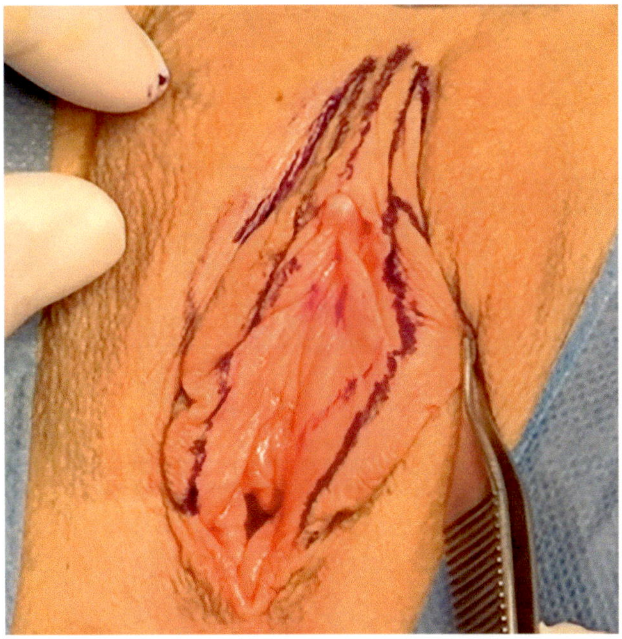

(b)

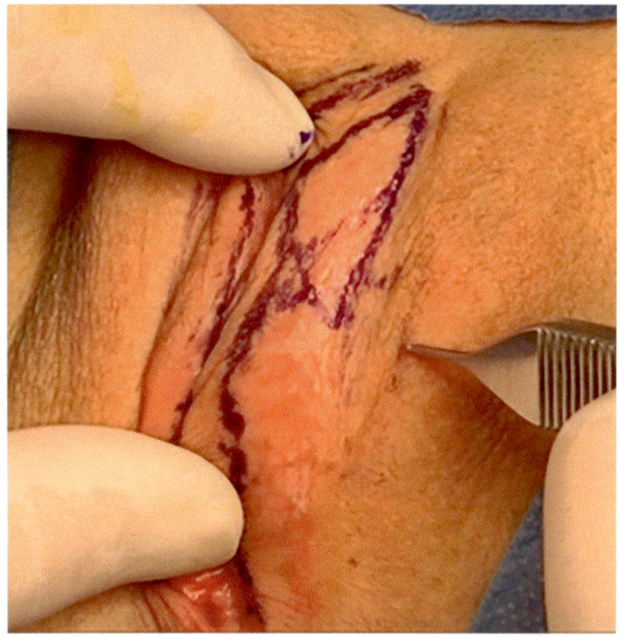

(c)

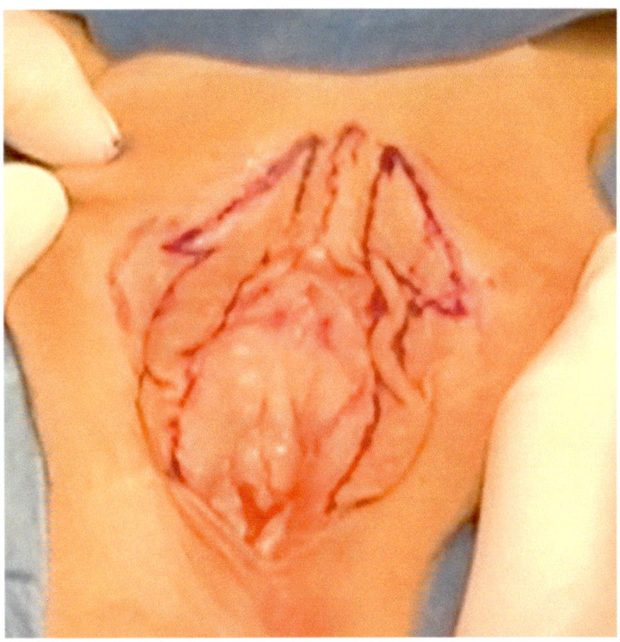

FIGURE 5.7 (a) Longitudinal line runs up from the fossa navicularis region towards the top of the clitoral hood (inside of the labia). (b) At the clitoral glans level, the diagonal line departs from the longitudinal one (outside of the labia), turns up and run towards the top of the clitoral hood. (c) Markings presented on both sides of the labia minora and clitoral hood.

resection seems to be the best way but a protruded clitoral hood causes a problem, the linear Z technique should be taken into consideration (Fig. 5.5).

A patient with protruded labia minora without clitoral hood protrusion should not be qualified for this surgical method; neither should a patient with “double labia minora” when “real labia” are not atrophic (Fig. 5.6). Such patients should proceed with the one-cut technique.

Patient evaluation and all preoperative procedures are the same as those described in Chapter 7 about the de-epithelialization technique.

TECHNIQUE OF SURGICAL PROCEDURE

As was described previously, the first important step is to determine the size of the labia minora and clitoral hood

(a) (b) (c) (d) (e) (f)

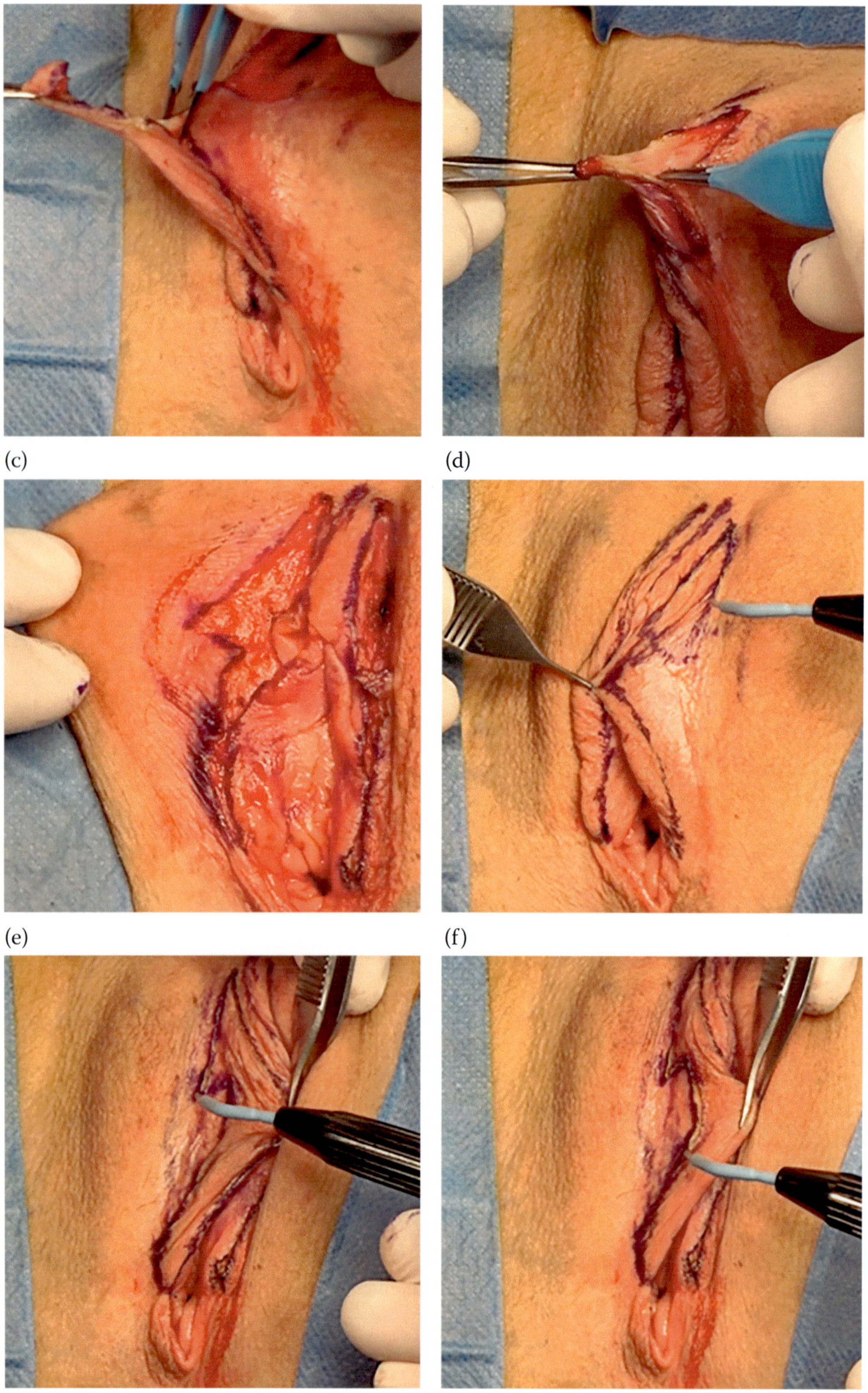

FIGURE 5.8 Labial skin is being cut inside (a, b) and outside (c) with a very straight cut line; (d,e) skin of the clitoral hood is also cut and (f) the letter "Z" has been created.

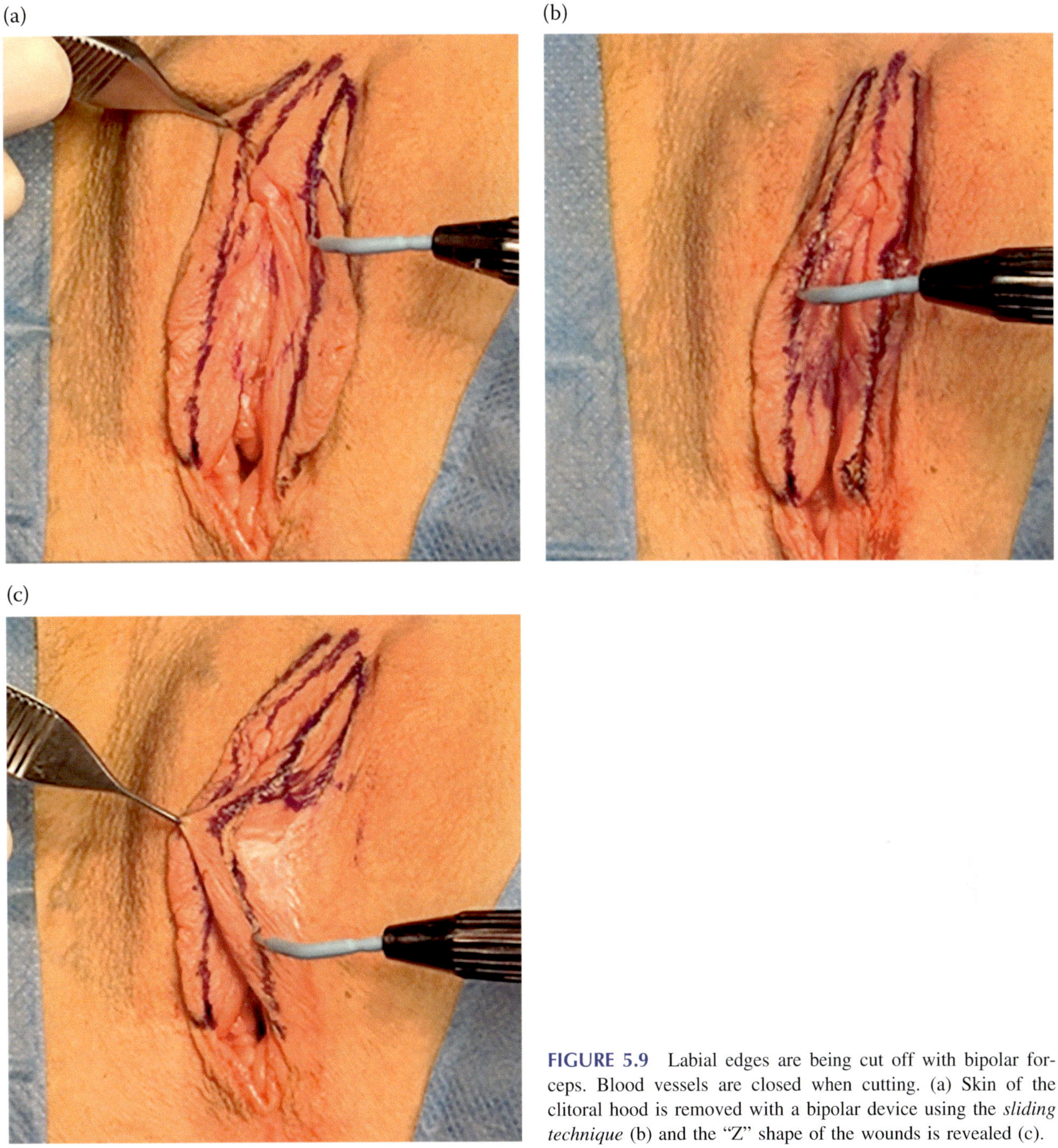

FIGURE 5.9 Labial edges are being cut off with bipolar forceps. Blood vessels are closed when cutting. (a) Skin of the clitoral hood is removed with a bipolar device using the *sliding technique* (b) and the "Z" shape of the wounds is revealed (c).

to be reduced. All margins of the future incisions need to be determined and marked. The longitudinal line runs along the edge of the labia from the region of fossa navicularis towards the top of the clitoral hood from inside and to the level of the clitoral glans from outside of the labia, where the diagonal line departs from the described longitudinal one and crosses the clitoral hood in a Z-shape to its base. At this point, the line turns up and then goes to the top of the clitoral hood, joining the previously drawn longitudinal line, forming a

(a) (b)

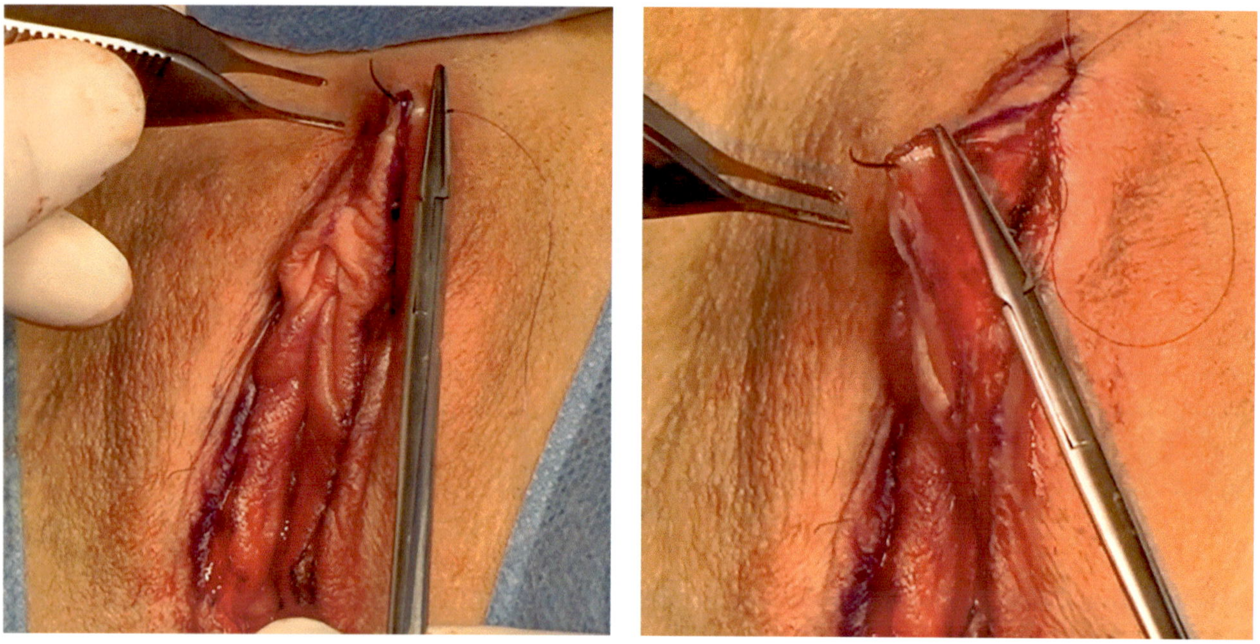

FIGURE 5.10 (a) Sharp end of the letter "Z" (a) is sewn to (b) the base of the periclitoral fold incision.

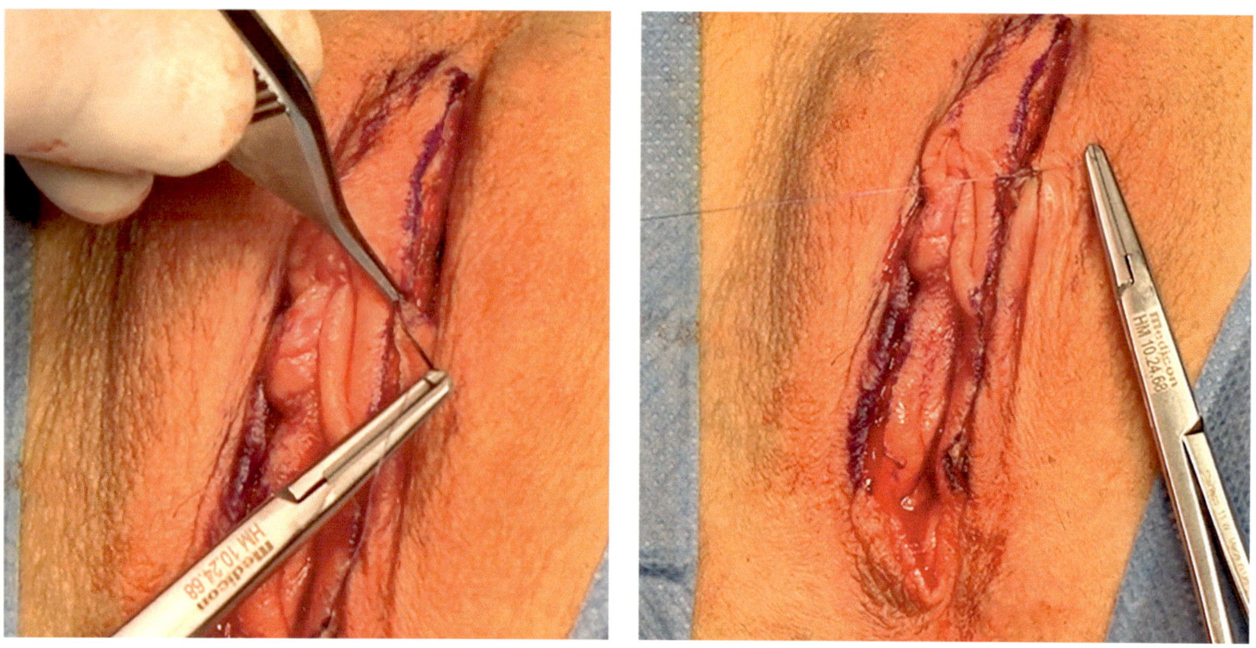

FIGURE 5.11 Wound edges are sewn with running suture, which starts at the top of the clitoral hood.

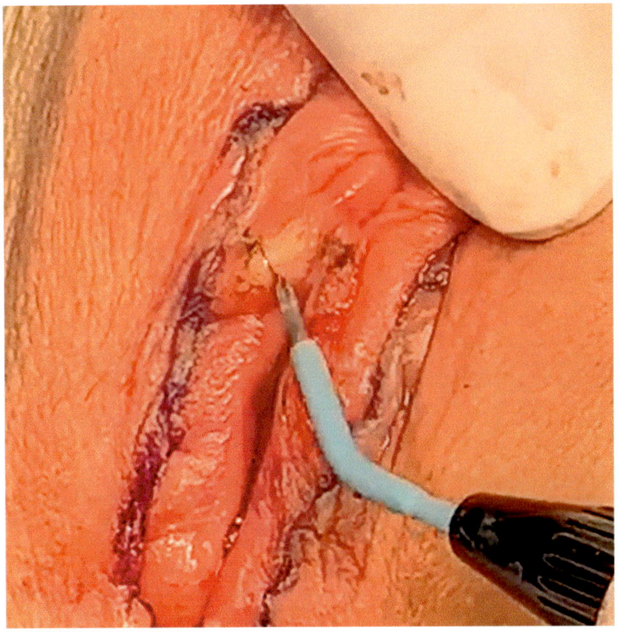

FIGURE 5.12 Feathering technique is the best method for removing remains of atrophic labia minora.

triangle (Fig. 5.7). The planning stage is one of the most important and determines the final aesthetic effect of the treatment.

The procedure is performed under local anaesthesia. The anaesthetic solution is the same as when the one-cut technique is being performed. Because this technique is very similar to curvilinear edge resection, the surgeon does not need to do the blockade of pudendal and inguinal nerves. It is enough when the injection is performed along the previously marked cut line of the labia, just below the markings. The clitoral hood is infiltrated like it is during the one-cut technique.

In technical terms, the surgeon cuts the skin of the labia from the inside along the previously drawn lines from the mons pubic towards the perineum (it is also possible to cut the opposite way – bottom to the top). A similar cutting direction is performed on the outer side of the labia, but at the level of the clitoral glans the incision runs diagonally backwards, forming the letter "Z". Next, from the top of the first incision the cut is made downwards towards the base of this letter "Z", closing the clitoral hood's skin triangle, which is cut out with bipolar forceps using the sliding technique. Similarly, with this tool, the edges of the labia are cut out. Thanks to the bipolar device, all blood vessels are being closed when cutting (Figs. 5.8 and 5.9). Cutting is performed with a radiofrequency knife. Thanks to this device, the incision line is very straight, regardless of the folds in the tissues; the depth of the incision is easy to assess; and the thermal injuries of the wound edges are minimal, which is crucial for proper healing without leaving visible scars.

In the next move the "sharp end" of the letter "Z" is sewn to the base of the periclitoral fold's incision, what became the beginning of the new labia minora (Fig. 5.10). The edges of the wound are sewn together with a running suture (Monocryl 5.0) in such a way that the skin of the clitoral hood is sewn to its base, creating a new hood with a smooth surface and "hidden" between the labia majora and new labia minora gain a new, regular edge (Fig. 5.11). Sewing runs from the top of the clitoral hood (mons pubic area) down towards the fossa navicularis.

When sewing ends, the surgeon needs to remove the remains of the atrophic labia minora. Alinsod's feathering technique seems to be the most adequate to achieve this effect [1] (Fig. 5.12). It should be done to make the inside of the new labia minora smooth.

The suture material used for the procedure is fully absorbable, and the use of intradermal, running suturing excludes the need to remove sutures in the postoperative period. Thanks to this technique, we achieve two goals simultaneously – reducing the labia minora and reducing the volume of the clitoral hood. The use of a single cutting line running along the edge of the labia minora and at the base of the clitoral hood allows for the natural appearance of the labio-clitoral complex. This technique, like the one-cut technique, treats the labia minora and the clitoral hood as one compartment, not as two separate ones, as happens in the case of the classic technique used so far, in which different cuts reduce the size of the labia minora and the clitoral hood. Using the "linear Z" technique, the result looks natural (Fig. 5.13).

POSTOPERATIVE CARE AND COMPLICATIONS

Post-op proceedings are similar to those described in Chapter 7, which describes the same situation with postoperative complications. (See Video 5.1: Hybrid labiaplasty – Linear Z.)

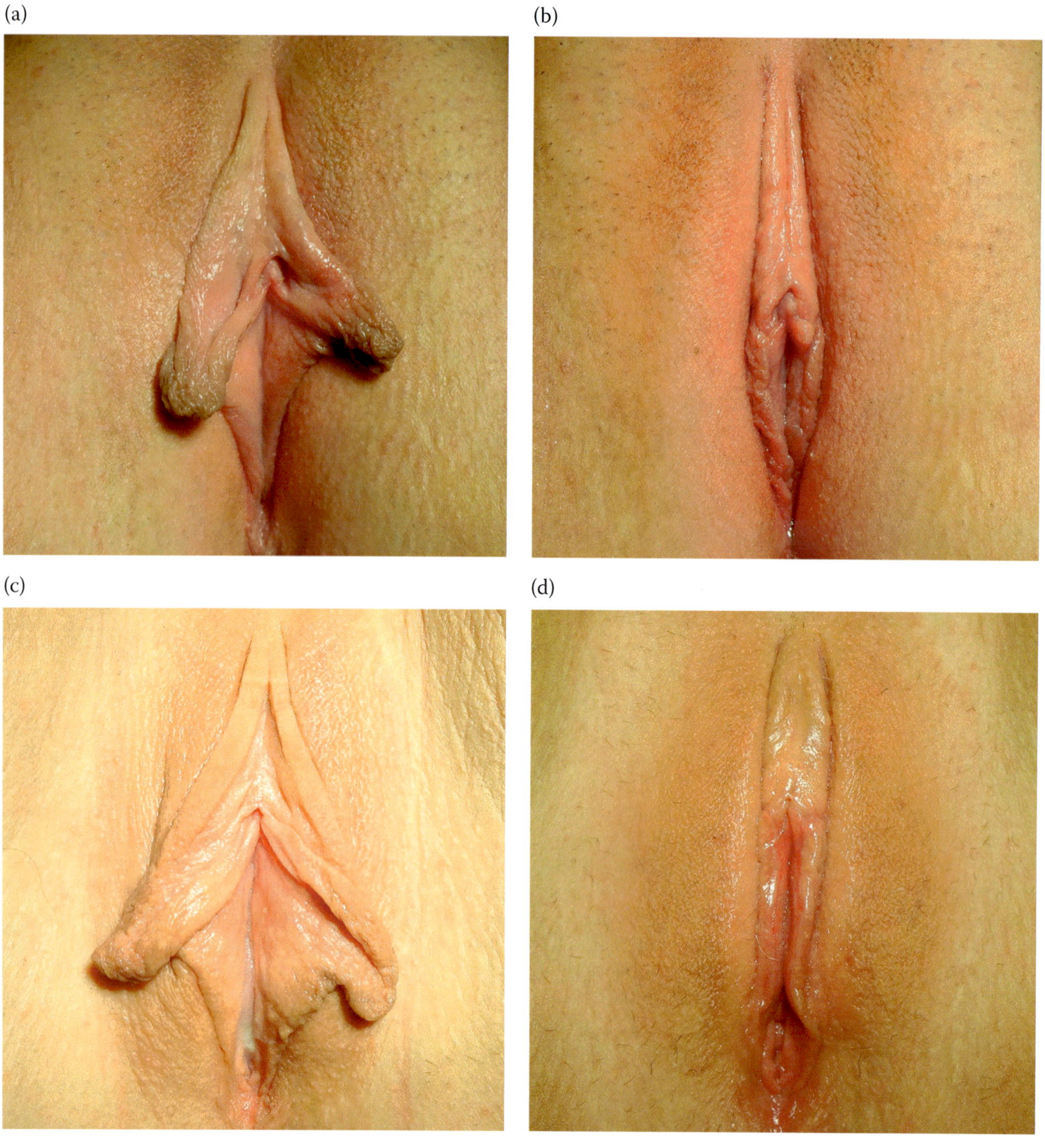

FIGURE 5.13 (a, c) Before and (b, d) after; the effect looks natural.

REFERENCES

1. Hammori CA, Banwell PE, Alinsod R. *Female Cosmetic Genital Surgery*. Thieme, New York, 2017:161–180.
2. Gress S. Composite reduction labiaplasty. *Aesthetic Past Surg* 37:674, 2013.
3. Alter GJ. Aesthetic labia minora and clitoral hood reduction using extended central wedge resection. *Past Reconstr Surg* 122:1780, 2008.

6 Deepithelialization Technique of Labia Minora Reduction

Rafal Kuzlik

Hypertrophic labia minora is a widespread problem nowadays, especially with sporty and sexually active women. The most common symptoms patients suffer from are persistent irritation with discomfort during physical activities or associated with rubbing while wearing close-fitting underwear, riding a bicycle or horseback riding; difficulties with maintaining hygiene; dyspareunia during sexual intercourse; and – critically – poor psychological condition caused by negative body image leading to decreased self-confidence, anxiety and social phobia, not only during female – male relations but also during other situations. The youngest group of patients usually claim to be ashamed of their intimate places and are sure it is (or could be in the future) a reason to avoid sexual relations. They also report shame when taking a shower at school with other girls – they feel different (like they "have a penis").

Many surgeons have performed labia minora reduction techniques in the past. However, the most popular are edge resection (direct excision) and wedge resection (with all modifications – Z-plasty, inferior resection and superior pedicle flap reconstruction) [1]. These two methods have one defect – all nerves and blood vessels are cut, so the sensitivity of the new edge of the labia can be worse than before the procedure. In this way of thinking, Choi and Kim described a new method – deepithelialization, which preserves neurovascular supply to the edge of the labia [2] (Fig. 6.1).

The next step in the way of labia reduction evolution was made by Ostrzenski, who described in 2014, a fenestration labiaplasty technique with inferior flap transposition [3]. Thanks to this technique, we reduce two dimensions of the labia minora – height and length. Except for symmetry, natural colour and contour of the labia is preserved, and the posterior edge of the fossa navicularis (labial frenulum) is restored. Alternatively, it could be created "de novo".

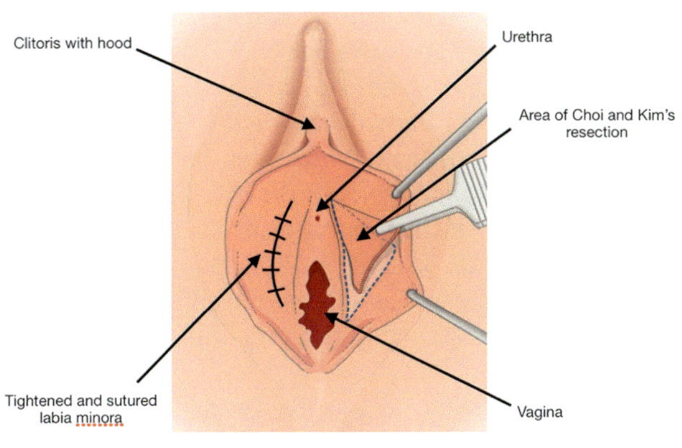

FIGURE 6.1 Choi and Kim's deepithelialization technique.

All the described methods apply only to the middle or the posterior part of the labia minora. Most surgeons treat the labia minora and clitoral hood as two different compartments. A new hypothesis is that we should view the labia minora and clitoral hood as one anatomical structure, which begins in the upper part of the vulva (periclitoral area) and ends as the frenulum. On the other hand, we should not talk about restoring labia minora size and shape without touching the clitoral hood (of course, if it is a protrusion – if not, we must not touch it at all).

Considering all the above, I designed a new method of simultaneous reduction of the labia minora and clitoral hood – the deepithelialization one-cut technique. It was presented for the first time in 2015. This method could also be considered a hybrid technique of labia minora reduction. This technique's description is in Chapter 6 of this book; the one-cut technique is a part of it.

Deepithelialization is one of the most crucial parts of the one-cut technique. Vascular and nerve-sparing surgery is the primary goal of this method. Complex restoration of the vulva with a natural look after surgery is another benefit achieved with this surgical technique.

INDICATIONS AND CONTRAINDICATIONS

A woman with hypertrophy of the labia minora connected to clitoral hood protrusion is the best example of a patient who should undergo a one-cut technique. Because of sparing the natural edges of the labia, we should consider it before surgical technique selection. Cases with smooth and pale edges are clearly candidates for this method (Fig. 6.2). In cases with edges that are dark, the patient needs to decide whether to keep them or not. Dark edges are not a contraindication for this surgery, but a lack of clitoral hood protrusion is a contraindication (Fig. 6.3).

DOI: 10.1201/9780429353079-6

(a) (b)

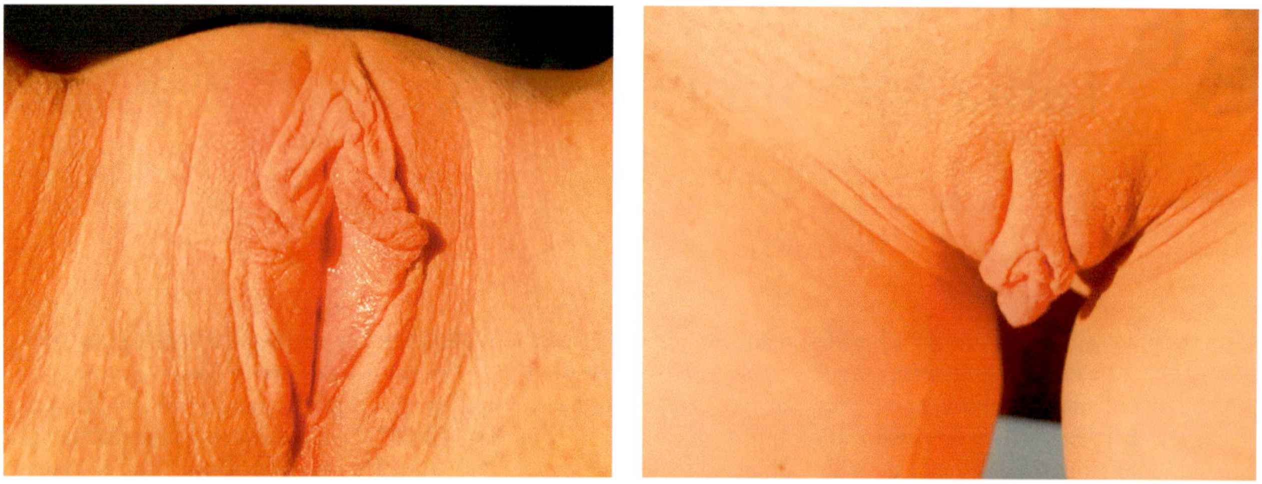

FIGURE 6.2 Properly qualified patient: (a) overgrown labia minora with pale and smooth edges and (b) protruded clitoral hood.

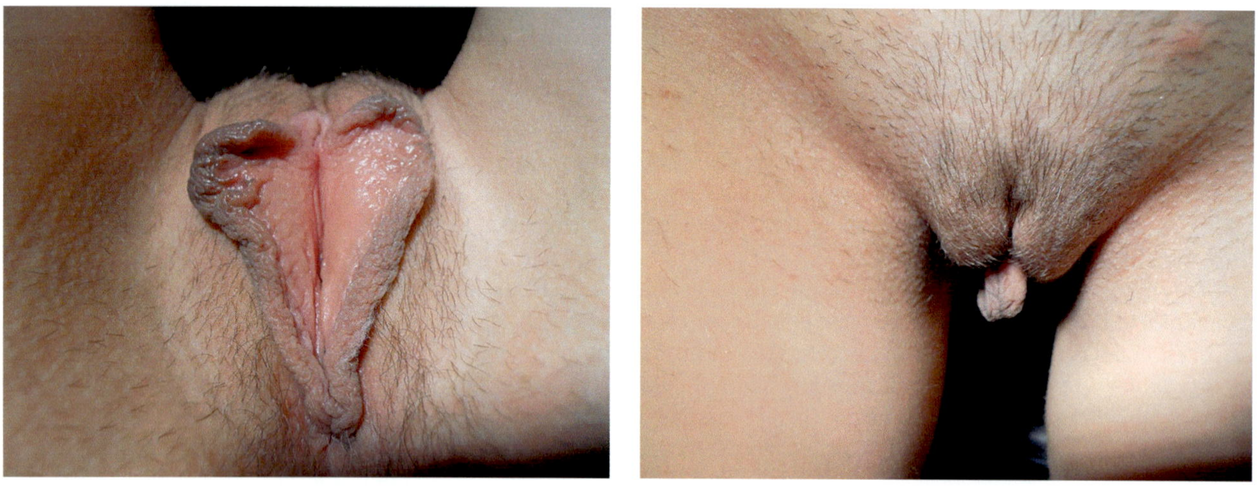

FIGURE 6.3 No proper qualification: labia minora with dark edges and no clitoral hood protrusion detected.

Before surgery it has to be clear that the patient is in good health, with proper PAP-smear and no pathology of the vulvovaginal region. Of course, she must not be in a current pregnancy.

PATIENT EVALUATION

Cosmetic patients seeking personal or social benefits such as confidence and acceptance must be completely healthy. The American Society of Anesthesiologists has developed a Physical Status Classification System (ASA) for surgical patients, which describes six categories: ASA I through ASA VI. Patients identified as ASA I and ASA II are well-chosen for surgery [4]. The initial conversation regarding the cosmetic request is an essential part of the patient evaluation process. Expectations and motivations need to be deeply explored. Besides cosmetic questions, psychological aspects need to be discussed to avoid patients who expect cosmetic surgery to remedy interpersonal conflicts. Individuals with body dysmorphic disorder (BDD) or with unrealistic expectations will never fulfil their needs, even if the surgical procedure is performed to perfection by any medical and aesthetic standard. They are examples of misguided personality types to be screened at the initial consultation. This preoperative consultation is also very crucial to reveal not

(a) (b)

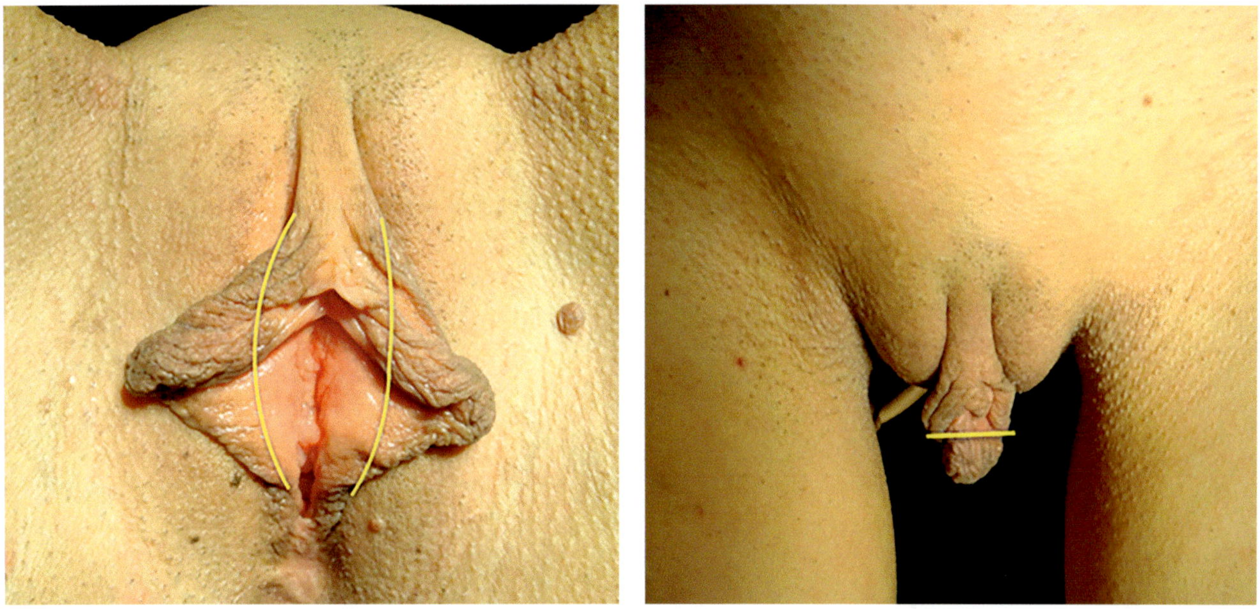

FIGURE 6.4 Planning in gynecological position (a) and possible effect – a "penis-like shape" (b).

only gynecological problems, but also problems in past medical history. The surgeon should conduct a physical examination in both positions – gynecologic dorsal lithotomy and a standing one – and should perform a speculum examination to identify any infection or other problems that could interfere with the surgical procedure. The patient might use a mirror during the whole examination when the surgeon is obligated to explain the vulvar reduction limits by palpating the target structures and displaying the anatomy. The surgeon should also show the patient the expected effect – during examination using fingers to help the patient visualize the degree of planned resection and reconstruction, and after examination using "before and after" photographs. These explanations of the degree of the vulvar area's changes expected after surgery are essential.

During the physical examination, proper photographs need to be obtained, and they should be taken in both positions: gynecological and standing. Otherwise, a crucial thing can be missed – clitoral hood protrusion. If the surgeon plans the procedure and chooses the technique only in the gynecological position, a "penis-like shape" can occur after surgery (Fig. 6.4).

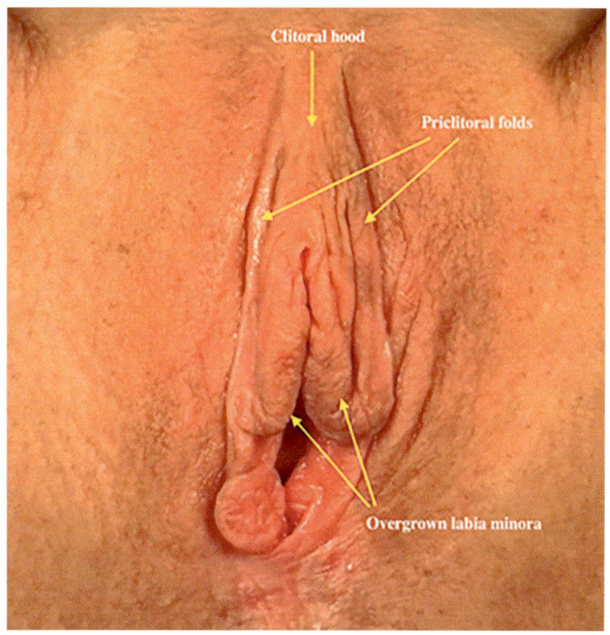

FIGURE 6.5 Overgrown labia minora and clitoral hood.

Preoperative Procedures

Preoperative preparing of the patient depends on the kind of anaesthesia we plan to proceed with. The majority of cases of labia minora and clitoral hood reduction can be performed under local anesthesia. In this situation, 2–3 weeks before the procedure the patient needs to do blood tests, like morphology and coagulatory (APTT and INR). On the other hand, if surgery is planned

(a) (b)

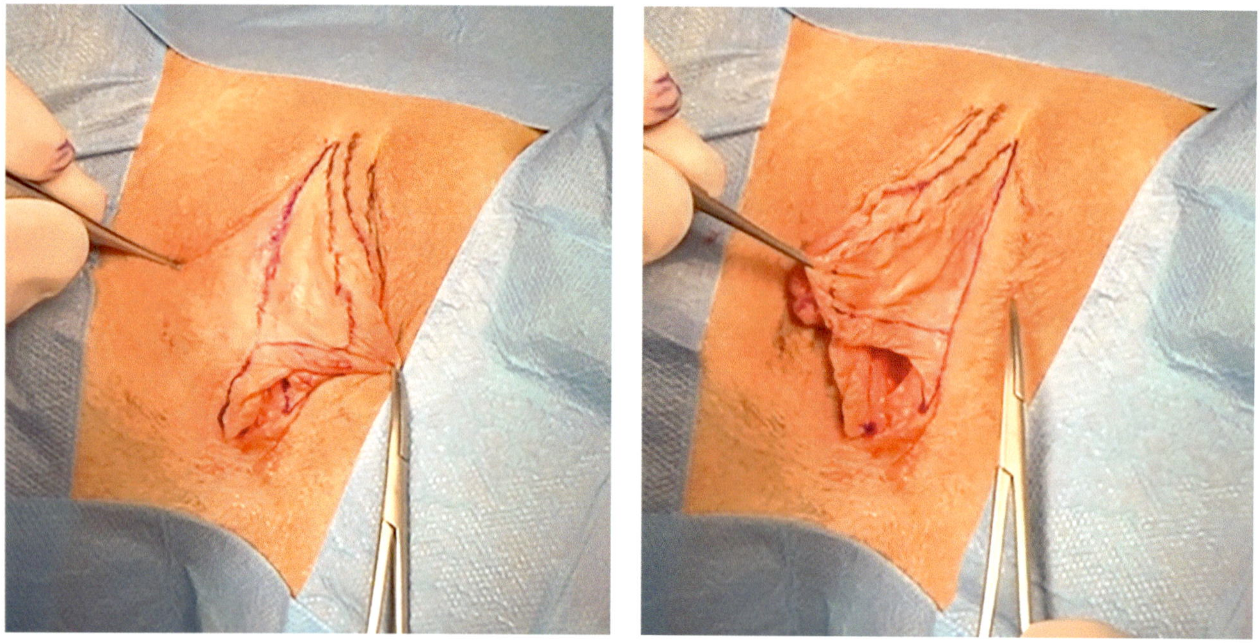

(c)

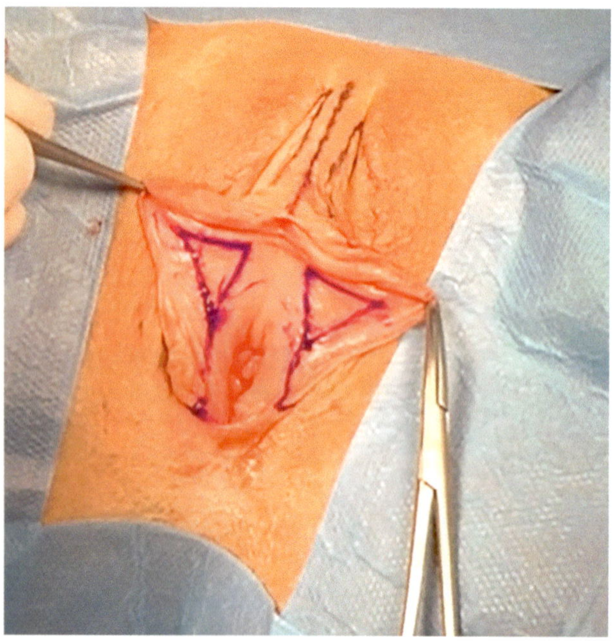

FIGURE 6.6 Markings: (a, b) right and left dermal part of the labia with periclitoral folds, (c) mucosal part of the labia.

to proceed under sedation, the patient also needs to do blood tests, but more parameters should be checked. Besides those described above, we should know the level of creatinine, Na^+, K^+, glucose, and TSH (in case of a thyroid gland problem). Regardless of the technique of anesthesia, the patient should be in the first part of the menstrual cycle or be given medicines (e.g., oral contraceptives) to block menstruation. Medications that could impair coagulation like ibuprofen, acetylsalicylic acid or statins should be discontinued 2 weeks before surgery. Cigarette smoking can impair the healing process, so it should be withheld 2 weeks in advance of

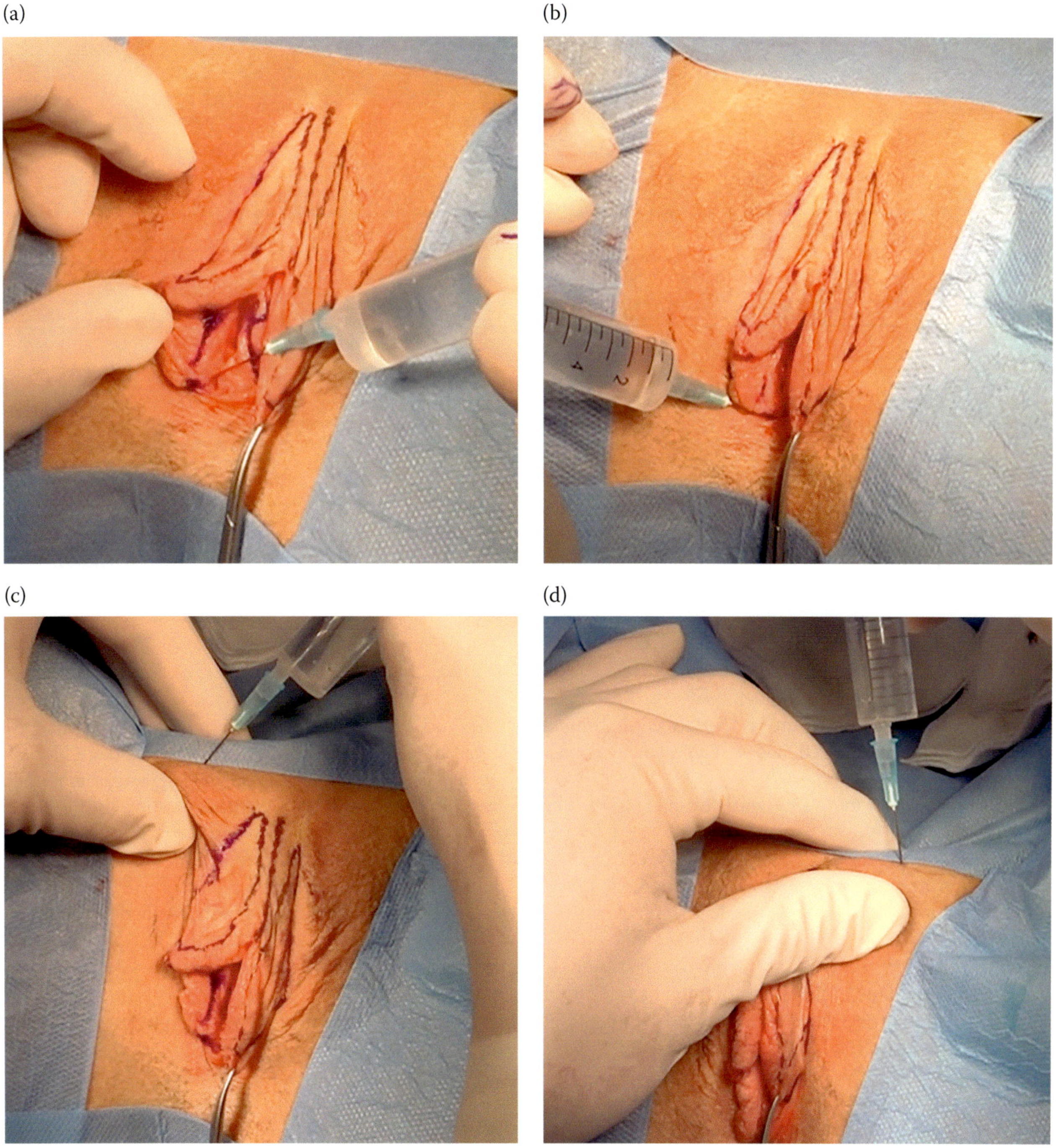

FIGURE 6.7 Pudendal nerve block (a, b) and inguinal nerve block (c, d).

surgery. If it cannot be discontinued or substituted, the patient needs to sign an informed consent, which is necessary because the risk of disturbances of the healing process is much higher among smokers than non-smokers. With general anaesthesia, the patient must not eat for 6 hours or drink for 3 hours prior to surgery. If local anesthesia is planned to be performed, then no restrictions are needed.

(a) (b)

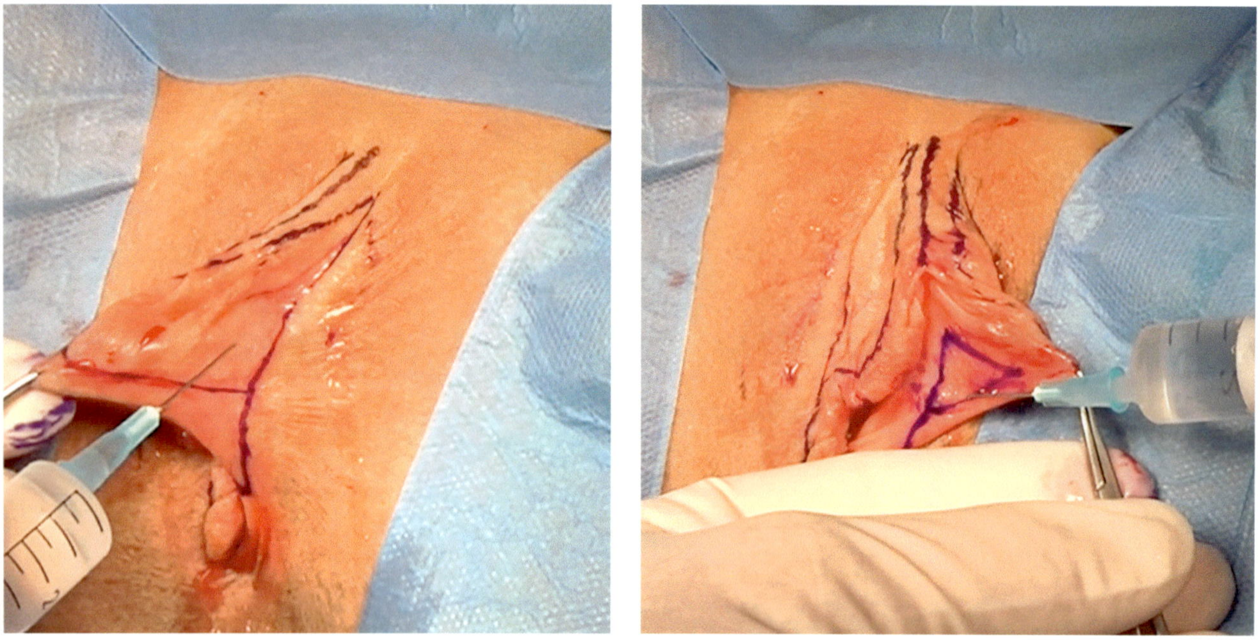

FIGURE 6.8 Dissection of the skin (a) and mucosa (b).

Preparing for Surgery

Before any surgical procedure is performed, informed consent needs to be obtained, and It should be signed just before surgery.

It is imperative to know what to prepare before surgery.

First is a surgical device that is used for cutting and coagulation. Labia minora and clitoral hood reduction can be performed with all available machines on the market, such as the CO_2 laser, radiofrequency (RF) knife or ordinary scalpel, although the last one is not very precise. One of the most common devices used for the procedure is the RF knife and bipolar tip. Thanks to this set, blood loss is minimal, and provides the highest cutting precision.

The **second** important thing is to prepare proper surgical tools (including surgical sutures) and collect them on the surgical table. The table should be set at an appropriate height, proportionate to the surgeon's height, how the operator is comfortable, and rest the operational hand's elbow on it. It is essential to stabilize the operational hand in which the surgeon holds the knife.

Third, proper anesthesia is essential to be prepared before surgery, if the procedure will be performed under local anesthesia. Usually, patients are given a local anesthetic. Tumescent local anesthesia (TLA) consists of lidocaine hydrochloride (800 mg/L), sodium bicarbonate (10 mEq/L), and epinephrine (1 mg/L) diluted in 0.9% saline solution [3]. It is an excellent anesthetic for all vaginal and vulvar surgery and possesses hemostatic properties [5]. Another anaesthetic solution that is being widely used is bupivacaine (50 mg/10 mL diluted in 10 mL of 0.9% saline solution) or ropivacaine 100 mg/10 mL diluted in 10 mL of saline.

Of course, in most cases of labia minora and clitoral hood reduction, there is no need to use TLA, and only the mix of medicines described above appears to be enough solution.

The **fourth** thing that should be prepared is perioperative medications. Prophylactic broad-spectrum antibiotics are given just before surgery, which are crucial for protecting against infection (second-generation cephalosporin 1–2 g i.v.). Dexamethasone (8 mg i.v.) is used as a prevention against intraoperative swelling of the surgical area. It is injected at the beginning of the surgery. After injection, the patient should be informed that she will feel a strange feeling in the vulvar or face area (like stinging).

It is also helpful to have the following on the surgical table (all must be sterile):

1. Marker
2. Gauze 10 × 10 × 10 cm

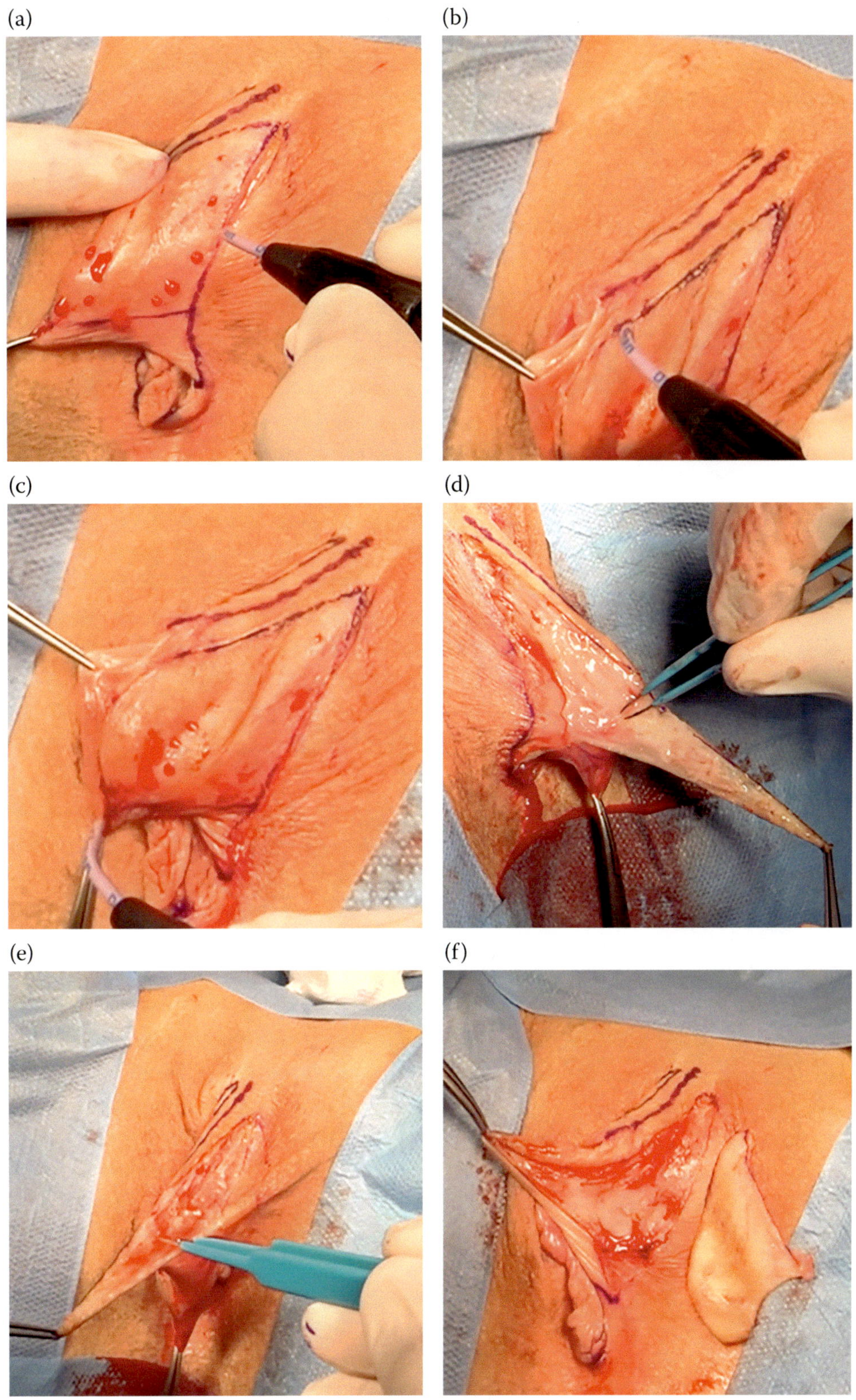

FIGURE 6.9 (a) The surgeon cuts labial skin along the furrow between the labia minora and majora from the top of the clitoral hood towards the frenulum; (b) the second cut line goes again from the top of the hood along the clitoris towards the top of the labia minora; and (c) turns down to the frenulum. (d, e, f) The skin is next separated from the underlying tissues using the *sliding technique* with bipolar pinceta.

(a) (b) (c) (d) (e) (f)

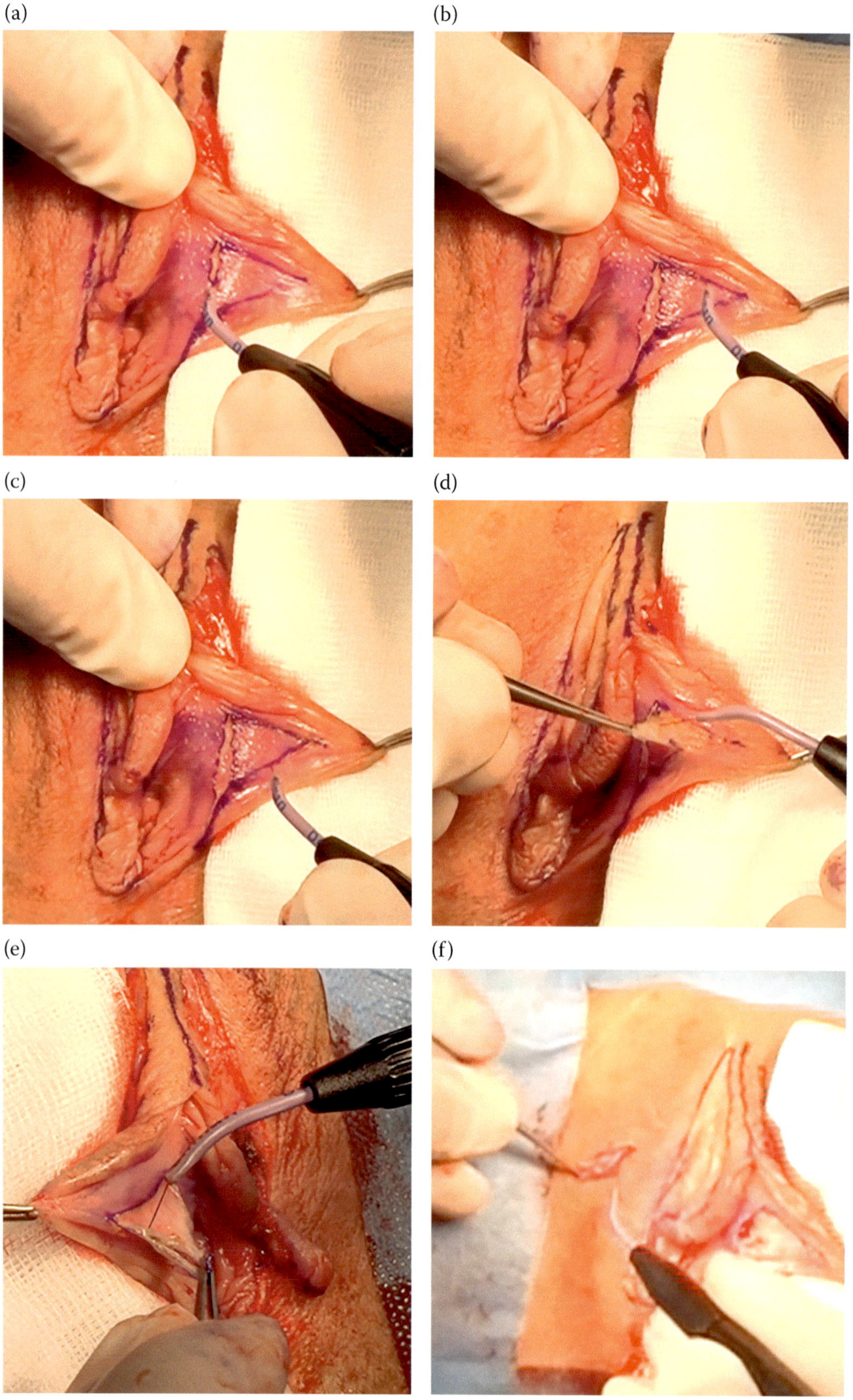

FIGURE 6.10 (a, b, c) A similar triangle is made on the internal side of the labia minora and (d, e, f) mucus is separated from submucosal tissue.

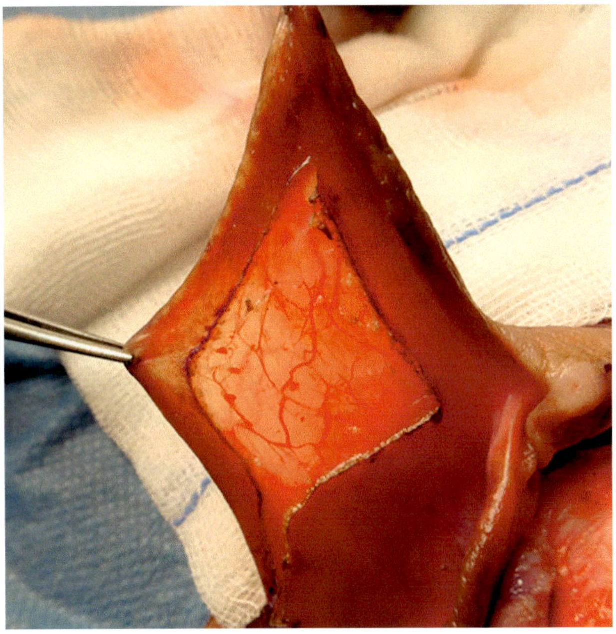

FIGURE 6.11 Deepithelialization with preservation of the neurovascular system.

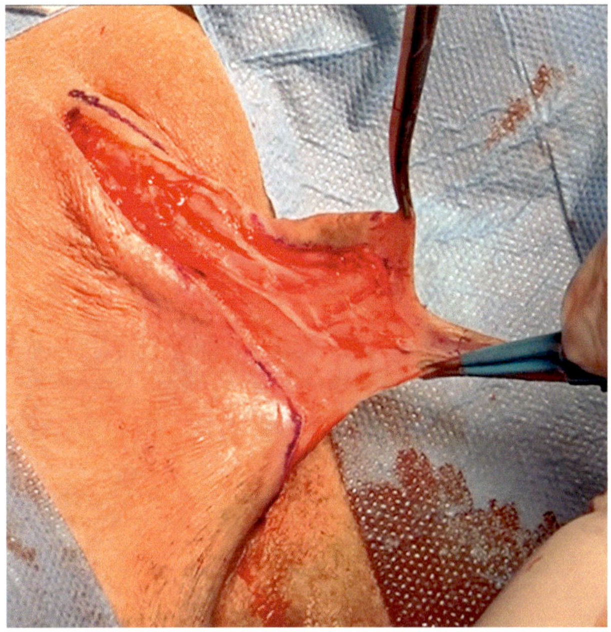

FIGURE 6.12 Labium minus is divided into two parts.

3. Knife (RF, CO_2 laser, scalpel)
4. Bipolar pinceta
5. Kocher clamp (small)
6. Surgical tip (small)
7. Scissors
8. Needle holder
9. Sutures: Vicryl coated 4.0 and Monocryl 5.0
10. Surgical sheets (four pieces or one with a hole in the middle with leg covers)

Technique of Surgical Procedure

The first critical step is to determine the size of the labia minora and clitoral hood to be reduced. All margins of the future incisions need to be determined and marked in the shape of a triangle on both sides of the labia (skin and mucus). In this simultaneous reduction of the labia minora and clitoral hood, periclitoral folds are also marked together with the dermal part of the labia (Figs. 6.5 and 6.6). Markings must be done before the injection of anesthesia.

The procedure is performed in local anaesthesia. The surgeon must do the blockade of pudendal and inguinal nerves (Fig. 6.7). Usually, these blockades are made with a solution of 0.9% saline, 1% lidocaine, and 0.01% adrenaline using a 22–24 G needle. For better and longer-lasting nerve blockade, together with lidocaine, I always use a solution of bupivacaine 0.5%–10 mL or ropivacaine 1%–10 mL with 10 mL of saline (1:1 proportion).

Next, dissection of the skin and mucus is performed with a solution of 0.9% NaCl, 1% lidocaine, and 0.01% adrenaline. Thanks to this action, the risk of bleeding is shallow. A 28–30 G × 1/2 inch needle and 10 mL syringe are used (Fig 6.8).

The "one-cut technique" involves the simultaneous excision of the mucus and skin of the labia minora, leaving nervation and vascularization intact (fenestration and deepithelialization). Periclitoral skin folds located on both sides along the clitoral hood are cut out simultaneously.

The incision is made with a radiofrequency device. This surgical device cut line is very straight, not too deep – only the dermal and mucosal part of the labia is cut. Damages of margins are minimal because the burning zone does not appear thanks to the tissue's vaporization.

Technically, the surgeon cuts the skin of the labia minora in the bottom (along the furrow between the labia minora and majora) from the top of the clitoris towards the frenulum.

The second cut line goes from the top of the clitoral hood along the clitoris (about 1 cm right and left below the middle line of peak margin) towards the top of the labia minora and turns down to the frenulum. This skin triangle is going to be deepithelialized with the bipolar tip using a sliding technique. With this unique technique, the surgeon separates the skin from the subdermal tissue without damaging underlying blood vessels and nerves (Fig. 6.9). A similar triangle is made on the inner side of the labia minora, and mucus is separated from submucosal tissue (Fig. 6.10). By doing so, the

(a) (b) (c)

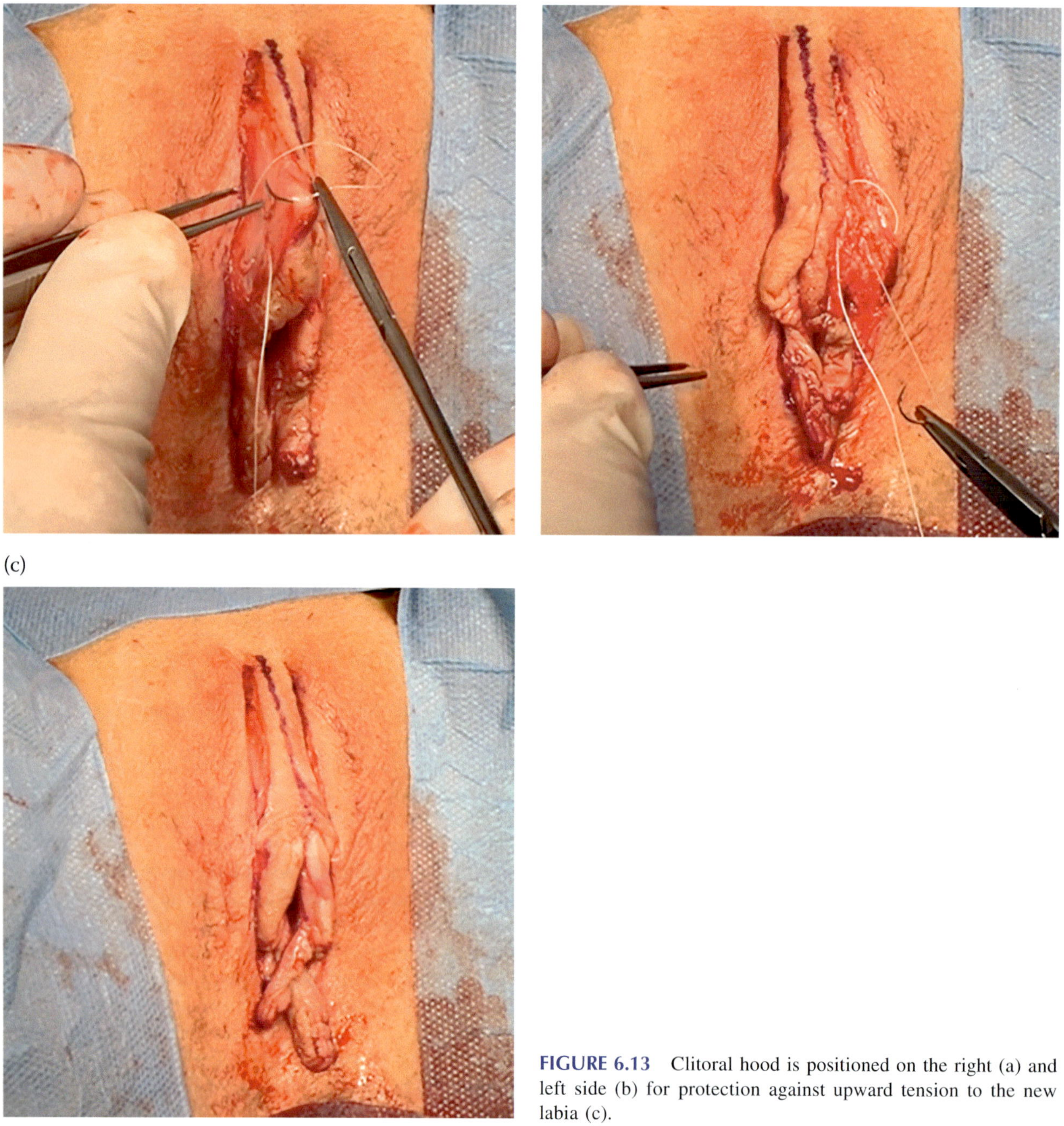

FIGURE 6.13 Clitoral hood is positioned on the right (a) and left side (b) for protection against upward tension to the new labia (c).

neurovascular system of the labia minora is spared because only skin and mucus are excised from the labial corpus (Fig. 6.11).

Next, the labia are divided into superior as a new top with preserved vascularization and nervation, and inferior at the base of the labia that will be excised (Fig. 6.11). Before excision of this part of the labia, the top of the clitoral hood with the clitoral gland within is situated in a new position with one stitch on both sides (Monocryl 4.0 coated) (Figs. 6.12, 6.13). Thanks to this action, there will be no upward tension for the new labia. It is an essential part of the procedure. If any tension persists, the healing process will be disordered and wound dehiscence could appear.

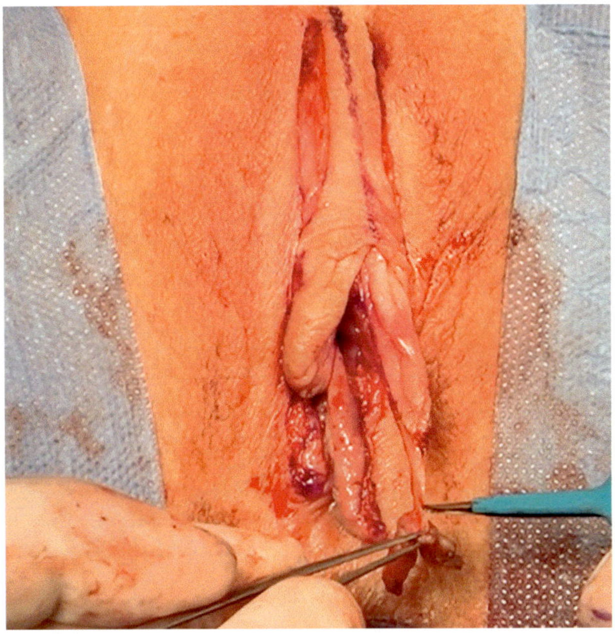

FIGURE 6.14 Leaving a small piece of tissue at the end of the new labia as a protection against necrosis.

It is vital to leave a small piece of the tissue at the end of the new labia from which new fossa naviculars will be created (Fig. 6.14). This significantly reduces the risk of necrosis of the ends of the new labia minora.

After creating a new diameter of the labia minora, the tips are situated in the perineal area. These parts of the labia are sutured with two to three interrupted stitches, and the fossa naviculars is created de novo (Fig. 6.15).

Next the external and internal labial laminas are sutured on both sites separately. First, the internal lamina is sutured with a few interrupted stitches (Vicryl 4.0 coated). Second, the external lamina is sutured with an intracutaneous, continuous stitch (Monocryl 5.0). The fundamental challenge is to bring the edges of the labia and clitoral hood together without any tension (Fig. 6.16).

In contrast to internal (mucosal) stitches, which are interrupted, the skin's external suturing is continuous. This means the beginning is evident, but the end is not. Usually, we start suturing from the top of the clitoral hood towards the fossa navicularis. The end of the stitch is made inside the vaginal vestibule (Fig. 6.17), which lowers the risk of infection.

Thanks to this technique we obtain two goals: first, it reduces the labia minora in two dimensions, and second is the reduction of the clitoral hood in its height and width (reduction of periclitoral skin folds). This method treats the labia minora and the clitoral hood as one compartment, so reducing this part of the vulva is performed with one cut simultaneously, not separately (labia and clitoral hood), as it is made in different techniques. By doing so, the shape of the new vulva looks natural (Fig. 6.18). (See Video 6.1: Deepithelialization technique of labia minora reduction – The one-cut technique.)

Postoperative Care

Postoperative pain or other discomfort can be controlled with oral or transrectal pain-relieving pills or suppositories (e.g., diclofenac 100 mg). Several days after the procedure, the patient is ordered to use ice packs (e.g., frozen 0.5 L bottle of mineral water) with two to three sterile gauze pads as protection against frostbite. This action is vital for the healing process to minimize oedema of the vulva, which is always present after surgery. For oedema, 1 mg of dexamethasone in oral pills with 20 mg of omeprazole (stomach protection) is also recommended. The patient is asked to take these medicines for the first 5 days after the procedure. During the first 7–10 days, patients may not wear underwear, and it is recommended that they use antiseptic solution after using the toilet. Taking baths and sexual intercourse are forbidden for 6 weeks. Ten days after surgery, patients can use micronized hyaluronic acid gel externally for a better healing process (Fig. 6.19).

Postoperative Complications

Statistically, the complication rate among patients after all plastic surgery is 21% among patients who underwent coordinated procedures compared with 5% in patients who had sequential procedures [5]. Smokers have significantly increased deep incisional surgical-site infections, incisional dehiscence, and reoperation, but superficial surgical-site infection rates are not significantly different between smokers and non-smokers [6]. Generally, the complication rate is observed in less than 0.5%. Hematoma and bacterial infection were the most common complications. Only ice packs being used for the first few days and compression were enough in the first one. Of course, if hematoma looks big and is growing, I recommend the regular strategy employed for every kind of hematoma. The surgeon should open the wound and close the bleeding vessel. If this is impossible, compression should be proceeded, and the wound needs to be closed with interrupted sutures and drainage performed. If no leakage is observed, drainage can be removed. This is why every bleeding needs to be stopped before the wound is closed, and only the dry wound can be sutured. I always respect this rule of "dry surgery", and thanks to it, I have had no significant hematomas during the past years.

(a)

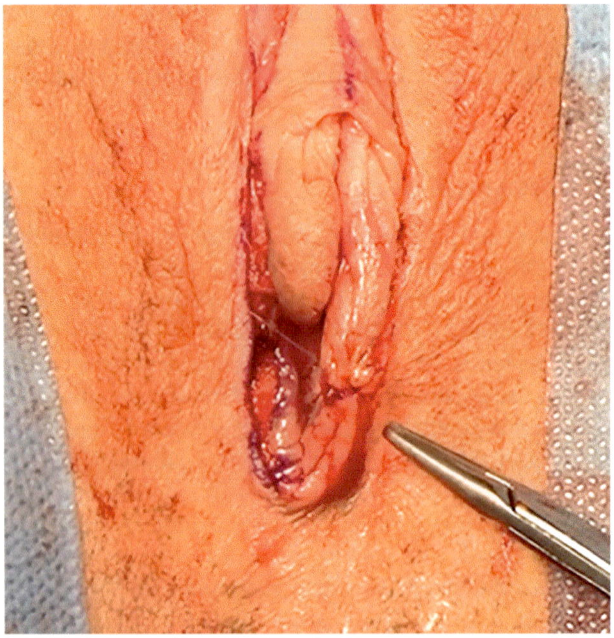

(b)

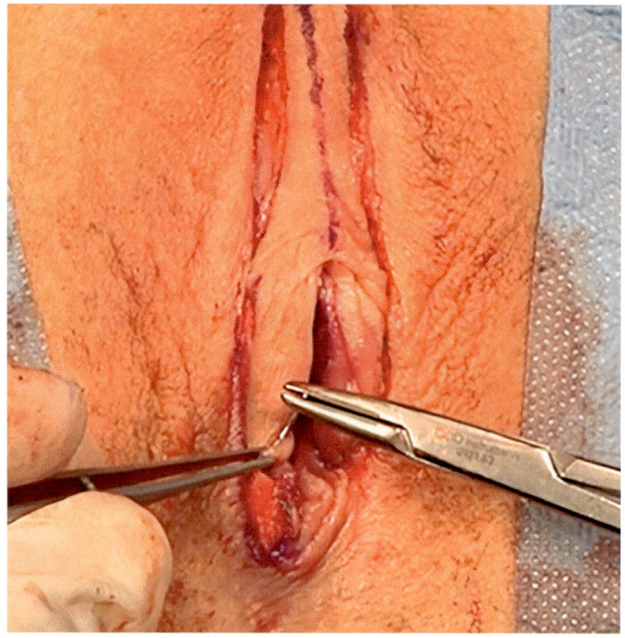

(c)

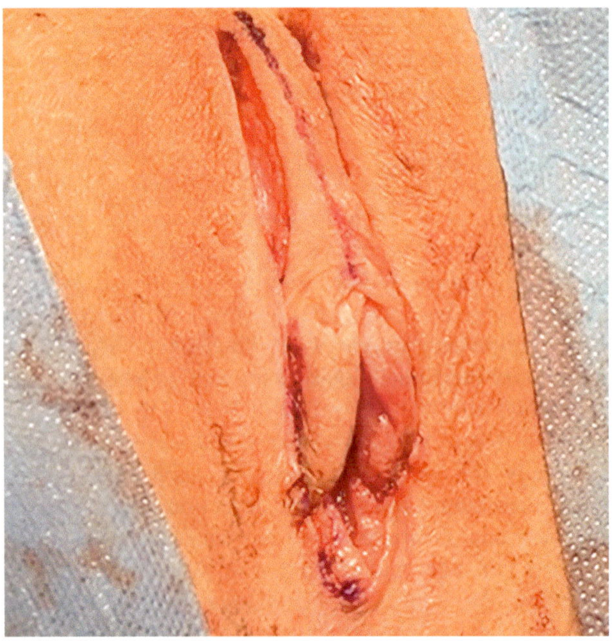

FIGURE 6.15 The tips of the labia minora are sutured with three interrupted stitches on the left (a) and right side (b). A new fossa navicularis has been created (c).

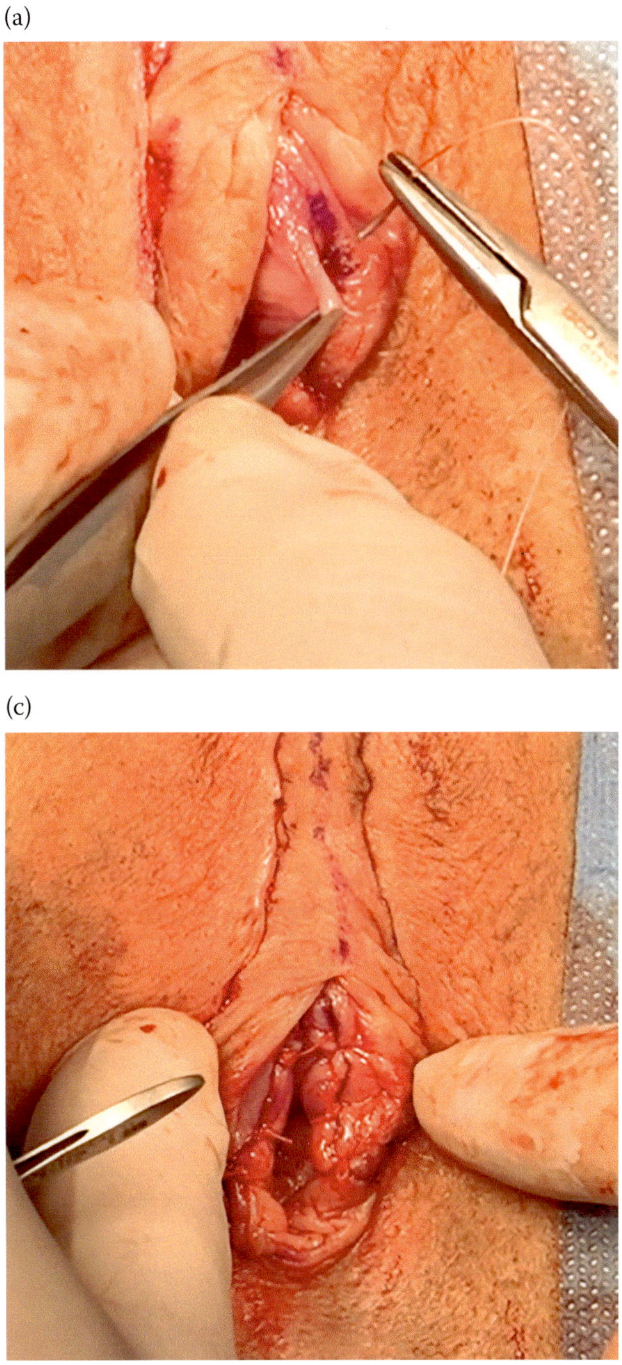

FIGURE 6.16 Internal lamina is being sutured with several interrupted stitches (a) and external with continuous intracutaneal (b). Labial edges are brought together without any tension (c).

(a) (b)

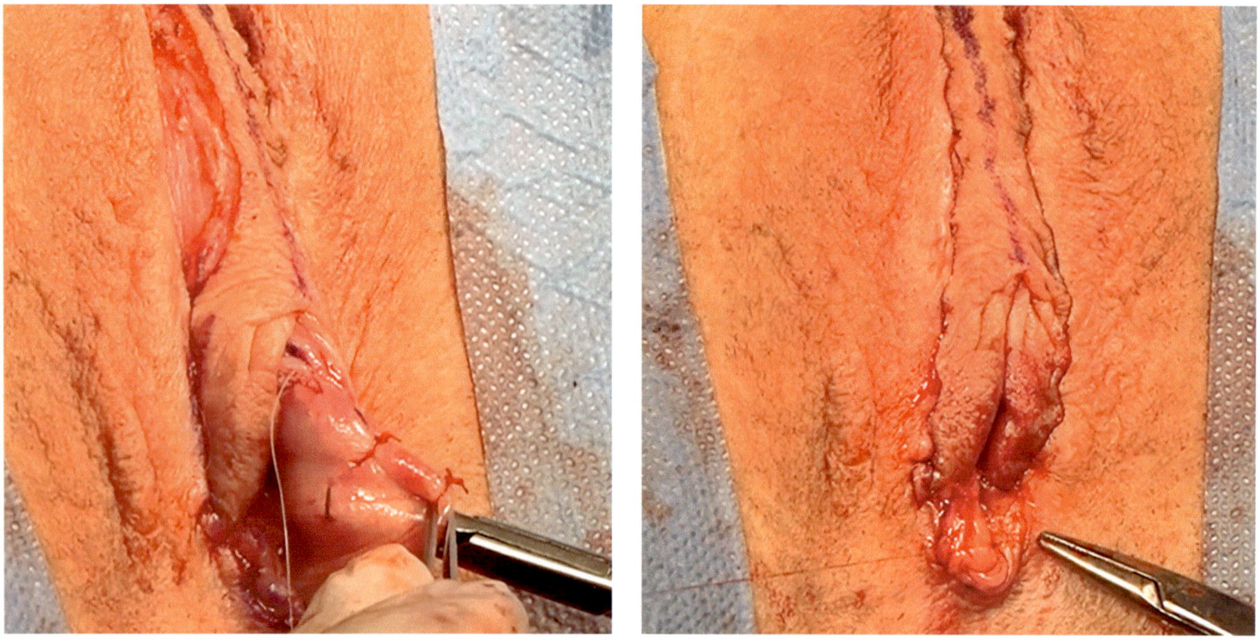

FIGURE 6.17 The end of the external continuous stitches are situated on both sides (left – a, and right – b) inside the vaginal vestibule.

(a) (b)

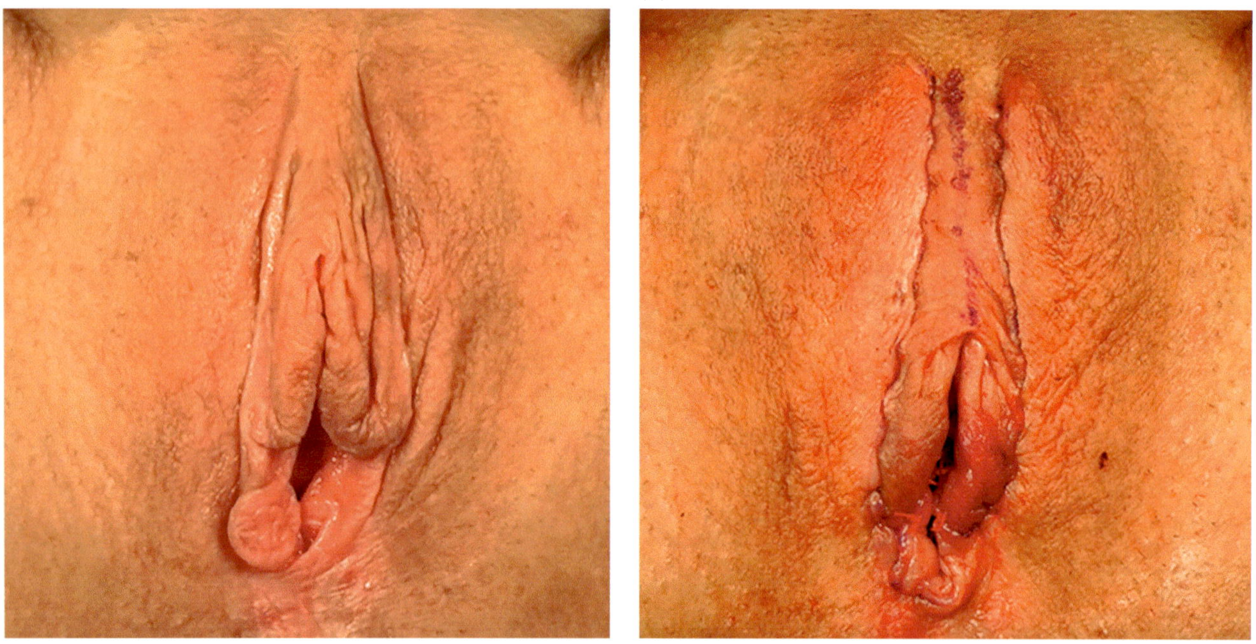

FIGURE 6.18 Before (a) and just after the procedure (b).

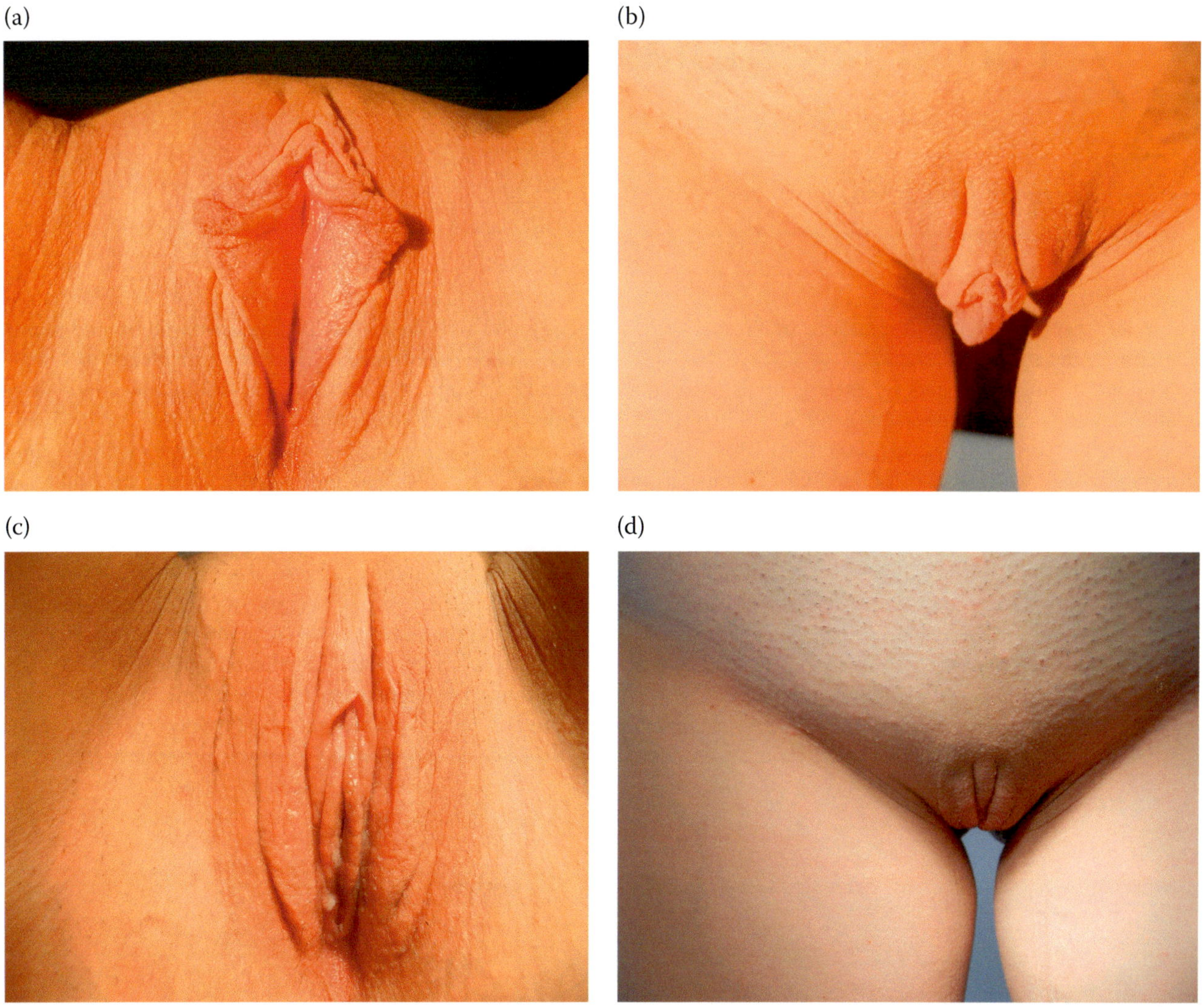

FIGURE 6.19 (a) Before in gynecological and (b) standing position; (c) after in gynecological and (d) standing position.

Despite the proximity of the anus and the bowel movements, a bacterial infection of the wound is quite rare, but it is the second most common complication. If infection happens, wound dehiscence can occur. Most often, it is partial. If it happens during the early healing phase, the best treatment is prompt surgical repair. If it happens more than 10–14 days after the surgery, PRP can be used as a booster to healing. The decision about eventual repairing can be made only after 6 weeks, and it can be performed only after 4–6 months, not earlier when angiogenesis has been completed. Pain is a usual symptom, and a complication should not be automatically suspected; it can last for 1–2 weeks and should decrease every 2–3 days.

REFERENCES

1. Kuzlik R (2018) "One cut technique" – simultaneous reduction of labia minora and clitoral hood. *Int J Gynecol Clin Pract* 5: 141.
2. Choi HY, Kim KT (2000) A new method for aesthetic reduction of labia minora (deepithelialized reduction of labioplasty). *Plast Reconstr Surg* 105: 419–422.
3. Ostrzenski A (2014) Fenestration labioreduction of the labium minus: a new surgical intervention concept. *ISRN Obstet Gynecol* 2014: 671068.
4. Hammori CA, Banwell PE, Alinsod R (2017) *Female Cosmetic Genital Surgery*. Thieme: New York, 161–180.
5. Tevis SE, Steiman JG, Neuman HB, Greenberg CC, Wilke LG (2019) Postoperative complications in combined gynecologic, plastic, and breast surgery: an analysis from National Surgical Quality Improvement Program. *Breast J.* 25(6): 1111–1116.
6. Toyoda Y, Fu RH, Li L, Otterburn DM, Rohde CH (2018) Smoking as an independent risk factor for postoperative complications in plastic surgical procedures: a propensity score-matched analysis of 36,454 patients from the NSQIP database from 2005 to 2014. *Plast Reconstr Surg* 141(1): 226–236.

7 Labiamajoraplasty

Piotr Kolczewski

There are surprisingly few descriptions of normal female genitalia in the medical literature.

In contrast, measurements for male genitals are widely available and were published as early as 1899 [1]. The study conducted by Lloyd in 2005 filled this gap and illustrated the wide range of genital dimensions in "normal" women. There are a variety of appearances in women's labia minora and majora, and there are no data indicating that one size or shape is more normal or preferable to others. When it comes to labia majora, the length ranges 7–12 cm with a mean of 9.3 cm [2]. This information should be considered by women and doctors when making the decision to have genital surgery.

With age and as a result of pregnancies and childbirths, the labia majora lose tension and become pendulous, saggy and wrinkled, thus posing an aesthetic and sometimes functional problem. Increasing incidence of female obesity has resulted in common complaints of a large mons pubis and labia majora consequent to unsightly fat deposits. Even with dramatic weight loss, these areas remain descended and bulky, with excess fat and skin. These unnatural fat deposits can also severely affect self-esteem [3] (Figs. 7.1a and 7.2a).

Unfortunately, only a few articles have appeared in Pubmed on the subject of labia majora hypertrophy and their reduction [4,5]; however, such deficiencies are addressed by three textbooks on cosmetic gynecology [6–8].

Although labiamajoraplasty in cosmetic surgery is a relatively young procedure, most gynecologic surgeons have repeatedly performed a similar procedure – a simple

(a) (b)

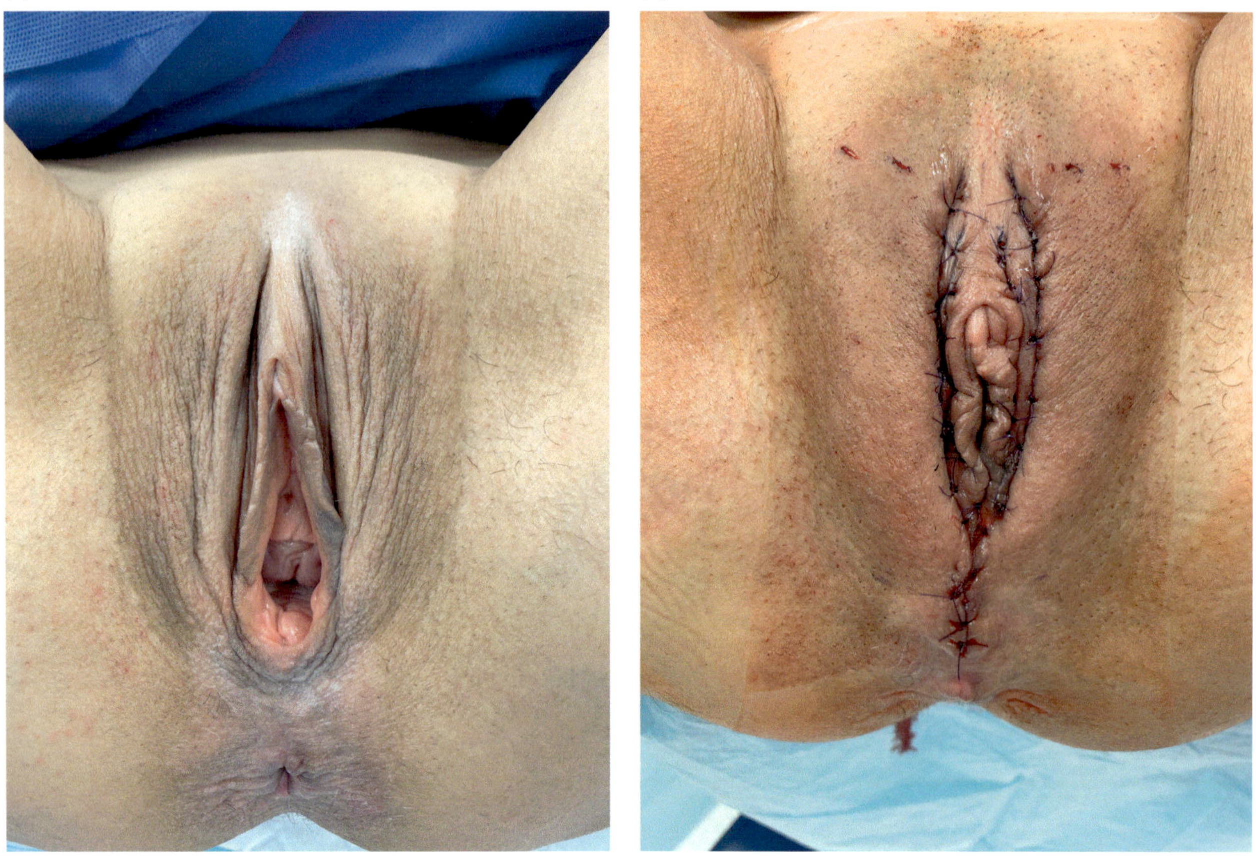

FIGURE 7.1 (a) Before and (b) after operation.

DOI: 10.1201/9780429353079-7

(a) (b)

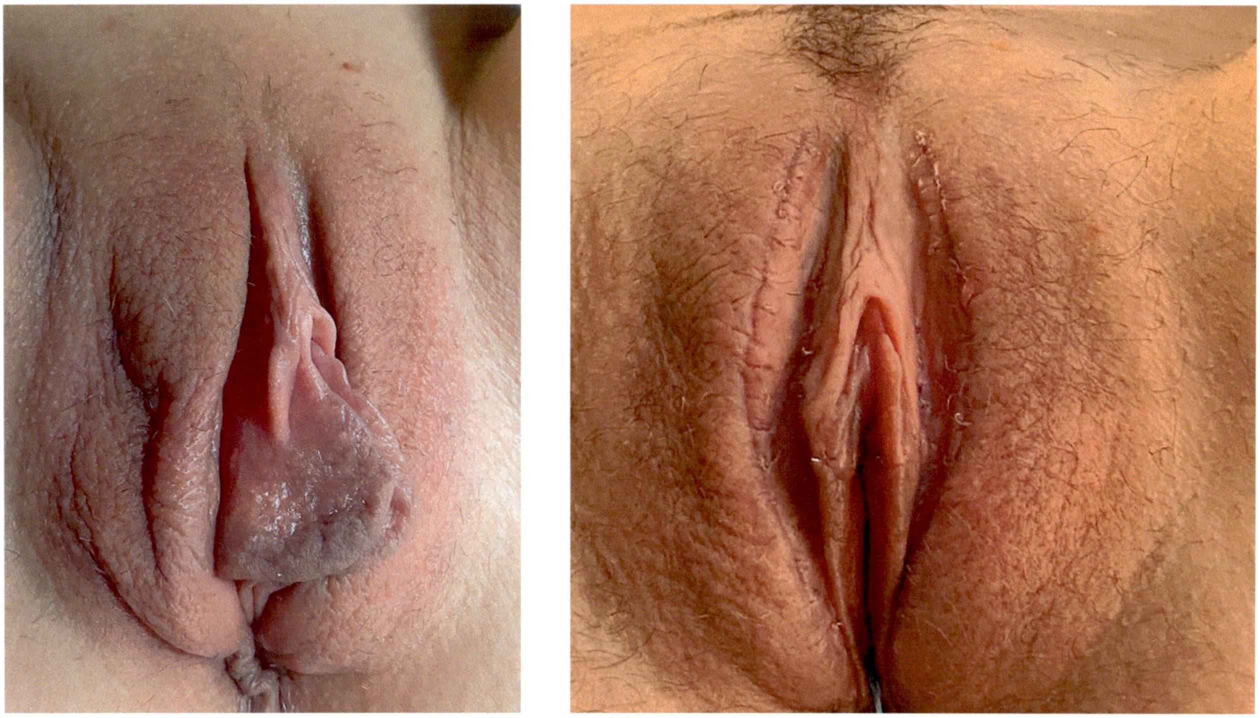

FIGURE 7.2 (a) Before and (b) after operation.

vulvectomy. Of course, the goals and the final result of these procedures differ significantly. Ablative surgery, although similar in technique, aims to save lives and does not pay much attention to aesthetics.

INDICATIONS AND CONTRAINDICATIONS

Labia majora hypertrophy can be primary or secondary.

Primary is due to excess fat in the subcutaneous layer of the labia majora, and affects younger women, while secondary is the result of loss of skin volume and flaccidity, and occurs in older patients or is the result of intense weight loss [6].

Similar to labiaminoraplasty, labiamajoraplasty can be performed for aesthetic or functional indications, and in practise these indications intersect.

Contraindications include undiagnosed vulvar skin pathologies and active viral, bacterial and yeast infections. Also, planned weight loss should be taken into account as a relative contraindication, and surgery should be scheduled after the patient has achieved the planned weight [6].

One should be cautious in patients with vulvodynia, as surgery of the vulvar region may exacerbate the patient's problem. Surgical repair should also be postponed in women who are planning to have vaginal delivery.

PATIENT EVALUATION

Cosmetic patients who are looking to improve their appearance and sometimes function, as in the case of labiamajoraplasty, should be healthy. Regardless of the aesthetic considerations and expectations of the patient, the doctor should take a thorough medical history.

Evaluation of the labia majora should take place in both the standing and gynecological positions [6–8] (Figs 7.2a and 7.3). Most patients evaluate their labia majora in the standing position, and often in this position by pulling their labia backward they show what effect they would like to achieve after surgery. Using mirrors and taking pictures are useful to help patients understand the issue and visualize the degree of planned surgery. Preoperative evaluations of the hypertrophic labia majora and planned surgery should also take into account two issues resulting from the specific anatomy of this region [6,7].

The first one is gapping of vaginal introitus. If too much labial skin is removed, it creates lateral skin tension, pulling the vaginal introitus open. It is better to perform under-resection out of caution and ensure that wound margins can be approximated without tension.

Another issue to consider in preoperative planning is the height of the labia minora. A surgical reduction of labia majora can lead to a volumetric confusion and labia minora protruding beyond their previous cover. We should warn the patient if this is to be expected.

All the data taken should be recorded, and the doctor should describe the planned procedure in a way that is understandable to the patient. The law provides that the patient should be given time to review and discuss detailed informed consent for the procedure.

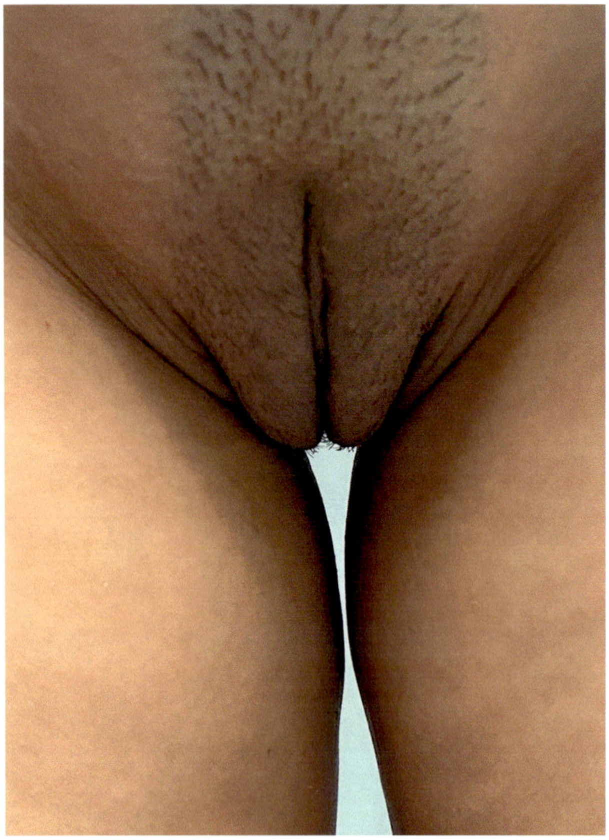

FIGURE 7.3 Labia minora in the standing position.

MEDICATION AND PREPARATION

Labiamajoraplasty is similar to other cosmetic surgeries of the external genitalia, and be performed under any type of anesthesia. However, given the scope of the procedure, local anesthesia seems to be most appropriate. The exceptions are bulky labia majora when lipectomy is necessary, which can be painful with local anaesthesia, and rather require general or spinal anaesthesia [6].

In my practise, 30 minutes before the scheduled surgery, an ointment with 15% lidocaine is applied to the skin of the labia majora. This makes local injection anesthesia with lidocaine or/and bupivacain almost painless. Adequate analgesia should be prescribed before every surgical procedure, and then continued depending on the patient's needs. Paracetamol and ketoprofen are most commonly used for this purpose. When peripherally acting analgesics are not sufficient, it is worthwhile combining them with central-acting agents.

The routine administration of antibiotics is to some extent disputed, but most surgeons in practise administer cephalosporine 1 hour before surgery as blanket antibiotic cover, and continue for up to 3–5 days.

PLANNING AND MARKING

The anatomy of the labia majora does not leave too many options open, especially if we want the scar to be concealed and inconspicuous. The spindle-shaped incision seems to be the best, if not the only, reasonable solution here. Figure 7.4 [*right labia*] shows a typical marking. The medial line should lie along the interlabial fold, except for the superior segment: at this point, i.e., along the clitoral shaft, the incision should run somewhat lateral to the interlabial fold, at a distance of about 2–3 mm, in order to maintain the curve of the medial origin of the labia majora [7]. Thus formed, the lateral line of the spindle dictates its width depending on the degree of hypertrophy and the patient's wish. The maximum width of the spindle should be located in the middle of the length of the labia majora.

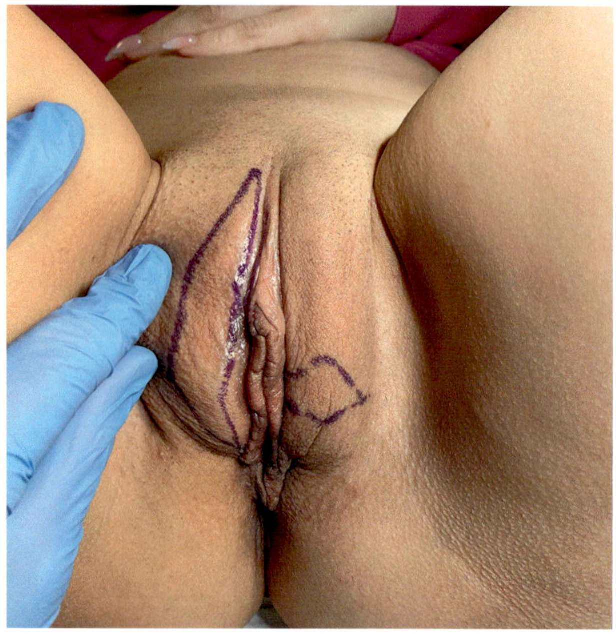

FIGURE 7.4 (Patient's right) Spindle-shaped incision; (Patient's left) spindle-shaped incision horizontally between interlabial and crural fold.

If the visibility of the scar is not a problem for the patient, the marks can be made also spindle-shaped but in the crural (genito-femoral sulcus) and vulvar creases. Apart from visibility, another disadvantage of this technique is that the scar is formed in a high-tension site, as is the crural crease, leaving it susceptible to wound dehiscence [9].

Another interesting option described by Barwijuk assumes that the spindle-shaped figure of the incision lies horizontally between the interlabial and crural fold [10] (Fig. 7.4, *left labia*).

TECHNIQUE

The patient is placed in the lithotomy position; 10% povidone-iodine is applied to the skin, and the patient is draped in a sterile fashion. Care is taken during positioning to pad all pressure points, so as to prevent iatrogenic injury. Compression stockings during the perioperative period and intermittent pneumatic compression devices are optional and should be considered in patients with risk factors or history of venous thromboembolism.

The incision can be made with any instrument of the surgeon's choice. The author of this chapter prefers a high-radiofrequency unit (2.2 MHZ), which allows cutting without burning and also mono- and bipolar coagulation. In most patients only a "skinning" incision that does not affect the fat pad is sufficient [6]. Lipectomy is recommended in the case of bulky fat deposits. Liposuction is also possible, but the results are unsatisfactory because of the limited amount of fat that can be extracted from the labia majora and often uneven healing of the subcutaneous layer. Moreover, liposuction alone does not address the saggy excess skin of the labia majora [6].

After excising excess skin, following the marked lines, wound margins should largely lie together with no tension. However, if this is not the case and tension-free wound closure is difficult, we can relax skin closure by subcutaneously mobilizing labial skin 1 cm laterally [7].

Multilayered suturing is recommended to reduce the risk of postoperative bleeding, close the open area and dead spaces, and increase the consistency of the labia. We can use interrupted or running delayed absorbable sutures, such as Monocryl 3-0 or 4-0 [6–8].

A running or interrupted absorbable monofilament 5-0 thread fits best for skin closure. According to Gress, intradermal suturing techniques are not advisable in labial surgery, as they are less able to withstand mechanical stress than over-and-over continuous skin sutures. An exception is the superior part of the wound parallel to the clitoral shaft. Using an intradermal suture here will prevent needle entry and exit sites to be visible later [7]. Nonetheless, it seems that applying intradermal barbed monofilament absorbable suture will eliminate the concerns described above.

Sometimes during closing the skin on the level of posterior commissure, especially when the skin herein is flaccid, a trap-door deformity can occur. In such a case, a triangle of the excessive inferior labial skin with the base placed on a lateral incision (Burow triangle) should be excised and sutured [7].

Labia majora changes in shape and tension can also be achieved by puboplasty, monsoplasty or modified abdominoplasty with upward traction. Patients should be warned that these procedures, although effective, can unnaturally pull the anterior commissure upwards. To strengthen the flaccid skin of the labia and to enhance the effect of labiamajoraplasty, the author of the chapter also uses lifting threads. (See Video 7.1: Lifting of the labia majora after labiamajoraplasty with barbed threads.)

It is also possible to perform a partial labiamajoraplasty to address the asymmetry of this region, especially after previous imperfect surgery (Fig. 7.5). (See Video 7.2: The full procedure of labiamajoraplasty.)

ANCILLARY PROCEDURES

Labiamajoraplasty can be successfully performed together with other genital cosmetic procedures, such as labiaminoraplasty and perineoplasty [6,11]. When a patient's dominant concern is skin excess, labiamajoraplasty can also be combined with volume augmentation with autologous fat graft. The sequence of procedures is significant. The labiamajoraplasty should be performed before labiaminoraplasty, which allows better evaluation of the degree of labia minora reduction. It is worth mentioning that according to Gress, labiaplasty of both the labia minora and the labia minora in one session is not advisable, as this hinders healing [7].

When it comes to perineoplasty, it is better to perform it as the first procedure. The reason behind it is that perineoplasty pulls medially lower parts of the labia majora and approximates them at the level of the perineum, thus changing the shape of the lower part of the labia majora and to some extent reducing the degree of the planned reduction in their lower segment.

POSTOPERATIVE CARE

The patient is instructed to place an ice pack on her vulva every 30 minutes for the first 24 hours. All patients return for follow-up on postoperative day 1. Patients are instructed to gently rinse the operated area with soapy water four times a day, and after every bathroom visit, so as to keep the area clean, minimize the risk of infection, and prevent scabs from forming along the incision. Soaking in a bath is discouraged. Patients return for follow-up appointments at the 1-week, 6-week, and 3-month time points. Patients are instructed to refrain from strenuous physical activity for 4 weeks, and sexual intercourse for 6 weeks. After 2 weeks, the patient can also apply fingertip pressure along the line of the scar to promote healing and obtain an optimal scar. Special silicon-based creams can also be used. Postoperative swelling after labia majora reduction goes down slowly and may take up to 1 year. It is important to provide the patient with the above information before surgery [7].

PITFALLS AND COMPLICATIONS

Since the region of the external genitalia is highly vascularized by the internal pudendal artery and inferior epigastric artery, a thorough hemostasis is necessary. One paper presented by Di Saia addressed the issue of postoperative hematoma. After its evacuation, there was no delayed wound healing or distortion, and the patient was satisfied with the aesthetic effect achieved after 6 weeks [12].

In his series of labiamajoraplasties, Alinsod reported 5% premature suture breakage necessitating resuturing [6].

(a) (b)

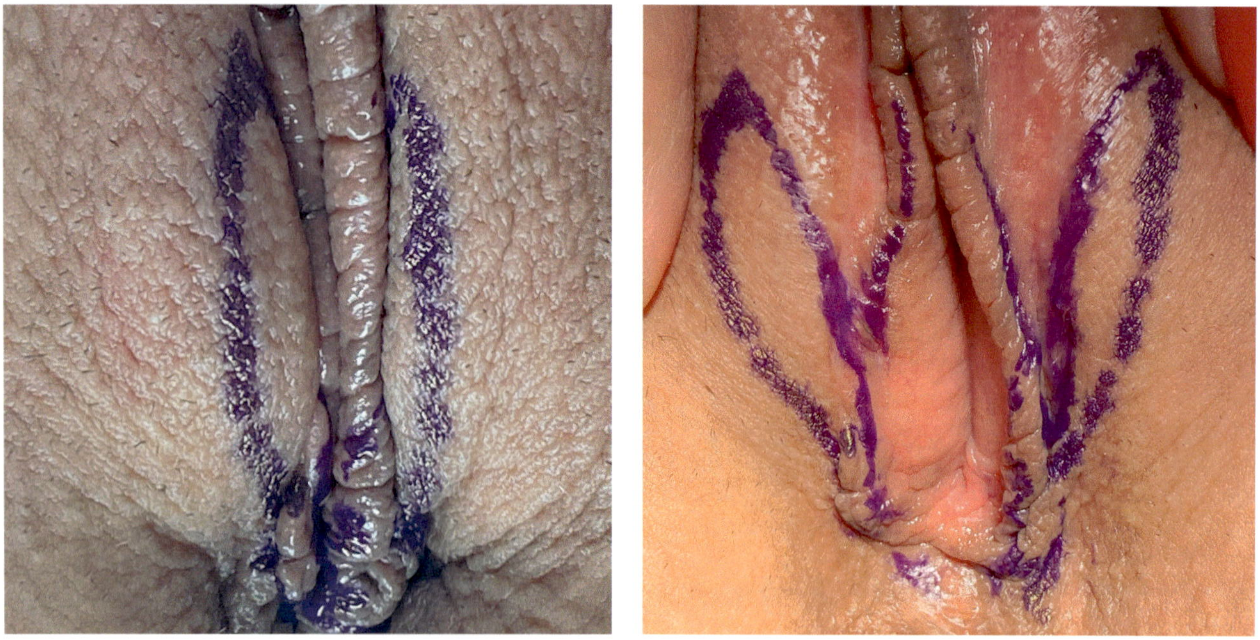

(c)

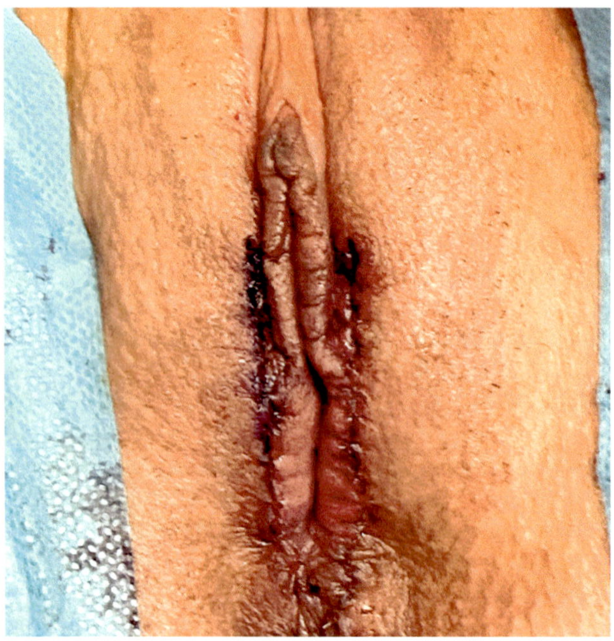

FIGURE 7.5 (a) A patient after labiaminoraplasty with asymmetry of trimmed labia minora, deformation of the region of posterior furchette and a minor hypertrophy and asymmetry of labia majora; (b) the same patient with a full drawing of the surgery planned; (c) after operation.

The author attributed it to physical activity that pulled the edges apart. Given that the perineal region is vulnerable to mechanical stress, free-tension closure of the wound is crucial for seamless wound healing. As already mentioned, too excessive skin incision can also lead to gapping of vaginal introitus.

Another pitfall specific for labiamajoraplasty, resulting from volumetry reduction, is the patient's perception of the labia minora, which may appear larger than before the procedure.

We must also be aware that tightening of the labia minora causes tension on the inner labia. If the labia minora have little height, they may become too flat [7].

REFERENCES

1. Loeb H. *Harnrohrencapacitat und Tripperspritzen Munch Med Woechenschr* 1899;46:1016.
2. Lloyd J, Crouch NS, Minto CL, Liao LM, Creighton SM. Female genital appearance: "normality" unfolds. *BJOG.* 2005 May;112(5):643–646.

3. Alter GJ. Management of the mons pubis and labia majora in the massive weight loss patient. *Aesthet Surg J.* 2009 Sep–Oct;29(5):432–442.
4. Lapalorcia LM, Podda S, Campiglio G, Cordellini M. Labia majora labioplasty in HIV-related vaginal lipodystrophy: technique description and literature review. *Aesthetic Plast Surg*. 2013 Aug;37(4):711–714.
5. Mottura AA. Labia majora hypertrophy. *Aesthetic Plast Surg*. 2009 Nov;33(6):859–863.
6. Hamori CA, Banwell P, Alinsod R. *Female Cosmetic Genital Surgery*. pp. 76–87, 2017 Thieme.
7. Gress S. *Aesthetic and Functional Labiaplasty*. pp. 95–99, 2017 Springer.
8. Goodman M. *Female Genital Plastic and Cosmetic Surgery*. pp. 92–97, 2017 Wiley.
9. Triana L, Robledo AM. Refreshing labioplasty techniques for plastic surgeons. *Aesthetic Plast Surg*. 2012 Oct;36(5):1078–1086.
10. Barwijuk A. *Atlas Ginekologii Plastycznej*. p. 133, 2017 PZWL.
11. Miklos JR, Moore RD. Simultaneous labia minora and majora reduction: a case report. *J Minim Invasive Gynecol*. 2011 May–Jun;18(3):378–380.
12. Di Saia JP. An unusual staged labial rejuvenation. *J Sex Med*. 2008 May;5(5):1263–1267.

8 Clitoral Plasty

Hood Lifting and Reduction

Rafal Kuzlik

The labia minora and clitoral hood should be considered together, not separately, as one organ, one region of the vulva. This is why clitoral hood reduction or lifting (more rarely) is most often performed together with labia minora reduction. It is very rare that only the clitoral hood alone needs to be reduced as primary surgical intervention, but it is quite common that if labiaplasty is botched, the remaining clitoral hood stays as a micro penis. In such cases, only the clitoral hood reduction can be done as an isolated procedure. Sometimes clitoral repositioning must be performed together with clitoral hood reduction but this problem will be described in the later section of this chapter on the double "O" technique. In this chapter, I present clitoral hood reconstruction techniques as primary procedures.

Historically, Graves et al. described removing the portions of the clitoral hood as an integral part of clitoral reduction techniques in the case of clitoromegaly treatment [1] (Fig. 8.1). I call this technique the *classic anterior technique*. Next in 2005, Alter presented his technique of labia minora and clitoral hood reduction (CHR). He described central wedge resection of the labia with lateral excision of the clitoral hood [2] (Fig. 8.2).

It is impossible not to mention CHR described by Gress [3]. In 2006, he presented his technique of composite reduction labiaplasty, which involved modification of the edge resection technique and transverse resection of the clitoral hood at its top – the level of anterior labial commissure (Fig. 8.3).

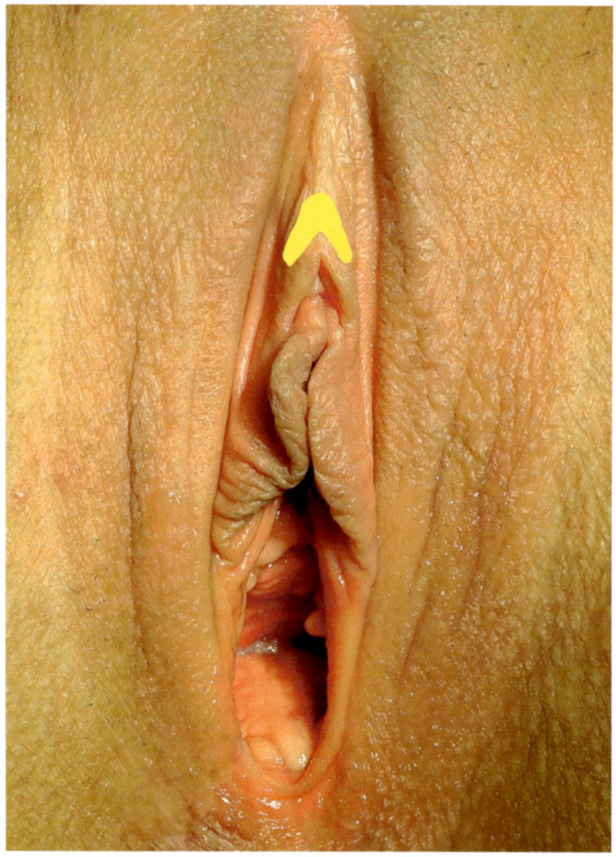

FIGURE 8.1 CHR described by Graves et al. [1] as a part of clitoromegaly treatment.

In 2007, Felicio discussed isolated CHR [3]. She performed a fusiform excision lateral to the clitoris in each side (Fig. 8.4). I call this technique a *classic lateral* one. It is simple excision of periclitoral folds and, in my opinion, should be proceeded with labia minora reduction (especially trim/edge resection technique) as one combined procedure. Felicio discouraged simultaneous CHR and labia minora reduction because of prolonged edema. I cannot agree with this opinion, especially if a small dosage of steroids (1 mg of dexametrhason) is being prescribed after surgery. It is very important to mention that one of the main goals she stressed was the importance of maintaining the middle orientation of the clitoris and preservation of the symmetry relative to the labia minora and majora and of achieving clitoral exposure [4].

Another technique of CHR was described in 2008 by Apesos et al. [5]. An inverted V resection of the clitoral hood is located high, at the superior extent of the anterior labial commissure (Fig. 8.5). Personally, I am not a supporter of this technique because of the transverse scar on the longitudinal organ and because of higher risk of wound dehiscence.

DOI: 10.1201/9780429353079-8

(a) (b)

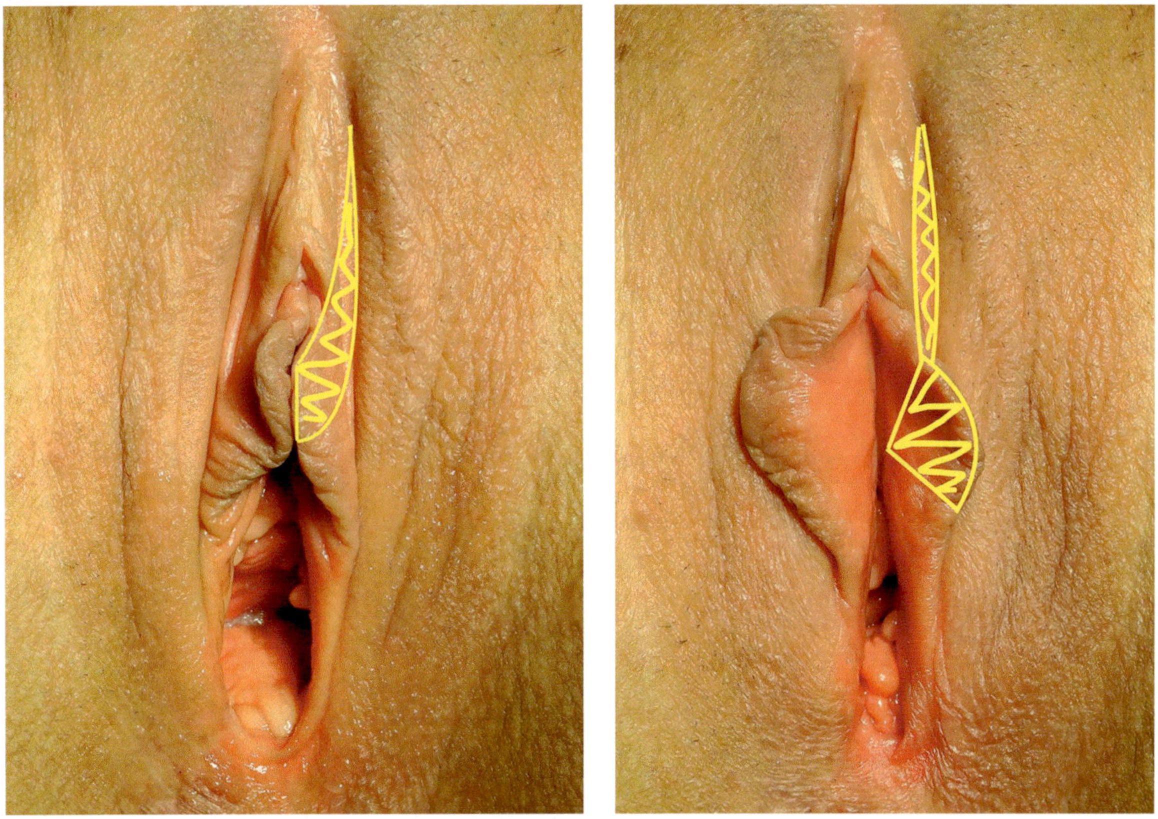

FIGURE 8.2 CHR described by Alter [2] as a part of his wedge labiaplasty technique, shown (a, b) from both sides of the labia.

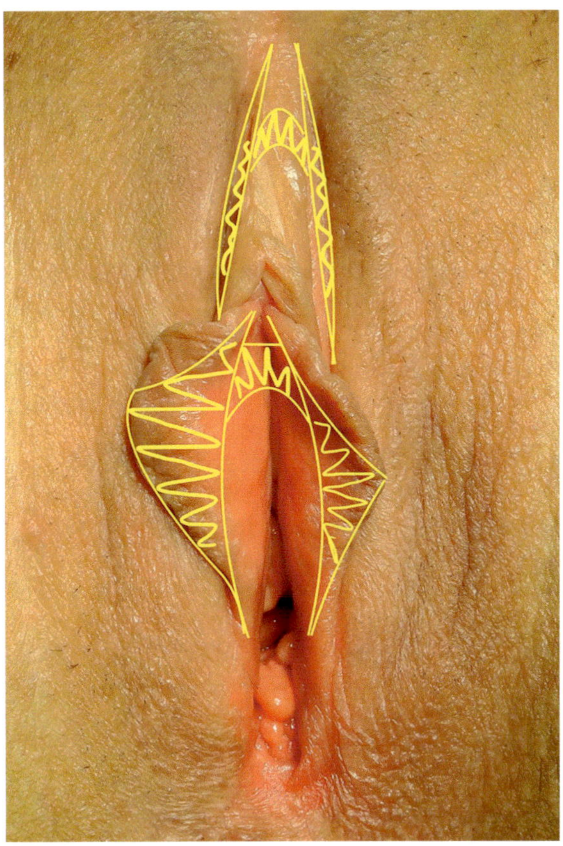

FIGURE 8.3 CHR described by Gress [3] as part of composite reduction labiaplasty.

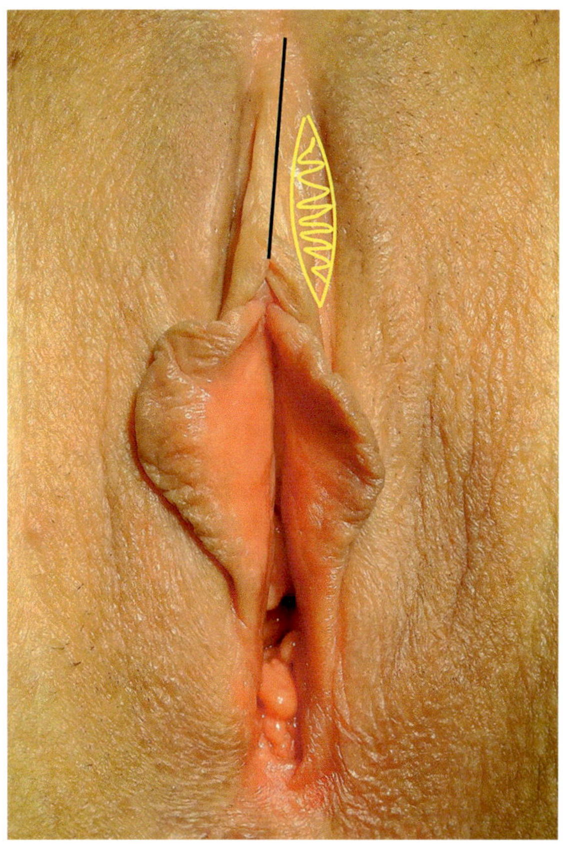

FIGURE 8.4 Isolated CHR described by Felicio [4].

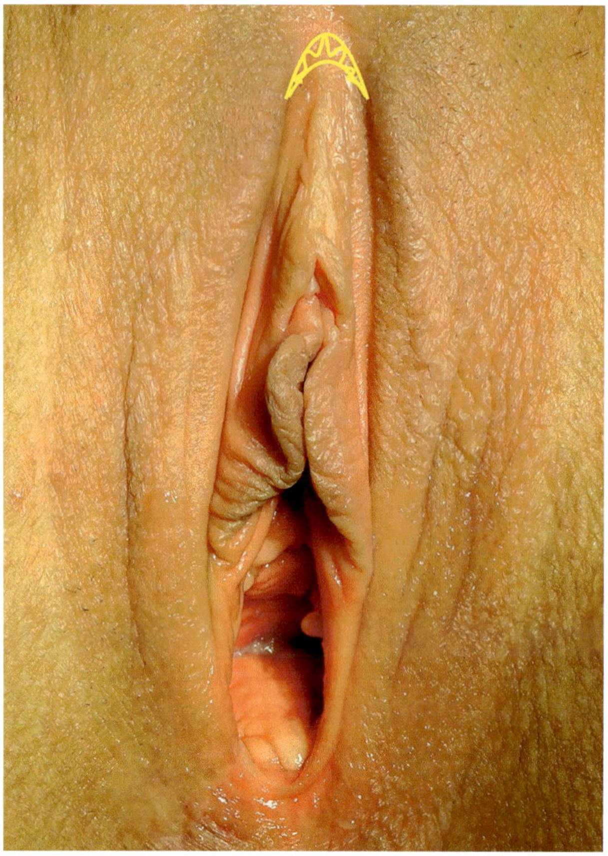

FIGURE 8.5 Isolated CHR described by Apesos et al. [5].

The clitoral hood itself, as well as the labia minora, looks different in different women. Sometimes it is smooth and thin, and other times it has folds situated on both sides. Sometimes it is long and the clitoral gland is totally covered, and other times it is very short with a visualized clitoral gland (Fig. 8.6). In the case of a smooth and short clitoral hood, surgical intervention is rarely undertaken. In the case of a long or folded clitoral hood, surgery is the most frequently chosen method of treatment. These types of clitoral hood shapes affect the choice of surgical lifting technique. The *anterior technique* should be planned in cases of smooth and long clitoral hoods. If the patient's clitoral hood is smooth but protruded, the *classic lateral technique* seems to be the best choice. In the case of folded clitoral hood (with periclitoral folds situated on both or one side), with protrusion of this region, which is very common, especially if the clitoral gland is visualized, in my opinion only the *deepithelialization technique* can be considered. When the clitoral hood type is mixed (e.g., too long and folded or smooth but too long) a mixed technique needs to be performed – the *anterior technique* together with *deepithelialization* or the *classic lateral* technique.

In my practice, I perform different kinds of clitoral hood restorations depending on the patient's type of clitoral hood. In the majority of cases, I use the following techniques: classic anterior or lateral, deepithelialization (one cut), linear "Z" and double "O".

Considering all the facts mentioned above, I created the *Clitoral Hood Classification.* It is very important to recognize the type of clitoral hood before surgery.

CLITORAL HOOD CLASSIFICATION TYPES

Type 1: Smooth
Type 2: Folded

Each type can be:

- Normal (clitoral gland is partially covered) – Subtype A
- Short (clitoral gland is fully uncovered) – Subtype B
- Long (clitoral gland is completely covered) – Subtype C
- Protruded (shown over the labia majora) – Subtype D
- Non-protruded (hidden between the labia majora) – Subtype E

A thorough assessment of a patient's relevant anatomy and treatment goals will guide the surgeon in choosing the optimal approach to the clitoral hood. However, to help the surgeon choose the appropriate method, I created a simple guide so that, depending on the type of clitoral hood, the proper technique can be chosen (Table 8.1).

My Techniques

In my experience, only a few surgeons prefer the inverted V or other transverse incisions of the clitoral hood to converge superiorly to treat vertical redundancy. I have found that most of them use the lateral approach.

However, as I mentioned, CHR is rarely performed as an isolated procedure. In the majority of cases it accompanies labia minora reduction.

In my practice, I usually perform the *classic lateral* or *anterior technique* for an isolated clitoral hood reduction. Sometimes I also perform the *double O technique* as an isolated procedure, but this method is definitely intended for botched labiaplasty treatment ("penis-like shape") or isolated protrusion of the clitoris and clitoral hood, which is very rare. However, it is also impossible not to mention the other two techniques that I perform in my practice: the *one cut* and *linear Z.* These two are combined techniques of simultaneous reduction of the

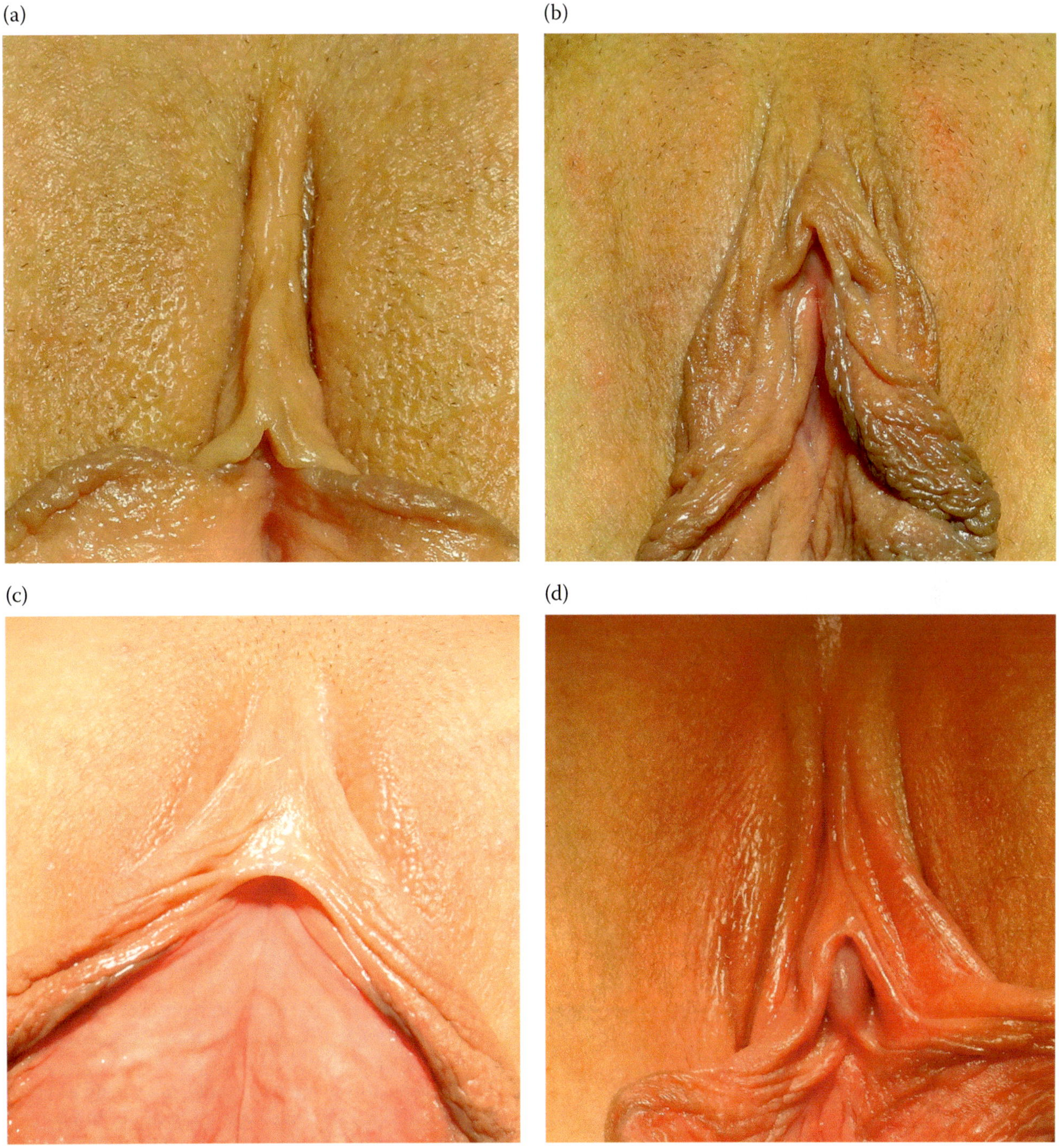

FIGURE 8.6 Different shapes of clitoral hood: (a) smooth; (b) folded; (c) long with covered clitoral gland; and (d) short with shown clitoral gland.

labia minora and clitoral hood, and as different techniques they are described in separate chapters (Chapters 6 and 7) of this book.

Patient evaluation and preoperative and postoperative procedures are the same as those described in Chapter 7 of this book on deepithelialization, where what the surgeon needs to have on the table (Fig. 8.7) is also described.

Anesthesia and Antibiotics

The type of local anesthesia depends on the technique the surgeon is going to perform. In the case of the *classic lateral* or *anterior technique,* 0.5% lidocaine with 0.9% saline seems to be a sufficient solution. On the other hand, if the double "O" technique needs to be done, 0.5% lidocaine may not be enough. In my practice, I always use

TABLE 8.1
Choice of Surgical Technique According to the Type of Clitoral Hood

<table>
<tr><th>Subtype of the Hood</th><th>A – Normal</th><th>B – Short</th><th>C – Long</th><th>D – Protruded</th><th>E – Non-Protruded</th><th>Type of Hood</th></tr>
<tr><td rowspan="2">A</td><td>X</td><td rowspan="2">X</td><td rowspan="2">X</td><td rowspan="2">Classic – lateral
Double “O”</td><td rowspan="2">X</td><td rowspan="2">S</td></tr>
<tr><td>Classic – lateral</td></tr>
<tr><td rowspan="2">B</td><td rowspan="2">X</td><td>Classic – lateral</td><td rowspan="2">X</td><td>One cut
Linear “Z”</td><td rowspan="2">Classic – lateral</td><td rowspan="2">F</td></tr>
<tr><td>x</td><td>Classic – lateral</td></tr>
<tr><td rowspan="2">C</td><td rowspan="2">X</td><td rowspan="2">X</td><td>Classic – anterior</td><td rowspan="2">Classic – lateral + anterior</td><td rowspan="2">Classic – anterior</td><td rowspan="2">S</td></tr>
<tr><td>One cut
Linear “Z” + Classic – anterior</td></tr>
<tr><td rowspan="2">D</td><td rowspan="2">One cut
Linear “Z”
Double “O”</td><td>One cut
Linear “Z”
Double “O”</td><td rowspan="2">One cut
Linear “Z”
Double “O”
+ Classic – anterior</td><td>One cut
Linear “Z”</td><td rowspan="2">X</td><td rowspan="2">F</td></tr>
<tr><td>Classic – lateral
Double “O”</td><td>Classic – lateral</td></tr>
<tr><td rowspan="2">E</td><td>X</td><td rowspan="2">X</td><td>Classic – anterior</td><td rowspan="2">X</td><td>Classic – lateral</td><td rowspan="2">S</td></tr>
<tr><td>Classic – lateral</td><td>One cut
Linear “Z”
+ Classic – anterior</td><td>Classic – lateral</td></tr>
<tr><td>TYPE OF HOOD</td><td>F – Folded</td><td>S – Smooth</td><td>F – Folded</td><td>S – Smooth</td><td>F – Folded</td><td></td></tr>
</table>

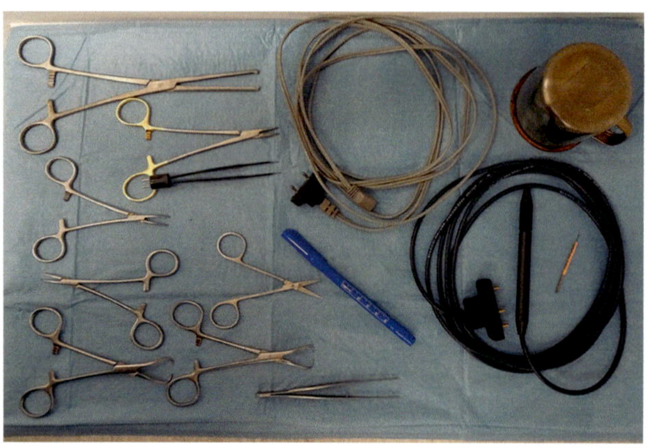

FIGURE 8.7 Typical surgical table.

bupivacaine (50 mg/10 mL) or ropivacaine (100 mg/10 mL) diluted in 10 mL of 0.9% saline. TLA also can be performed in such cases.

Prophylactic broad-spectrum antibiotics should be given just before surgery, and they are the same as in cases of labia minora surgeries – second-generation cephalosporin 1–2 g i.v.). Dexamethasone (8 mg i.v.) also needs to be injected as a prevention against intraoperative swelling of the surgical area.

Markings and Positioning

The patient always should be positioned in gynecologic dorsal lithotomy with legs fully open. It is important to have full access to the area of interest. Markings of

(a) (b)

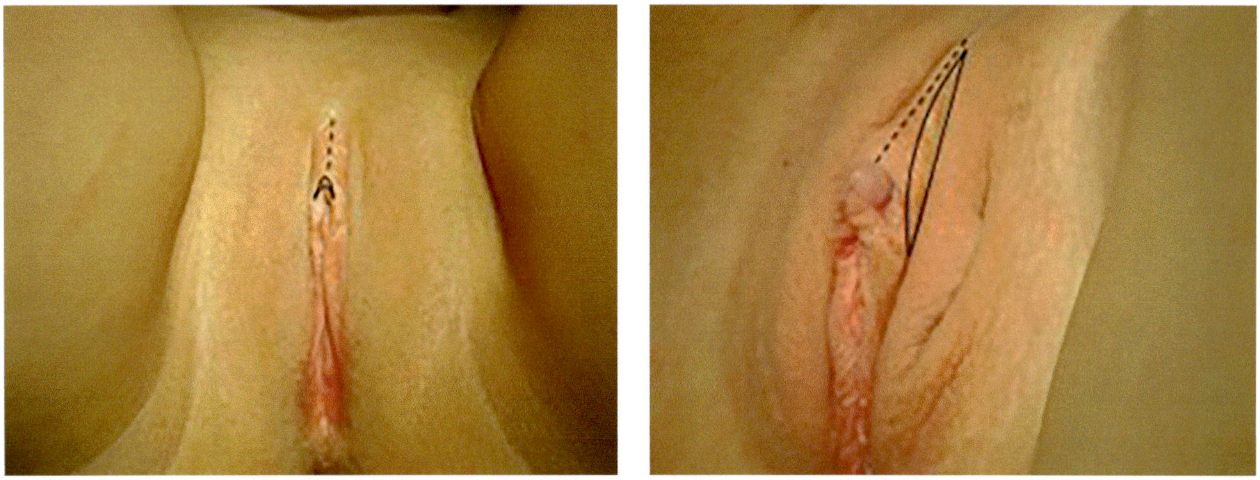

FIGURE 8.8 CHR – anterior (a) and lateral (b) approach.

(a) (b)

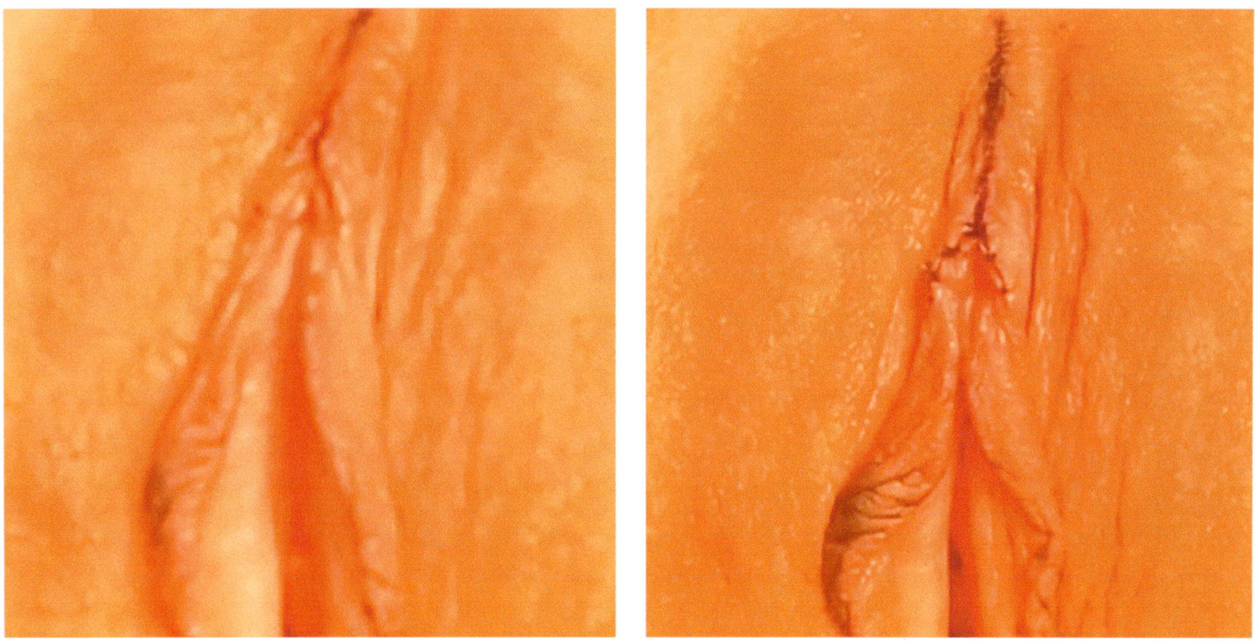

FIGURE 8.9 Classic anterior hood reduction: (a) skin removal and (b) wound suturing.

course depend on the technique that is going to be performed. In the case of the *classic anterior* approach, they are very small or sometimes we don't need any (because the area to be reduced is too small to be marked). When classic lateral or double "O" techniques are planned, markings are situated on both sides of the hood ("eyedrop" shape) (Fig. 8.8).

Classic Anterior Technique

Technically in the classic anterior approach a small amount of anesthesia is injected into the tip of clitoral hood and 2–3 mm of the skin is resected. It is important to remember the rule: a bigger piece of resected skin should be cut off from outside than inside of the hood.

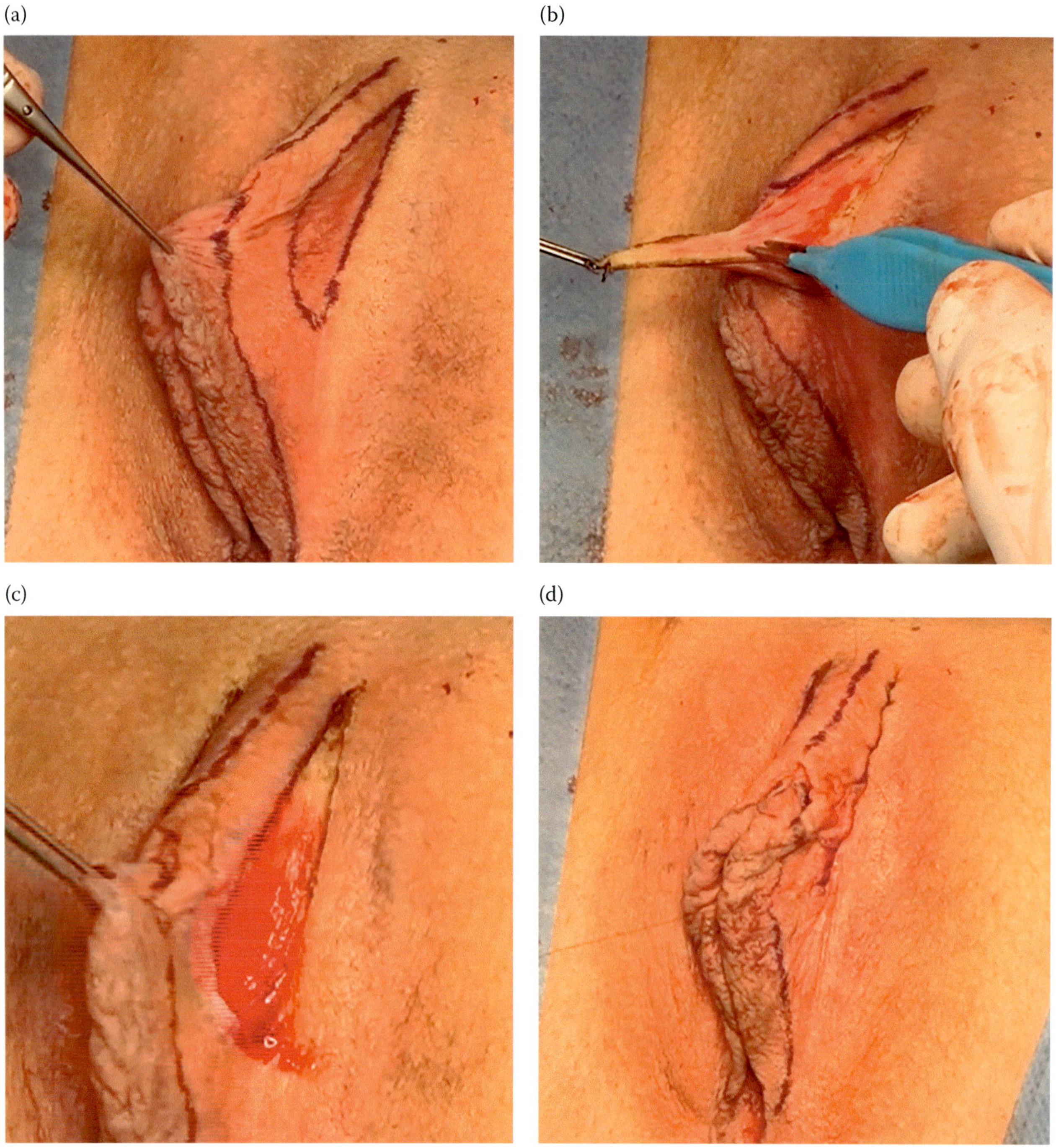

FIGURE 8.10 Classic lateral hood reduction: (a) markings; (b) skin removal using the sliding technique; (c) removal of the "eye-drop"-like part of the skin of the hood; (d) wound closure with running suture.

The difference is not big (1 mm generally should be enough), but it needs to exist to prevent clitoral irritation by the skin, which could be rolled in if the surgeon proceeds the opposite way (cut piece bigger from the inside). Next, three to five singular stitches (Monocryl 5.0) need to be done (one in the centre and one or two on both sides of the middle line) (Fig. 8.9).

Classic Lateral Technique

The surgeon cuts the skin after previous infiltration of the "eye-drop" area with regular solution of lidocaine, adrenaline and saline. Next this small eye-drop-like piece is cut off with bipolar forceps using the sliding technique. After control of the hemostasis, the wound is

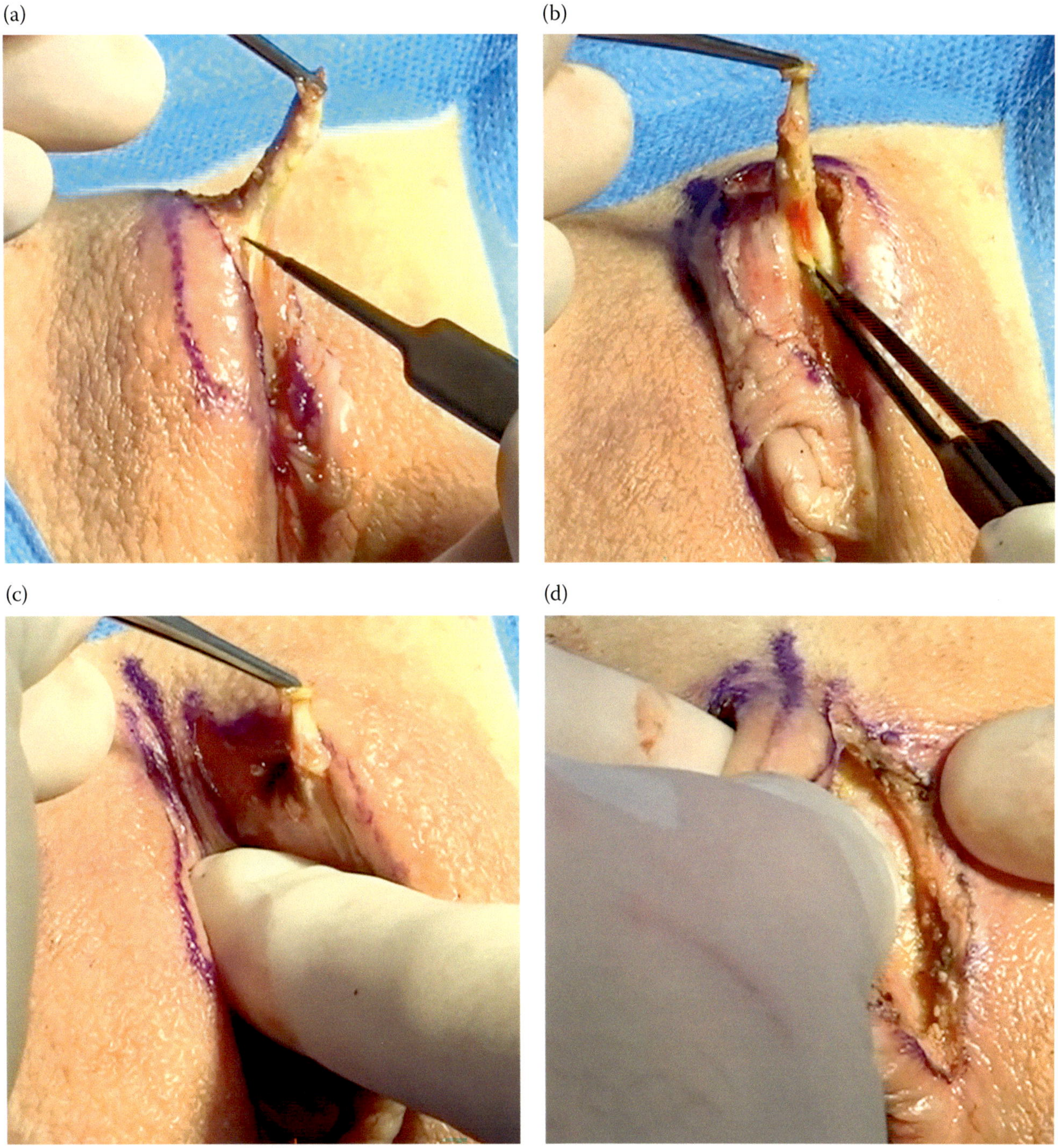

FIGURE 8.11 The surgeon "digs" layer by layer and removes loose tissues lying under the skin on both sides of the clitoral body (a, b). It is important to know the exact position of the clitoris – the surgeon touches it with one finger and between 2 fingers (c, d).

closed with an intracutaneous running suture (Monocryl 5.0) (Fig. 8.10).

Double "O" Technique

In the case of big primary clitoral protrusion, or post-operative side effects ("penis-like shape"), the regular techniques described above can appear inadequate for the problem. Of course, sometimes autologous fat transfer to the labia majora can be helpful, but if the patient doesn't want to have bigger majora, only hood reduction and repositioning of the clitoris appears to be the best solution.

The surgeon who wants to perform the double "O" technique needs to know the anatomy, of course, but the most important thing is to remember that clitoral

(a) (b)

(c) (d)

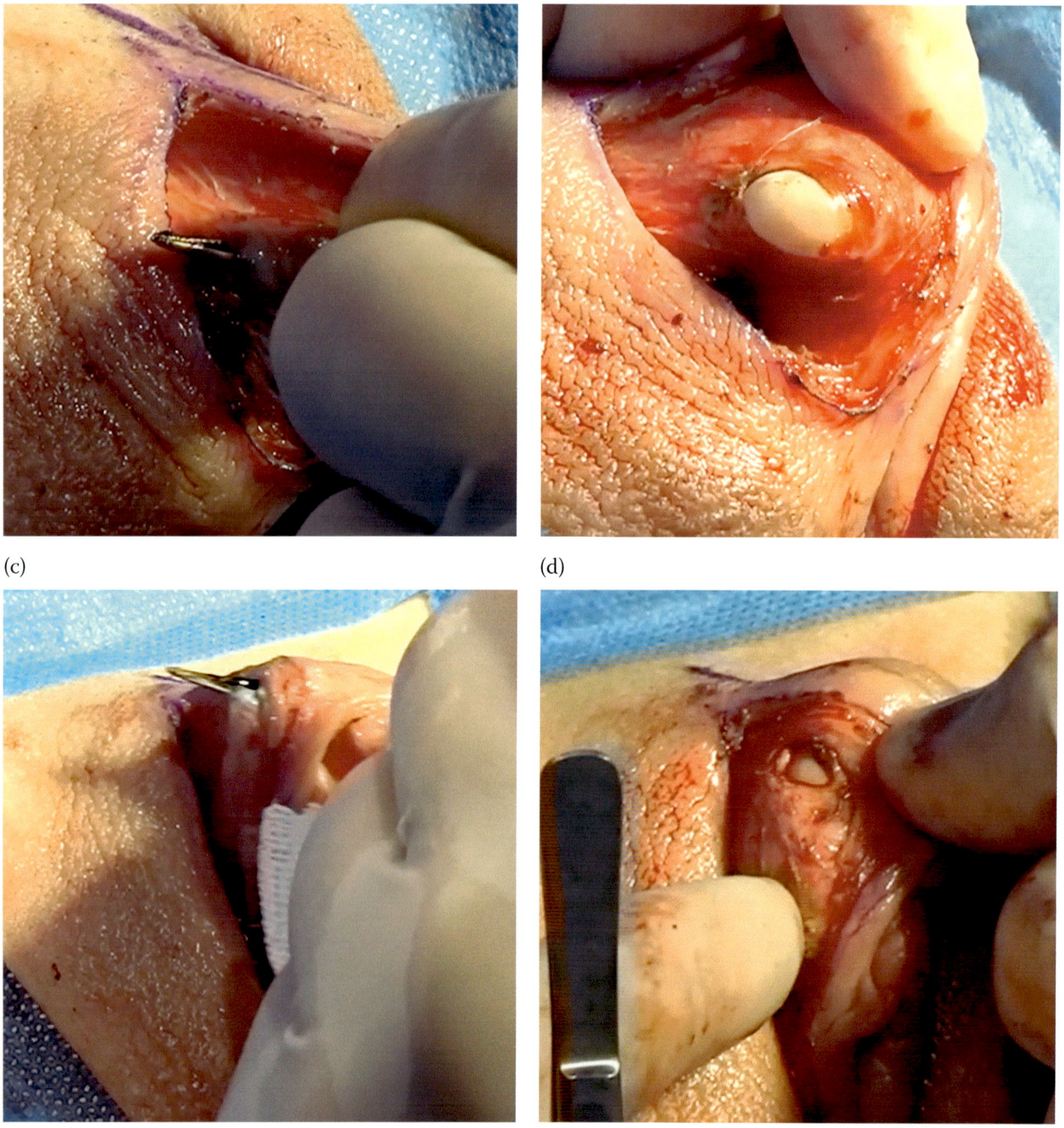

FIGURE 8.12 Two "O"s have been completed: below the clitoris (a, b) and over it (c, d).

vascularization and innervation are situated on the top of clitoral body. This knowledge is crucial because during this procedure the clitoral body is being uncovered on both sides – the top and the bottom. The risk of complication in the form of vascular and nerve damage is quite high. This is why this technique is designed only for severe cases, when none of the other techniques would hide enough the clitoris and its hood between the labia majora. Only a properly trained surgeon should do this procedure.

(a) (b)

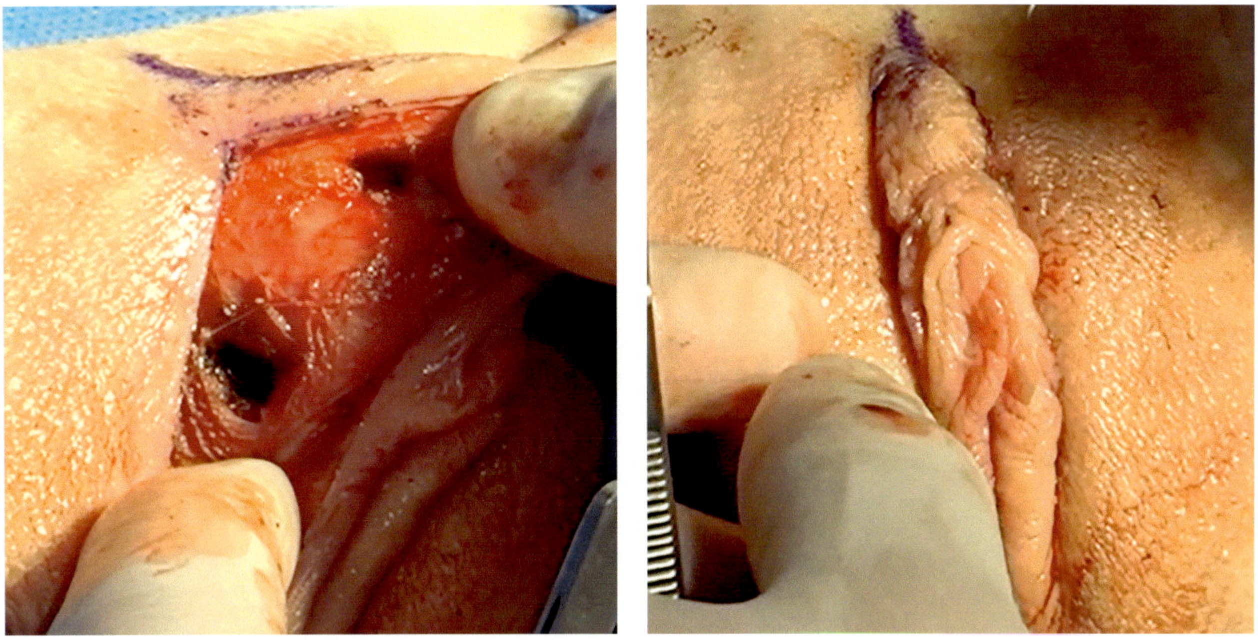

(c)

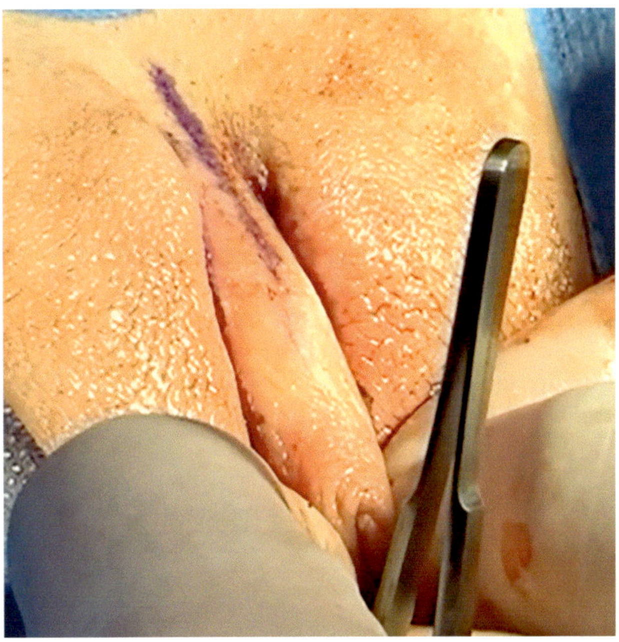

FIGURE 8.13 (a) Two holes have been created with the speared vascular-nerve bundle laying over the clitoral body. (b, c) Thanks to these holes, the clitoral hood is hidden between the labia majora, and proper mobility of the hood's skin has been achieved.

The Technique

Markings are the same as those described above (for the lateral approach). Anesthesia is infiltrated deeper than during the classic lateral hood reduction technique, and an inguinal block needs to be performed. Skin cutting and the flap removal technique are identical to that mentioned above. When the skin flap has been removed, part of the loose tissue lying under is also cut out. The surgeon "digs" under the clitoral body by removing these loose tissues layer by layer, but still needs to know where the clitoral body is situated. During the procedure you must know the clitoral positioning by touching it with a finger and sometimes holding it between two fingers (Fig. 8.11).

(a) (b)

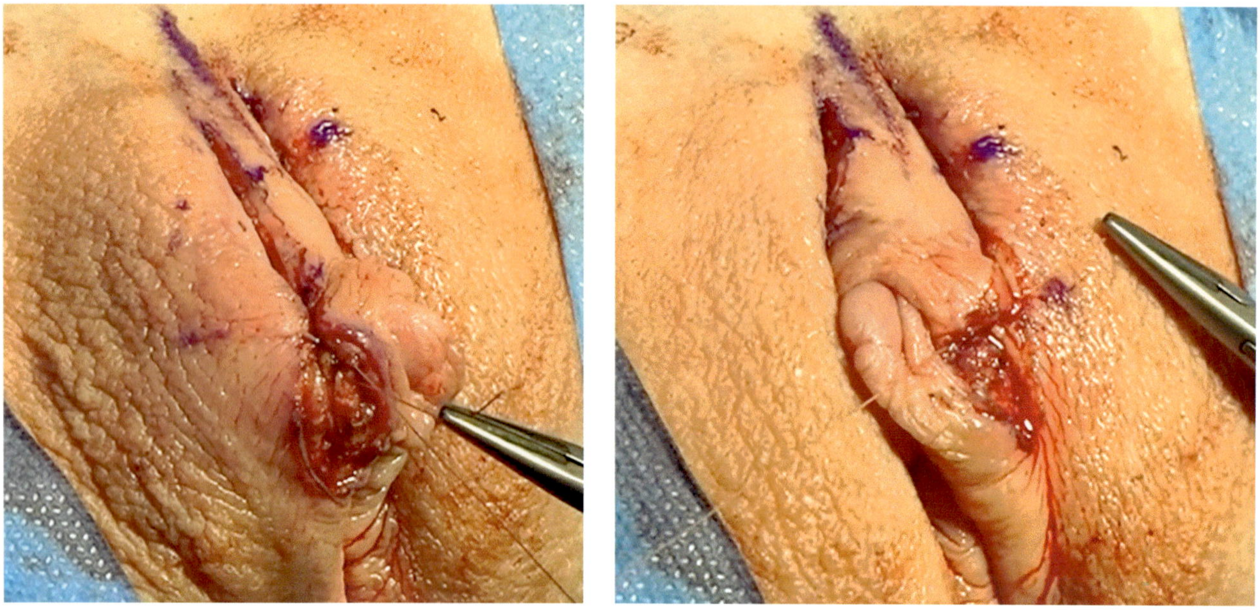

FIGURE 8.14 First layer of the stitches – (a) positioning of the clitoris and (b) clitoral hood.

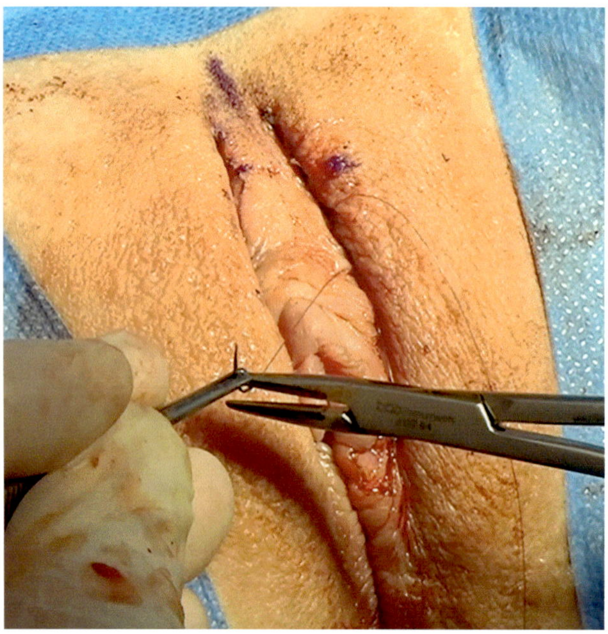

FIGURE 8.15 The wounds are being closed with resorbable running sutures.

After this initial activity, the lower "O" has been completed. It is important to be very careful during this procedure because there is a risk of bleeding at the bottom. Next, the upper "O" is undertaken. The technique of "digging" is similar to the previous one (Fig. 8.12).

The next step is to create adequate holes under and over the clitoral body. The main goal of creating these two holes is first, making the space under the clitoris (the lower "O") to hide the clitoral hood with the clitoris within and second, causing better mobility of the hood's skin. It is crucial not to damage the vascular-nerve bundle, as mentioned previously (Fig. 8.13).

The next step is positioning of the new clitoral hood with the clitoris within. This is a very important step of the procedure. Positioning is achieved by the first layer of two to three singular stitches (Vicryl 4.0) (Fig. 8.14).

Closing the wound is the last procedure. Unresorbable running sutures are used. The last notches are situated inside the vestibulum (Fig. 8.15).

The expected results need to achieve a clitoral hood to be hidden between the labia majora (Fig. 8.16).

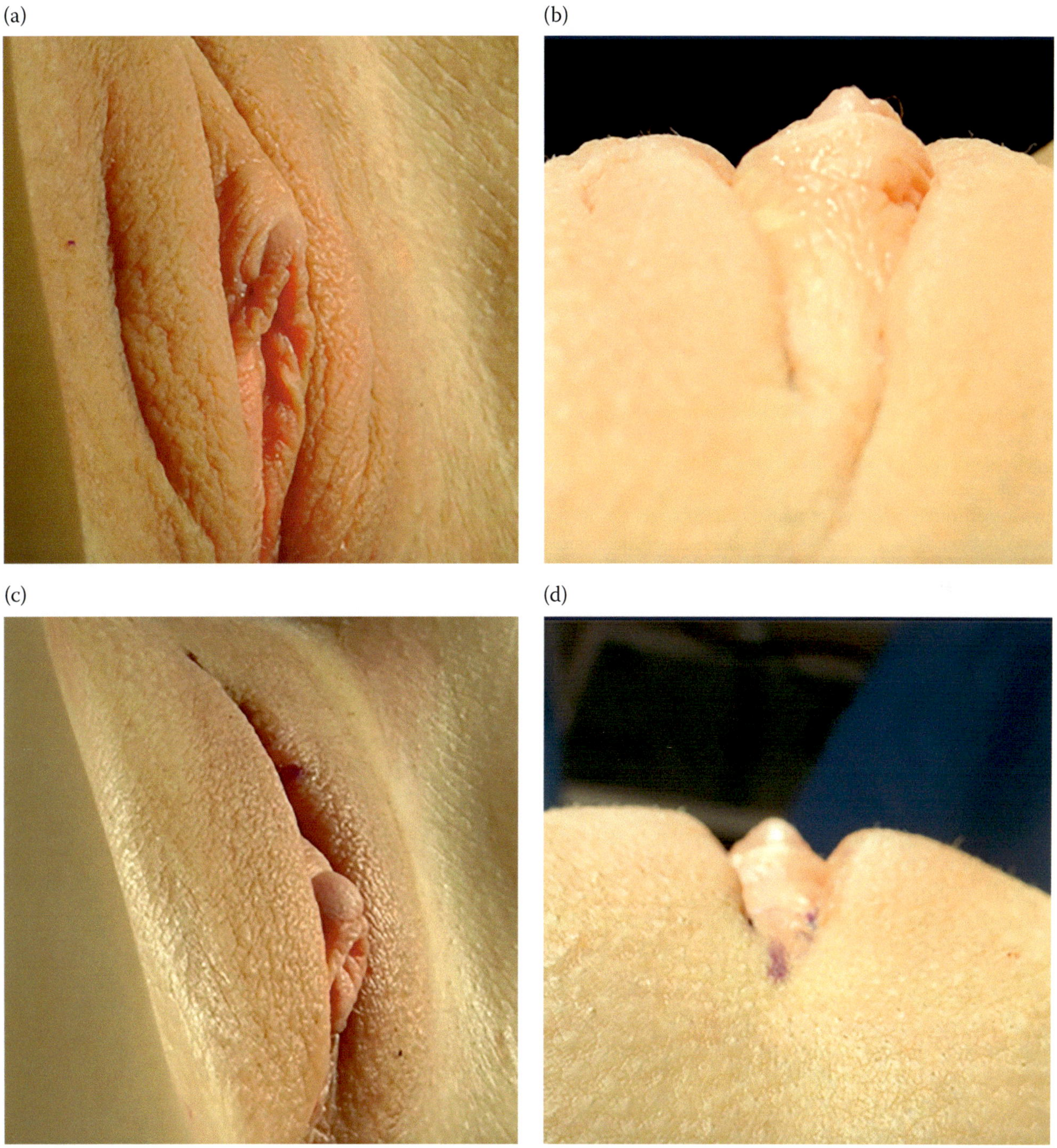

FIGURE 8.16 (a, b) Before and (d, e) results after the procedure.

Postoperative Care

Postoperative care is identical to that required after labia minora reduction. Airing the wound and keeping it clean and dry are the most important activities.

REFERENCES

1. Graves KL, Wilson EA, Greene JW Jr. Surgical technique for clitoral reduction. *Obstet Gynecol* 59:758, 1982.
2. Alter GJ. Central wedge nymphectomy with a 90-degree Z-plasty for aesthetic reduction of the labia minora. *Plast Reconstr Surg* 115:2144, 2005.
3. de Alencar Felicio Y. Labial surgery. *Aesthet Surg J* 27:322, 2007.
4. Hammori CA, Banwell PE, Alinsod R. *Female Cosmetic Genital Surgery*. New York: Thieme, 2017:161–180.
5. Apesos J, Jackson R, Miklos JR, et al, eds. *Vagina Makeover & Rejuvenation*. Cape Town: MWP Media, 2008.

9 Single Thread Vagino–Perineoplasty

Alexander Bader

INTRODUCTION

One of the most common surgical interventions in the vaginal canal is the anterior–posterior repair, often called "colporrhaphy" (anterior/posterior). The main indication of this intervention is what is referred to as vaginal prolapses. The term can include prolapse of the bladder "cystocele", prolapse of the rectum "rectocele", and prolapse of the bowel "enterocele". On many occasions, a combination of two or all three types of prolapse can be observed in the same patient. The main reason is the lack of anatomical support by the pelvic floor muscles and ligaments. As a result, the patient usually suffers several symptoms, including:

- A bulge near or at the vagina opening
- A pressure sensation in the pelvic area and or lower abdomen
- A sensation of fullness
- Urine leakage symptoms
- Increase of frequency
- A sensation of the inability to empty the bladder with urination
- Difficulty to start urinating
- Minor bleeding due to continuous rubbing of the exposed organ
- Constipation
- Lack of sexual sensation
- Trapped air inside the vaginal cavity which frequently produces sound
- Excessive vaginal discharge

The above symptoms can worsen the quality of life. A simple gynecology examination can make the diagnosis of the above anatomical defects. However, repairing the above situations is usually surgical, and surgery can be extensive and radical.

In recent years and due to lifestyle and less frequency of pregnancies, fewer women are suffering from significant degrees of prolapse. However, women significantly younger are suffering from vaginal wall relaxation without prolapse. The vaginal wall is elastic, and the superficial muscles are weak due to lack of exercise or even damage during delivery, and the situation could be described as a minor prolapse. Many suffer the same when they lose significant weight. These patients have as a primary concern the lack of sexual sensation and therefore pleasure. Rarely do they suffer the bulge and pressure sensation. Urine leakage or streaming is not an issue. The patients are particularly looking to improve their sexual function alongside the appearance of the surrounding external tissues, including but not limited to the perineum. Female sexual dysfunction is defined as a disorder of sexual desire, sexual arousal, orgasm, and sexual pain contributing to personal distress [1]. Sexual dysfunction is a multifactorial disorder; biological, psychosocial, and relational factors can contribute to female sexual dysfunction. Among these factors, the pelvic floor appears to have a significant influence. Dysfunction of vaginal support leading to incontinence, prolapse, and sexual dysfunction is highly prevalent [2].

The posterior vaginal wall repair sounds like the most likely procedure to improve the overall vaginal function, tighten the vaginal canal and repair the anatomical defects at the perineal area. Recently, vaginal rejuvenation and cosmetic vaginal surgery have been increasingly popular in gynecology. With the term "vaginal rejuvenation", many refer to the overall improvement of function and shape. However, the term referred to as vaginoplasty sounds more accurate and is most likely related to the surgical intervention performed to improve the function and appearance of the female genital area. Vaginoplasty comes from the combined words "vagina" (female genitalia) and "plasty", a word descending from the Greek word "platho", which means to create a form or give a shape – giving the vagina a form to improve the shape and consequently the function.

The chapter describes a new technique to perform perineo-vaginoplasty with a single barbered thread. The technique aims to tighten the entire vaginal canal and repair the perineal body in a much less invasive way.

CONSULTATION AND EVALUATION

The physical examination is the first step to determining the patient's needs. The visual and physical examination entails a classical gynecology assessment. In lithotomy position, the surgeon must look into the details of the area and work out the anatomical variation that has been created by a specific event such as a vaginal delivery, an

DOI: 10.1201/9780429353079-9

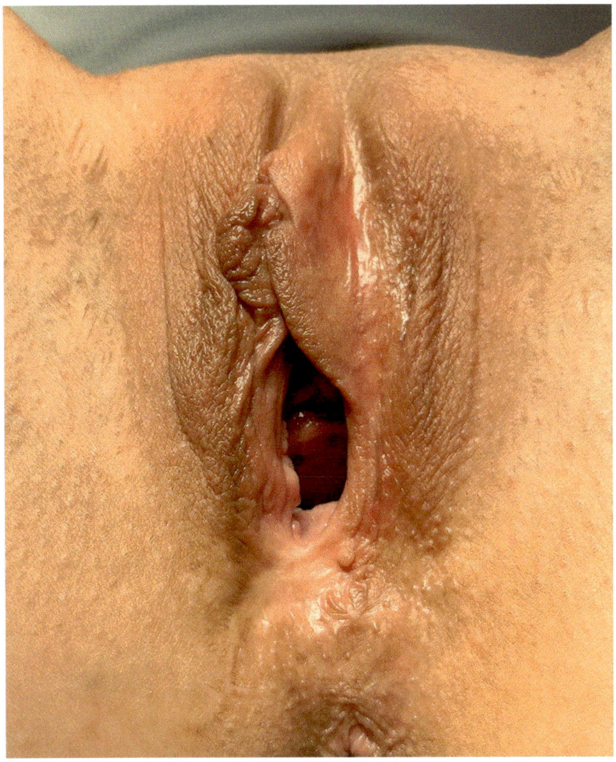

FIGURE 9.1 Perineo-vaginal damage after birth.

accident or even a previous surgery (Figs. 9.1 and 9.2). A speculum insertion, manual examination, vaginal muscle assessment and classification based on the Oxford scale, cough test and standing position examination would all be considered to have a complete picture and opinion over the patient's requests and needs. Since the goal of the vaginoplasty is not only functional but also cosmetic, an external assessment is mandatory. A perineal body examination has to be done, and a discussion with the patient over other anatomical aspects such as the labia minora or majora has to be established. It is advisable for the patient to hold a mirror during the external assessment. An interactive discussion over the appearance between the surgeon and the patient must be established. The patient must point out what she does not like and how she imagines the area will look after a procedure, and the surgeon must be able to provide options and show potential outcomes to their patient. Marking the area during the examination frequently solves many endless discussions.

PRESURGICAL PREPARATION

The admission process shall include a general health screen and a pregnancy test. The patient has been advised to come with the area very well shaved. Bowel preparation is advisable the night before the surgery. The patient is advised to bring a loose outfit, so she feels comfortable going home after the surgery. The patient is to sign consent

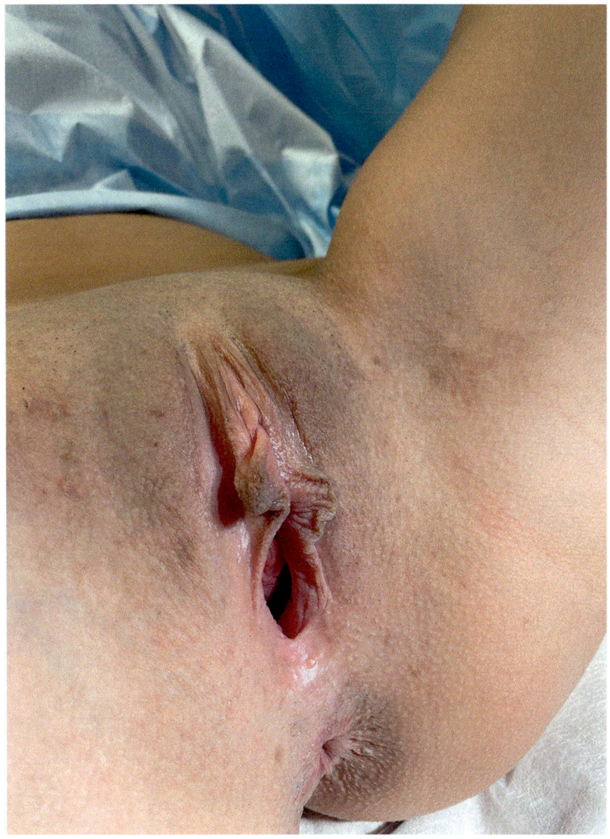

FIGURE 9.2 Perineo-vaginal damage after birth.

procedure informed risks forms and photography consent forms and get prepared for photographs and marking the area. Photography is taken before prepping the area. You could consider lithotomy capture, ensuring that the photos clearly show the vaginal situation, the perineal defects, and any other anatomical area you plan to operate on. The standing position is considered only in case an external cosmetic intervention is to be done. The last step before starting the surgery is prepping the area with an antiseptic solution while the patient is comfortable in a lithotomy position.

TOOLS AND INSTRUMENTS

To perform a single thread vagino-perineoplasty, the surgeon must have prepared the surgery table well. The standard set for minor procedures, such as colporrhaphy, includes needle holders, forceps, and scissors. The table should also include:

- 2 Edna Lorna towel clamps "4 in length" (Fig. 9.3)
- 4 Pratt T-shape clamps "6 in length" (Fig. 9.4)
- Alinsod A1 scissors, S-curved, shape/sharp tips "9 in" (Fig. 9.5)
- Double-needled 2-0 monofilament synthetic absorbable barbed suture with 30 cm × 30 cm

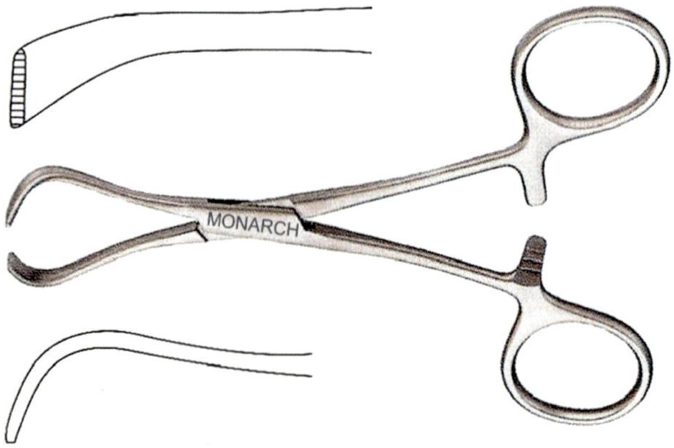

FIGURE 9.3 Edna Lorna towel clamp.

configuration. Reverse cutting 3/8 circle 18 mm needles (Fig. 9.6)
- Lone Star retractor and 4–6 elastic hooks with sharp tips (Fig. 9.7)
- Radiofrequency cautery attached to surgical pencil and RF Colorado tip (Fig. 9.8)
- Diathermy attached to surgical pencil and Colorado dissection needle tip (Fig. 9.9)

SURGICAL PERFORMANCE (STEP BY STEP)

Anesthesia

Local Anesthesia

Thirty minutes before surgery, the patient places numbing cream (compounded topical anesthetics of Benzocaine,

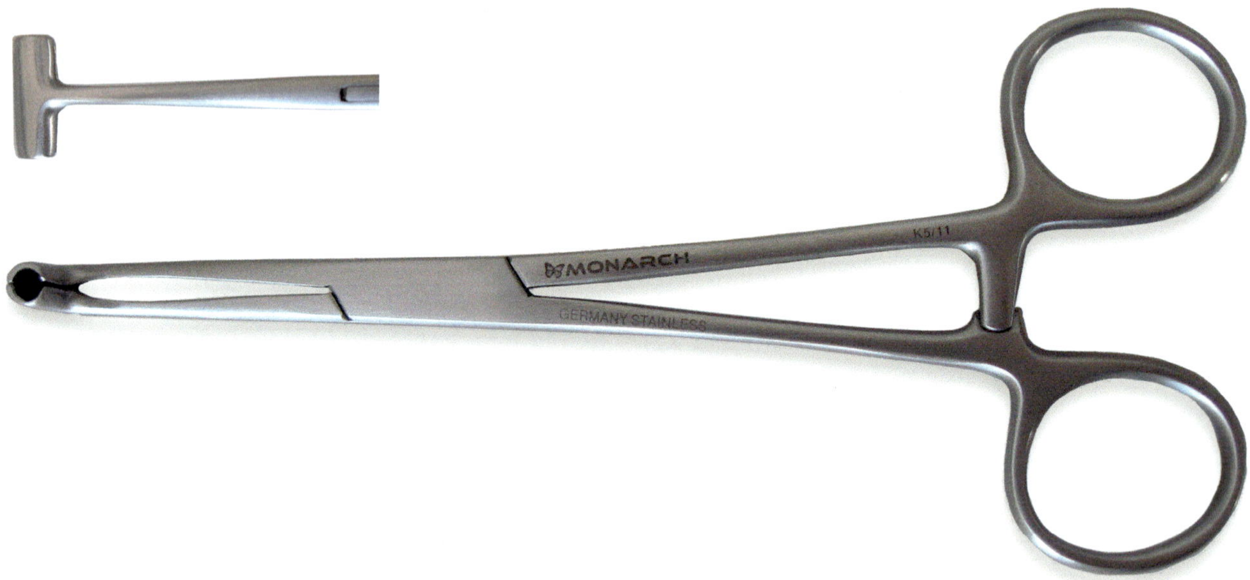

FIGURE 9.4 Pratt T-shape clamp.

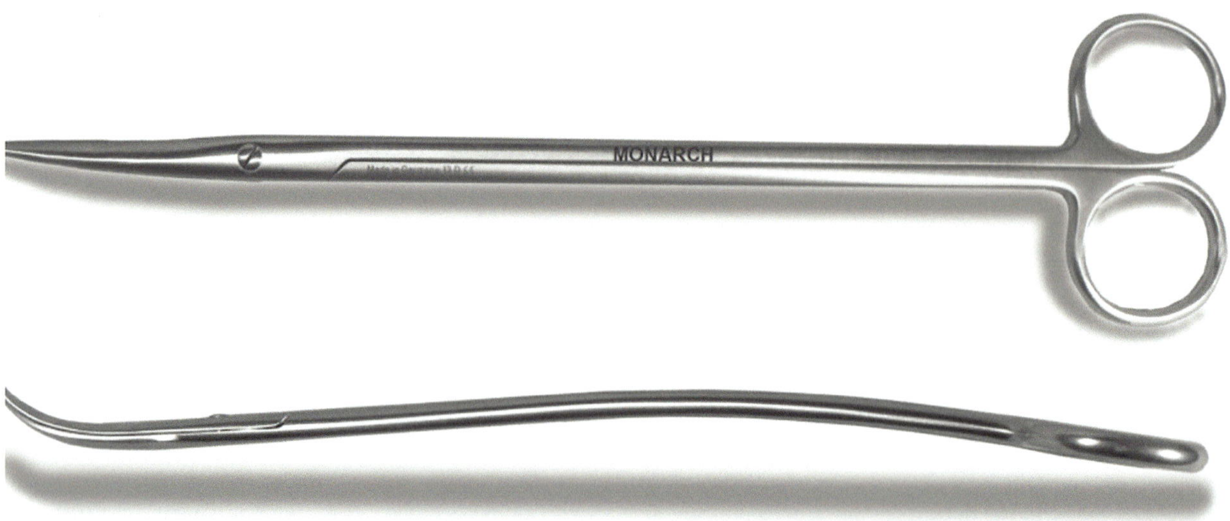

FIGURE 9.5 Alinsod scissor/Monarch curved.

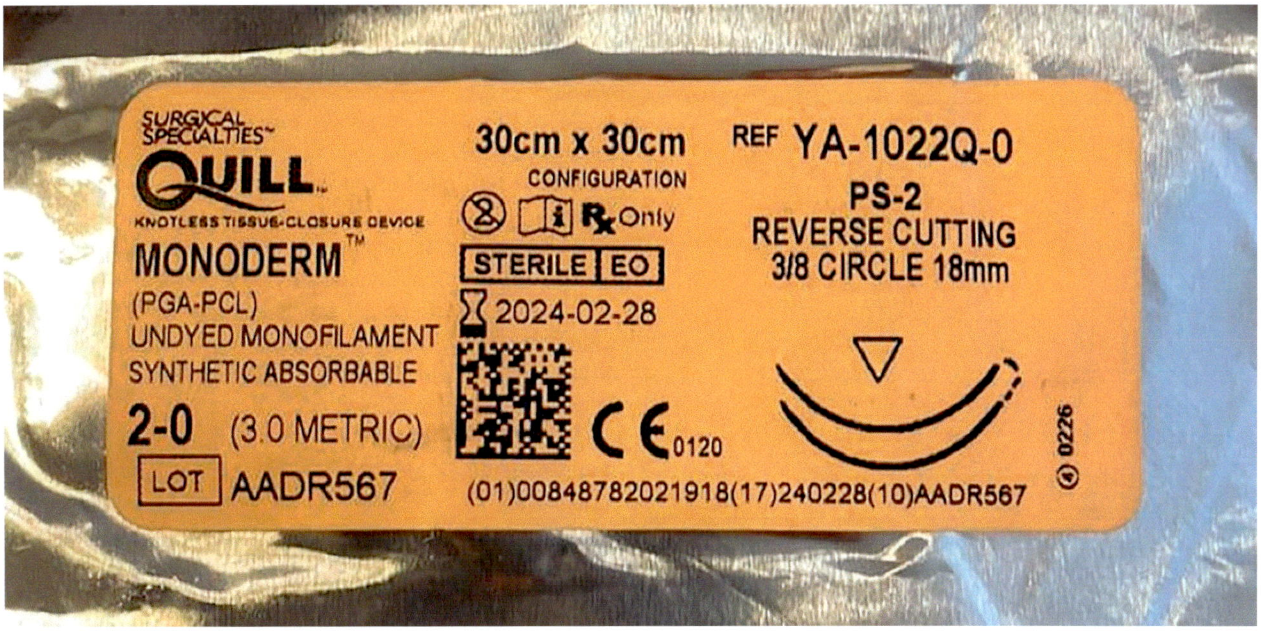

FIGURE 9.6 Double needle barbered thread.

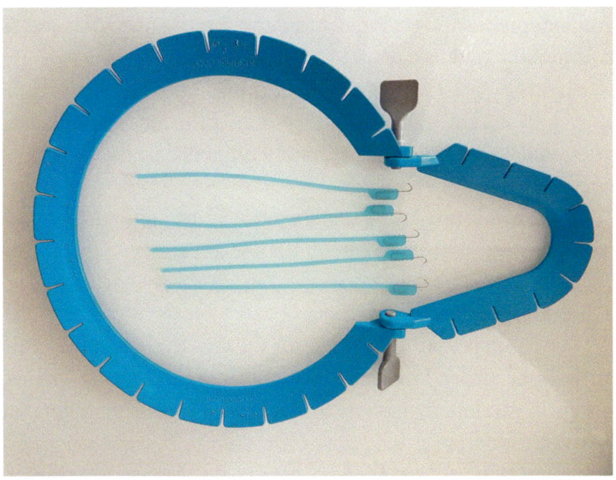

FIGURE 9.7 Lone Star retractor with elastic hooks.

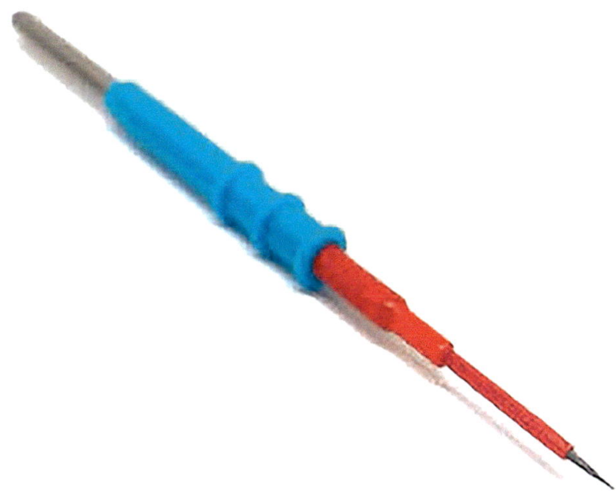

FIGURE 9.8 RF Colorado cutting needle.

Lidocaine, and Tetracaine) directly on the labia and directly at the clitoral body. Local anesthesia is administrated directly to the labia. Marcaine 0.25% is injected unmixed. The injections are done under the marking lines using a 30 G needle. The area will appear slightly swollen but not prohibited to intervene. The marking redefining sometimes is necessary as it might disappear while injecting the local anesthesia. Therefore, it is highly recommended to anesthetize and directly operate on the same side. The other side is to be done separately.

Pudendal Nerve Block [3]

A pudendal nerve block aims to block the nerve as it enters the lesser sciatic foramen, 1 cm inferior and medial, relative to the attachment of the sacrospinous ligament to the ischial spine (Fig. 9.10). Different anatomical approaches are utilized to achieve successful pudendal nerve blocks. They may be unilateral or bilateral. The syringe is not attached until the needle has reached its final position immediately before the injection of the anesthetic agent.

The transvaginal approach to a pudendal nerve block is common for obstetric and gynecological procedures. Typically, 10 mL is used per side, but this is variable (Fig. 9.11).

The female patient is placed in the lithotomy position, and the vaginal area is prepped.

The ischial spines can be identified by palpation along the posterolateral vaginal sidewalls. If, for any reason, the ischial spines cannot be palpated directly, the tight band of

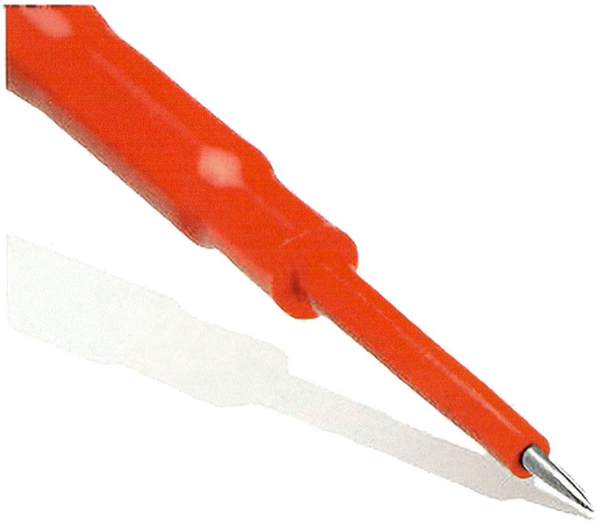

FIGURE 9.9 Colorado dissecting needle.

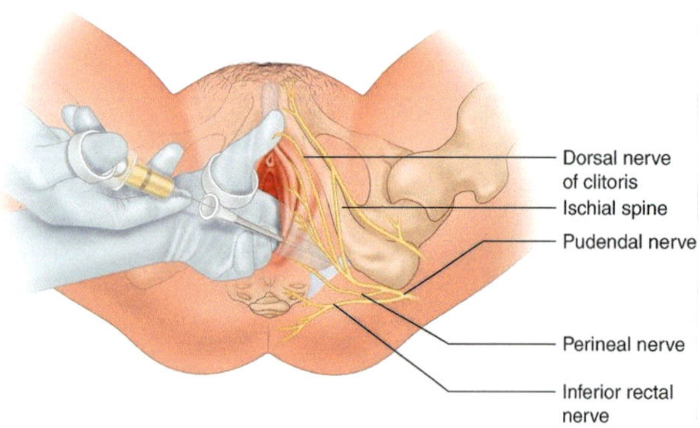

FIGURE 9.10 Transvaginal pudendal nerve block. (From Ref. [4], with permission.)

the sacrospinous ligament should be identified. This can be followed laterally from the sacrum to the respective ischia spine.

A needle guide is gently introduced so it lies on the vaginal mucosa along the sacrospinous ligament, approximately 1 cm medial and inferior to the ischial spine. A needle guide such as the Iowa Trumpet is recommended to limit penetration depth and minimize tissue injury.

The sacrospinous ligament is punctured.

Injecting 3 mL of a local anesthetic directly into the sacrospinous ligament near its ischial insertion before advancing the spinal needle to its final position is optional but suggested to minimize patient discomfort.

The needle is passed 1 cm caudal from the ischial spine until noticing a loss of resistance or confirmed by imaging [5].

Upon negative aspiration, the local anesthetic is injected posteriorly to the ischial spine at the attachment of the sacrospinous ligament.

Alternatively, the injection can be performed just medial to the ischial spine [6]. The nerve is located just behind the loose areolar tissue ligament. This area can be identified by imaging and the loss of resistance to the advancement of the needle as the ligamentous tissue is completely penetrated.

Aspiration to confirm positioning outside a vascular space is again performed as the inferior gluteal and pudendal vessels are immediately adjacent to the pudendal nerve.

A pinprick or similar sensory test in the anogenital area is performed to ensure adequate anesthesia.

The procedure is repeated on the opposite side to achieve a bilateral block.

The transperineal approach is used for anorectal and urological procedures and pudendal neuralgia in males. Imaging guidance, such as ultrasound, is recommended for this approach (Fig. 9.12).

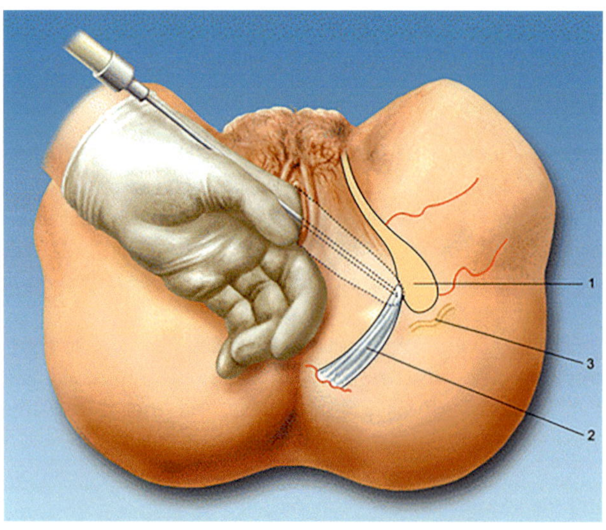

FIGURE 9.11 Transvaginal approach for pudendal nerve block anesthesia. (From Ref. [7], with permission.)

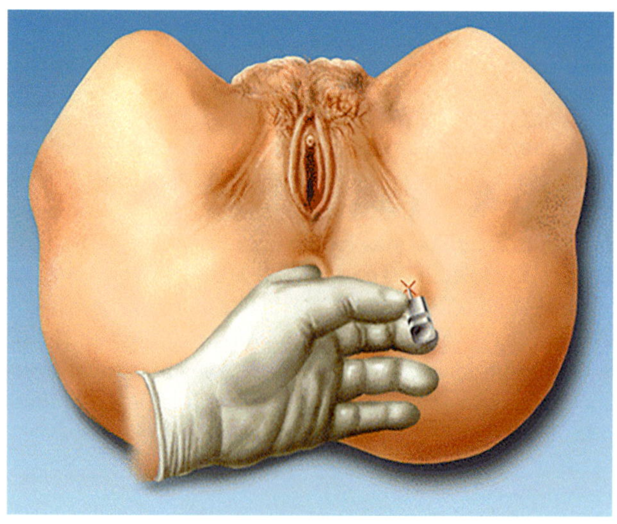

FIGURE 9.12 Transperineal approach for pudendal nerve block anesthesia. (From Ref. [7], with permission.)

The male or female patient will be placed in the lithotomy position.

The skin is prepped.

The clinician's index finger is inserted into the rectum (or vagina) to palpate the ischial spine.

The skin entry point is selected 1 inch (2.5 cm) posteromedial to the ischial tuberosity as determined by palpation or imaging.

After identifying the ischial spine, the needle will puncture the skin transperineally, medial to the ischial tuberosity.

The needle is advanced lateral to the clinician's finger in the posterolateral direction until it reaches the ischial spine.

Injecting 3 mL of a local anesthetic directly into the sacrospinous ligament near its ischial insertion before advancing the spinal needle to its final position is optional.

The needle is then advanced through the sacrospinous ligament 1 cm medial and inferior to the ischial spine.

The final position of the needle can be identified by imaging or by the loss of resistance to the advancement of the needle as the ligamentous tissue is completely penetrated.

After negative aspiration, the local anesthetic of choice is injected.

A pinprick or similar sensory test in the anogenital area is performed to ensure adequate anesthesia.

The procedure is repeated on the opposite side to achieve a bilateral block.

A perirectal approach to a pudendal nerve block has also been described using a nerve stimulator to elicit contractions of the external anal sphincter [6].

The patient is positioned in a recumbent position.

The skin is prepped.

The clinician's index finger is inserted into the rectum (or vagina) to palpate the ischial spine.

The needle is advanced lateral to the rectum and the clinician's finger in the posterolateral direction until it reaches the ischial spine [8].

Injecting 3 mL of a local anesthetic directly into the sacrospinous ligament near its ischial insertion before advancing the spinal needle to its final position is optional.

The needle is then advanced through the sacrospinous ligament 1 cm medial and inferior to the ischial spine.

The final position of the needle can be identified by imaging, by maximal anal sphincteric tone on nerve stimulation of the needle, or by the loss of resistance to advancement of the needle as the ligamentous tissue is completely penetrated.

After negative aspiration, the local anesthetic of choice is injected.

A pinprick or similar sensory test in the anogenital area is performed to ensure adequate anesthesia.

The procedure is repeated on the opposite side to achieve a bilateral block.

A transgluteal approach has also been described and is similar to the techniques reviewed above [9,10].

A pudendal block test injection directly into Alcock's canal is sometimes performed using contrast under image guidance to help indicate if surgical decompression surgery is likely to be successful [9,11].

The effect of a pudendal nerve block is usually immediate, within 5 minutes, but it may take up to 20 minutes to be fully effective [12]. Depending on the clinical symptoms and type of procedure, a pudendal nerve block is either unilateral or bilateral. Pudendal nerve blocks can take place with or without ultrasound guidance in females. However, in male patients, pudendal nerve blocks are typically performed using ultrasound guidance due to challenges in identifying the anatomical landmarks [13]. Pudendal nerve blocks under MRI, fluoroscopy (C-arm), or CT guidance have also been described but are less commonly used methods. Ultrasound also avoids ionizing radiation exposure to the patient and is ideal for patients needing repeated nerve blocks.

The most common cause for failure of the pudendal block is not giving sufficient anesthetic time. If a bilateral block is only effective on one side, an additional 5 mL of anesthetic can be administered to the unaffected side. Up to 50% of all pudendal nerve blocks may fail on at least one side, although the median failure rate averages about 20% [14,15]. This is often from poor technique due to a lack of physician training or experience [15–17].

Pudendal nerve blocks can effectively anesthetize the posterior perineum, the anus, the lower vagina, the vulva/scrotum, and the penis [18]. However, successful pudendal nerve blocks will not affect sensation in the anterior perineum, supplied by branches of the genitofemoral and ilioinguinal nerves. They will also not affect the cervix or upper vaginal vault and are ineffective in controlling pain from uterine manipulations [5,19].

The upper vaginal, cervical and lower uterine sensation is through the ureterovaginal plexus, which can be anesthetized through a paracervical nerve block [20,21]. Local anesthetics are given submucosally, just posterolateral to the uterocervical junction [22]. This effectively blocks sensory and pain nerve transmission at the paracervical ganglia [23]. As it may cause fetal bradycardia, paracervical blocks are not generally performed in the United States; epidural and other pain control methods are also widely available [24,25].

Long-term use of intermittent (typically monthly or as-needed) pudendal nerve blocks can be successfully used to relieve pudendal neuralgia. Still, there is evidence that it may lose efficacy after 2 years [26]. At that point, alternative therapies, such as decompressive surgery, can be utilized.

IV Sedation/General

This is a process that an anesthetist usually performs. However, this is beyond the scope of the current chapter.

MARKING

To achieve precise symmetrical results, marking should start from the perineal area – a "V"-shape drawing should be made (Fig. 9.13). The higher wing of each side should be at the lower level of the labia minora, and the lower tip should be enough to remove any scar or wrinkle skin from the perineum. For safety reasons, we need to maintain at least 1.5 cm between the lower tip of the "V" and the anus.

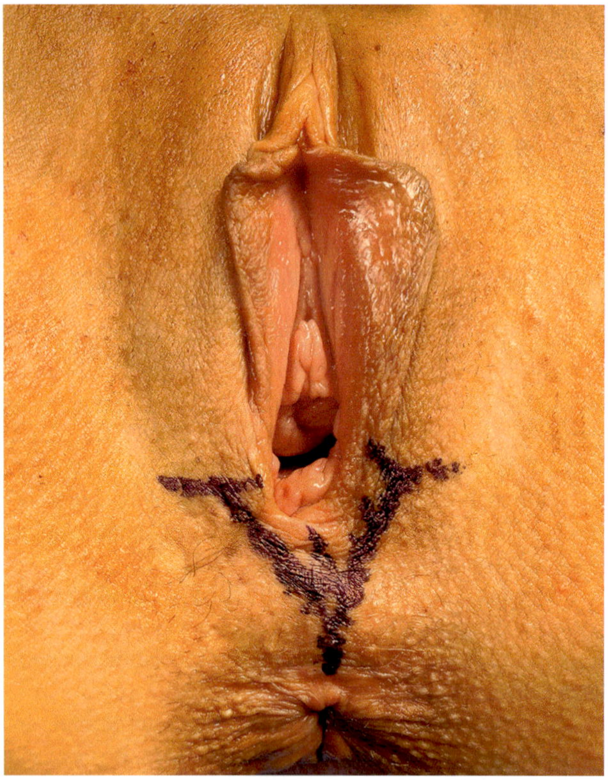

FIGURE 9.13 Perineal marking.

The skin marker used is a sterile type for surgical marking use (Fig. 9.14). You can complete the marking by drawing a line from the tip to the upper edge of the anus and

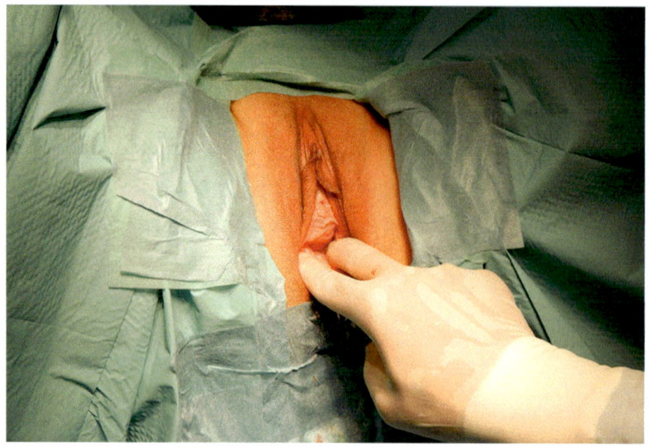

FIGURE 9.15 Clinical review of the surgical field.

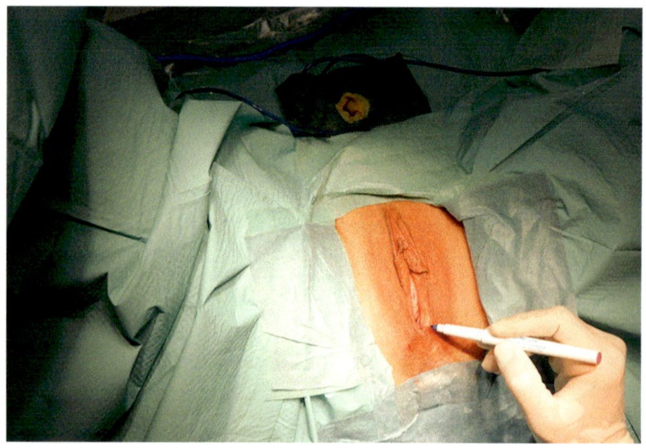

FIGURE 9.16 Start drawing from the lower edge of the labia minora.

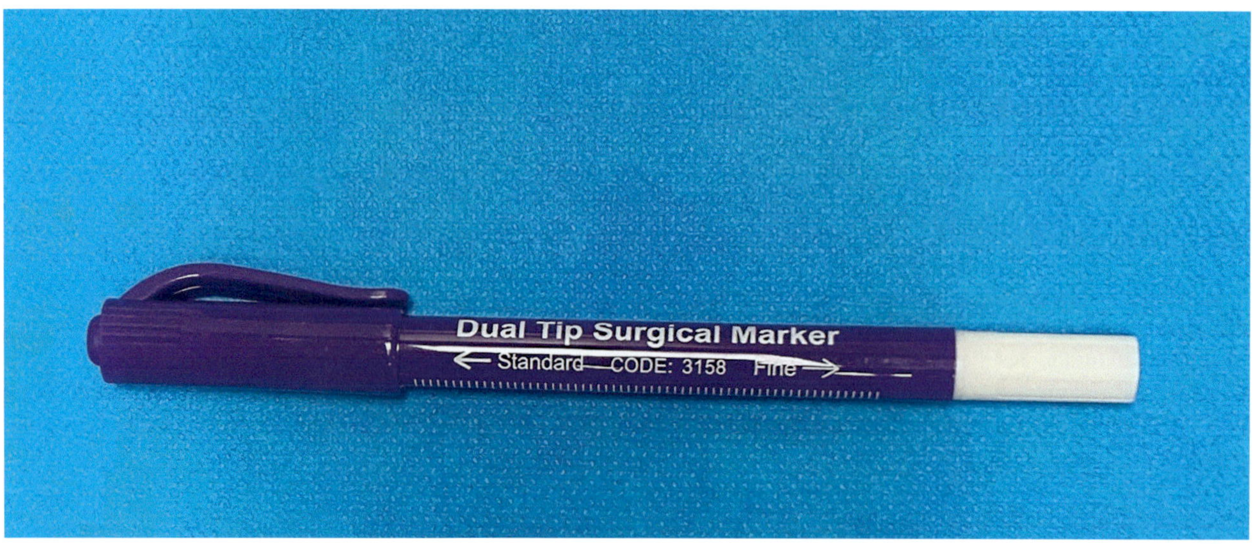

FIGURE 9.14 Skin marker.

drawing lines towards the groin. In this way, you will have more control of the incisions when you start performing them.

TECHNIQUE

The technique includes a review of the area prospect for the surgical intervention. Examine with one or two fingers to assess the laxity and the anatomical aspects of the perineum, introits, and posterior vaginal wall (Fig. 9.15). Mark the prospect surgical area. A "V" drawing should be done, making sure that the upper edge of the wing is just under the lower edge of the labia minora (Fig. 9.16). Complete drawing the V on both sides (Fig. 9.17). A superficial dissection on the marked area leaves a free flap (Fig. 9.20). An adjustment of the Lone Star

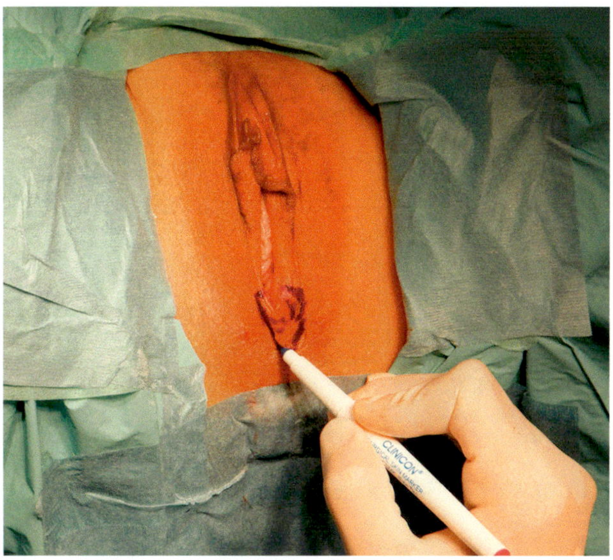

FIGURE 9.17 Completing the area marking.

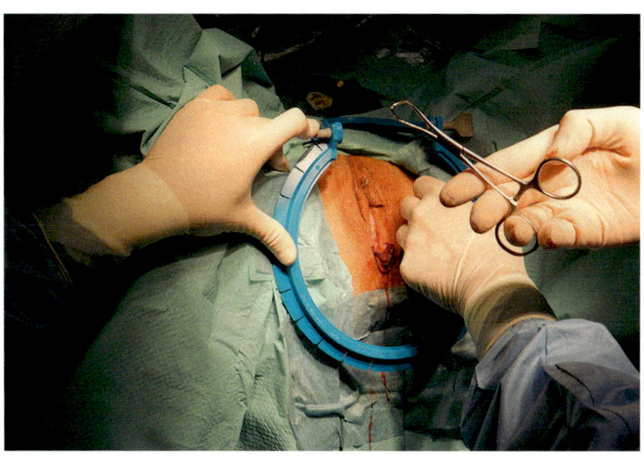

FIGURE 9.18 Adjusting the retractor.

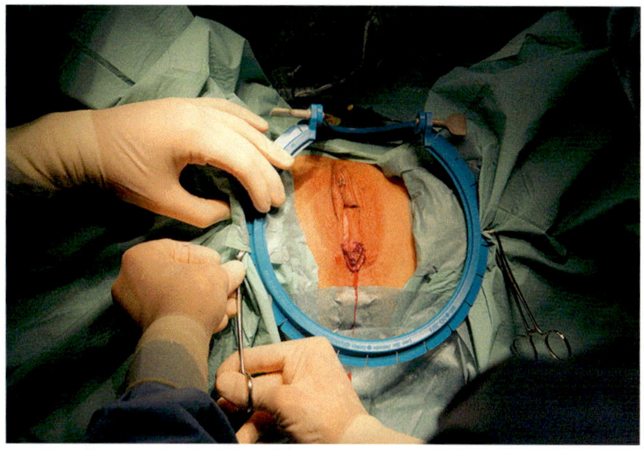

FIGURE 9.19 Adjusting the retractor.

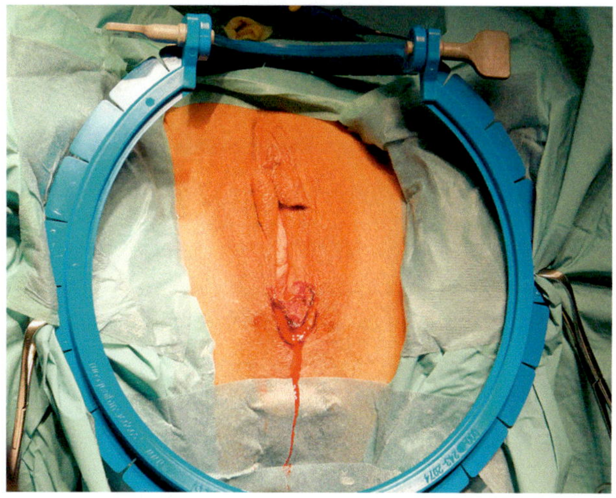

FIGURE 9.20 Free flap after introital skin dissection.

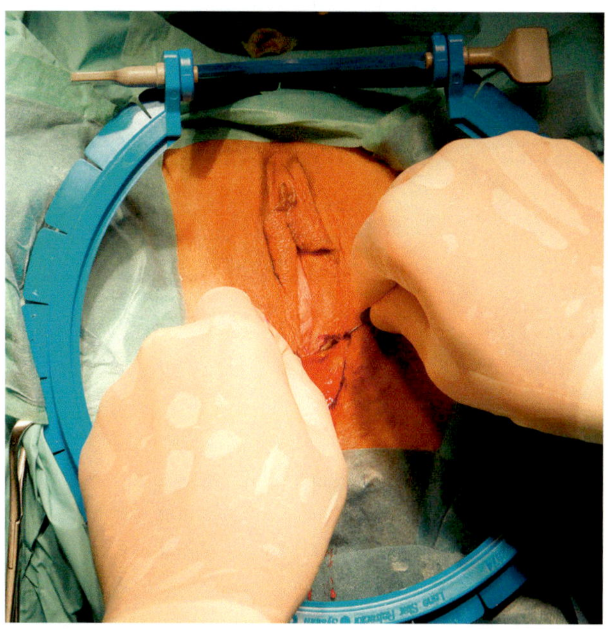

FIGURE 9.21 Placing the elastic hook.

retractor will be done. The small tail will be laid on the pubic area of the patient once the lithotomy has been perfectly done. The large tail is adjusted to include the surgical field. The retractor is stabilized by the Edna Lorna towel clamps (Figs. 9.18 and 9.19). Four elastic hooks are placed at the corners to allow full separation of the vaginal entrance: two are hooked on the top of the "V"-shape drawing to retract and separate the posterior part and the other two in the inner top of the labia minora to retract the anterior part (Figs. 9.21–9.25). Now we should be able to observe the entire vaginal walls and the vaginal canal up to the cervix. The next step is infiltrating 20–30 mL of NaCl 0.9% to the posterior vaginal wall straightaway under the mucosa (Fig. 9.26). This is done to assist in the next step of dissection. You can also mix the fluid with local anesthesia to add more comfort to the patient 24 hours after the surgery. The recommended mixture is 10 mL of lidocaine 2% and 10 mL of NaCl 0.9%, all mixed with a dilute vasoconstrictor. A 23 G needle (Blue) can perform the infiltration.

The next step is holding the far top of the posterior vaginal wall (vaginal apex) using an Allis clamp. Elevation is important to allow easy access under the mucosa during the next step (Fig. 9.27). Metzenbaum scissors are used to create a posterior tunnel under the mucosa (Fig. 9.28), and a longitudinal cut is done starting from base towards the vaginal apex (Fig. 9.29).

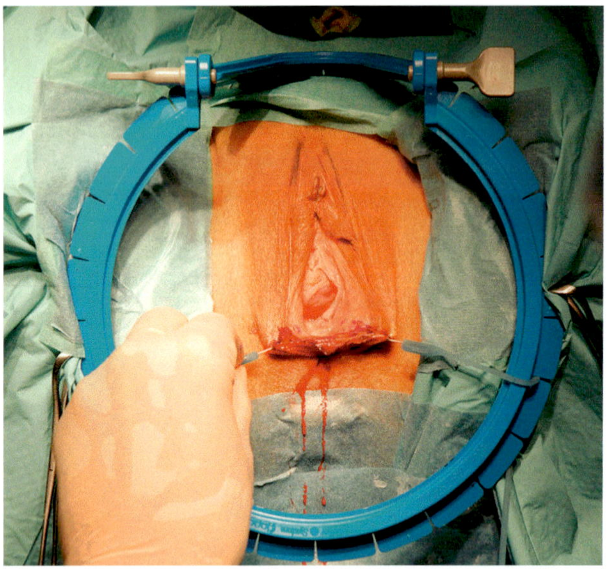

FIGURE 9.22 Placing the elastic hook.

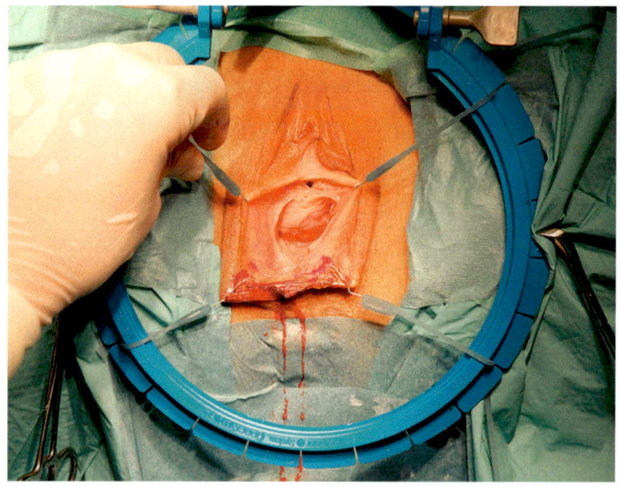

FIGURE 9.24 Placing the elastic hook.

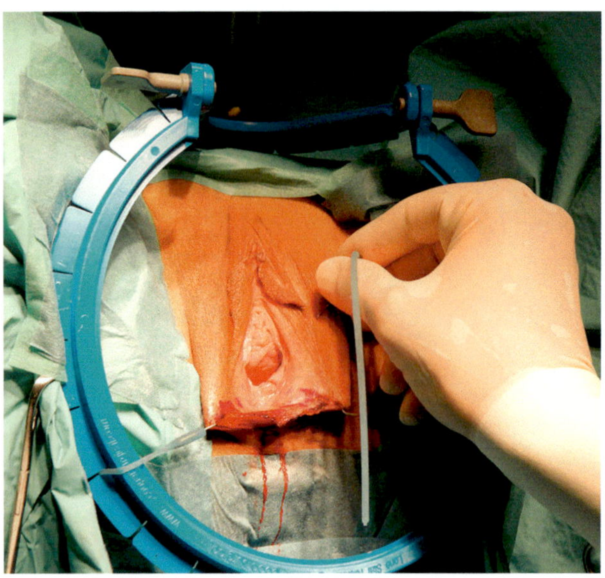

FIGURE 9.23 Placing the elastic hook.

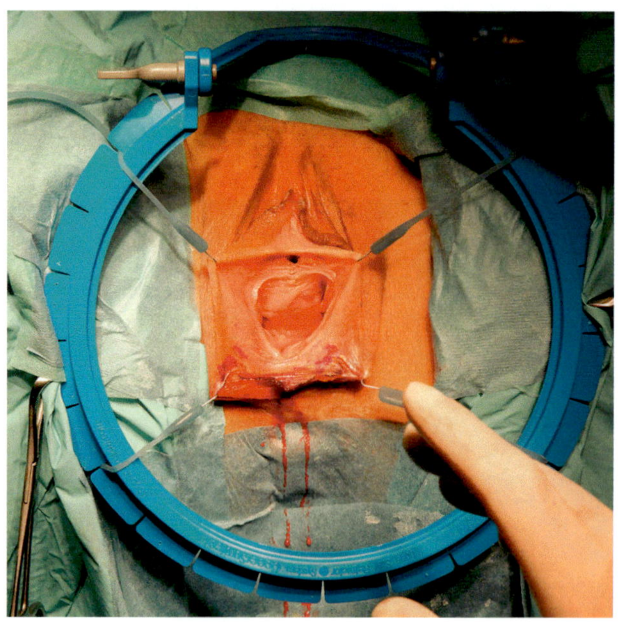

FIGURE 9.25 Placing the elastic hook.

This stops where we have the Allis clamp placed. The procedure continues initially by clamping the lateral free vaginal wall flaps using the Pratt T-shape clamps (Fig. 9.30). The dissection of the vaginal epithelium of the posterior vaginal wall is performed next. Typically, this could be done with wet sponges, laser, RF, or even simple diathermy. The dissection must

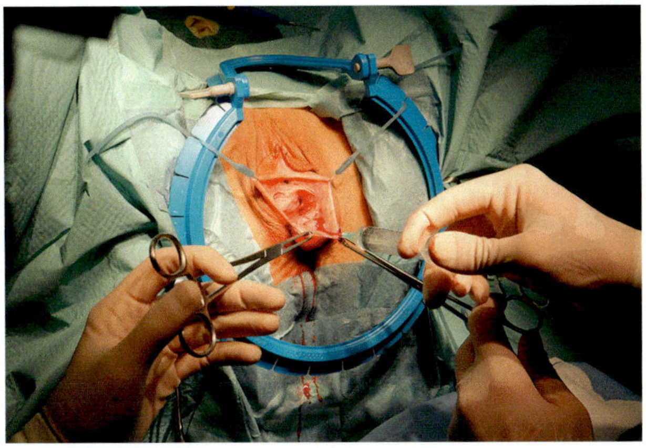

FIGURE 9.26 Submucosal infiltration with NaCl 0.09%. A 23 G needle is used.

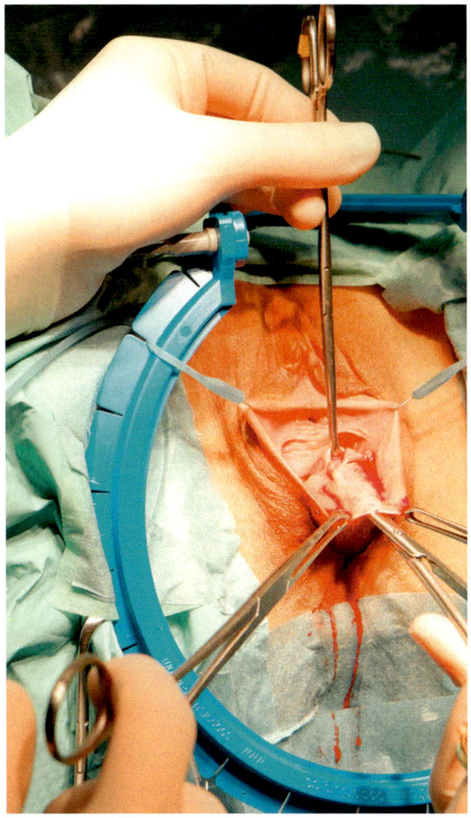

FIGURE 9.28 Tunnel creation.

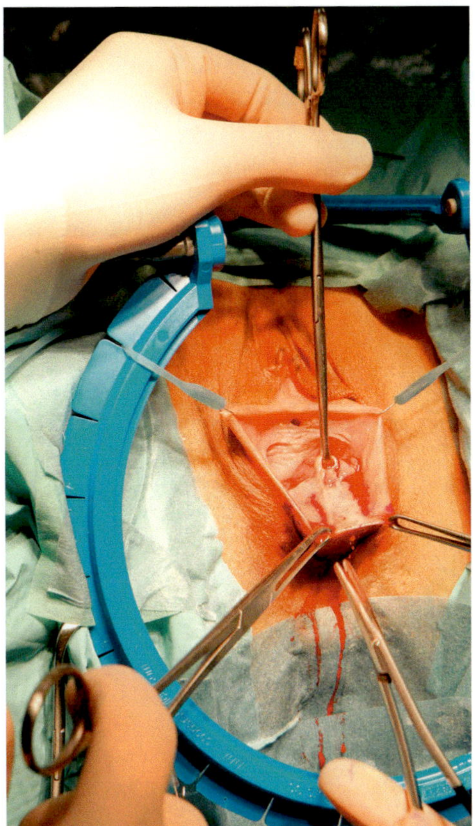

FIGURE 9.27 Apex elevation.

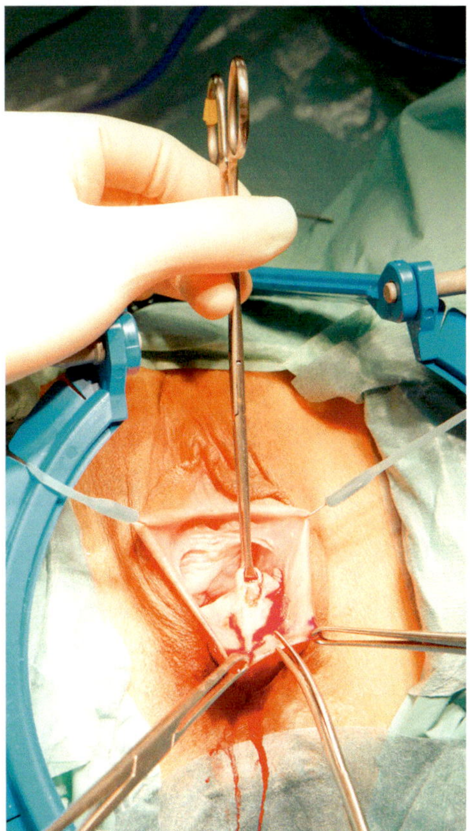

FIGURE 9.29 Posterior incision.

include the vaginal epithelium and the underlying rectovaginal fascia. It must reach the apex of the vagina, allowing the complete repair of the vaginal posterior wall in the following steps (Figs. 9.31–9.34). Once the dissection has been completed, we remove a generous size of the vaginal mucosa. We use Alinsod curve scissors, or any curve scissors if you do not have access to Alinsod scissors. The starting point is the corner at the lower hooks level (corners) with a line to the vaginal apex (Figs. 9.35 and 9.36); we make sure the mucosa removal is done symmetrically. The last step of this procedure is closure. This is done by using a double-needled barbered suture (Figs. 9.37 and 9.38).

We start the closure from the vagina apex by passing both needles at the submucosal level and locking the thread (Fig. 9.39). Now we have a 15 cm thread to repair the rectovaginal fascia and another 15 cm thread to repair and close the vaginal mucosa. We start repairing the rectovaginal fascia by performing small steps that pass continuously and unlock from one side to the other. Passing the needle in a half circle move is crucial to take the full thickness of the fascia (Figs. 9.40, 9.41).

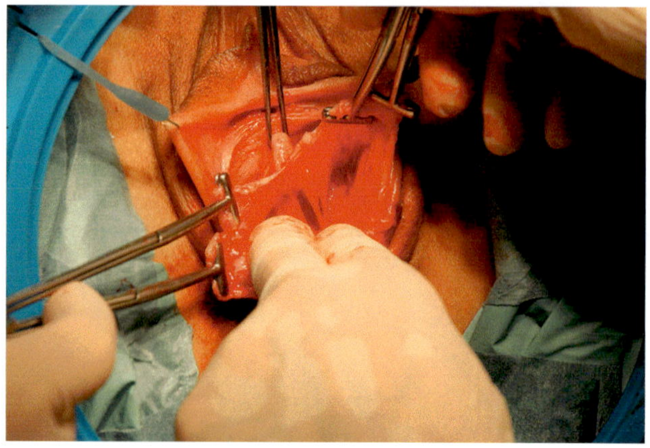

FIGURE 9.32 Epithelium and rectovaginal fascia dissection.

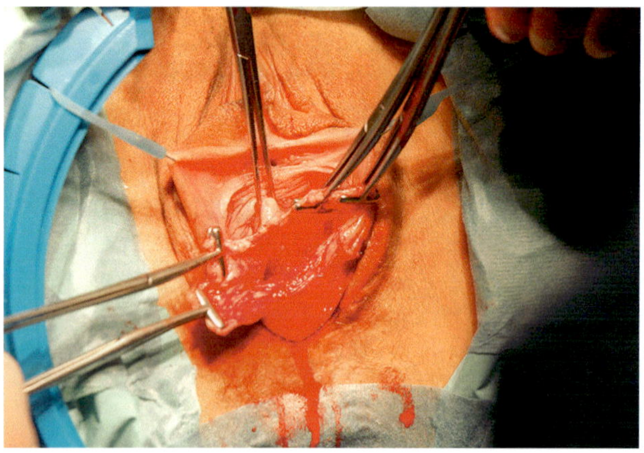

FIGURE 9.30 T-shape clamps holding the lateral vaginal free flaps.

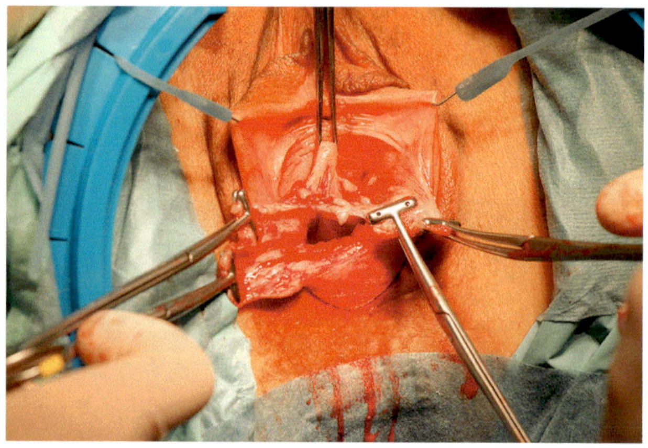

FIGURE 9.33 Epithelium and rectovaginal fascia dissection.

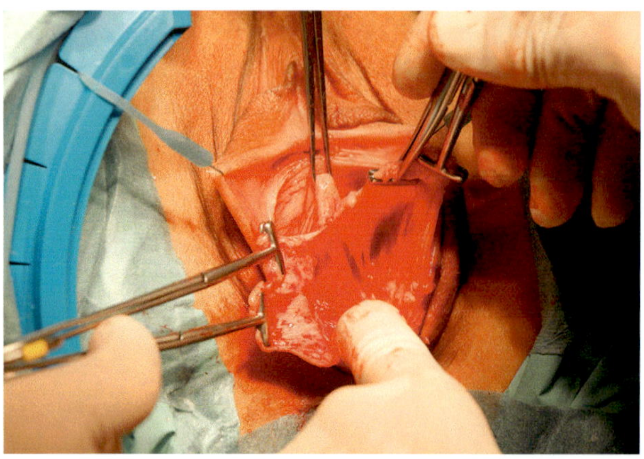

FIGURE 9.31 Epithelium and rectovaginal fascia dissection.

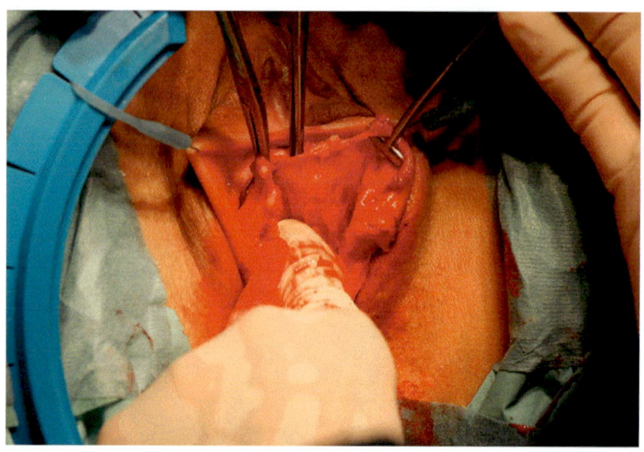

FIGURE 9.34 Epithelium and rectovaginal fascia dissection.

Once the rectovaginal fascia has been approximated, we go back to the other half of the thread and perform the mucosa-to-mucosa approximation continuously without a lock. At one point, both needles will meet at the introitus (Fig. 9.42). At that stage of the procedure, we dive both needles at the submucosal level and keep closing the perineum in a subdermal-to-subdermal approximation without locking the suture. Once the perineum approximation has been completed, we just cut the thread leaving 1 cm free (Fig. 9.43). We follow by massaging the posterior vaginal wall and perineum, allowing the barbs to stick and hood at the tissues.

We have completed a full posterior vaginal wall repair using one thread. The surgical wound has been closed without locking the suture, minimizing the possibility of necrotic and fibrotic tissues. In addition, the vaginal canal has been significantly tightened with less damage possible. Usually, these cases are treated as day cases with no overnight stay at the hospital. The pain level is very acceptable, and the patient can move around and conduct everyday activities relatively fast after the surgery.

Figures 9.44–9.47 show before and after cases. See also Video 9.1: Single thread vagino–perineoplasty.

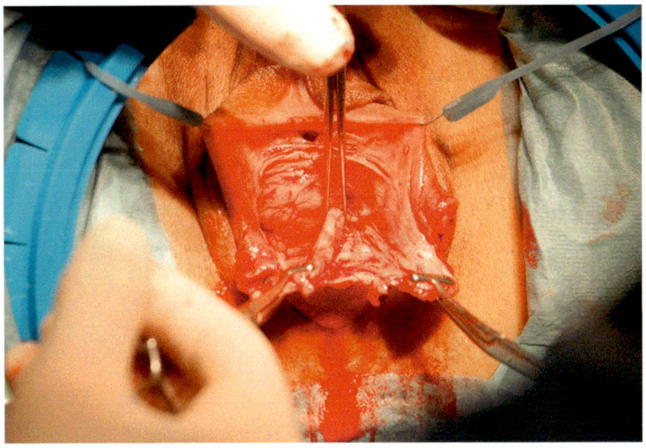

FIGURE 9.35 Removal of excess mucosal tissues.

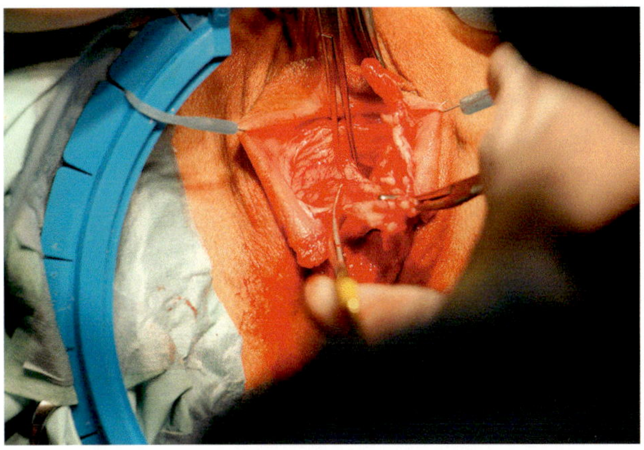

FIGURE 9.36 Removal of excess mucosal tissues.

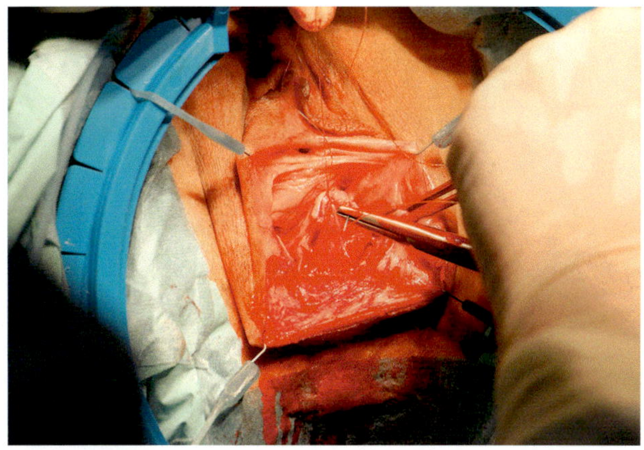

FIGURE 9.38 First step of passing both needles at the apex with locked thread.

(a)

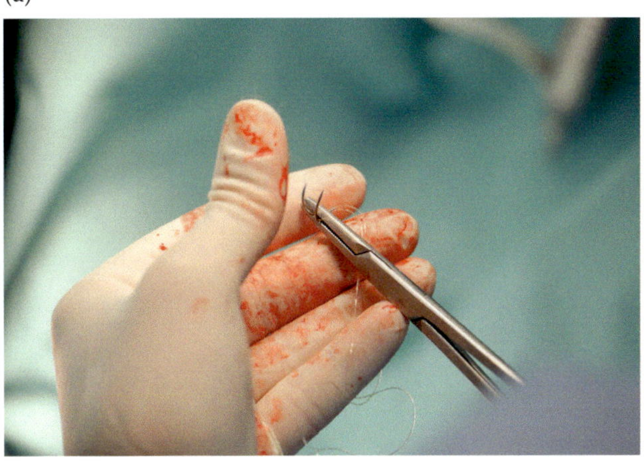

(b)

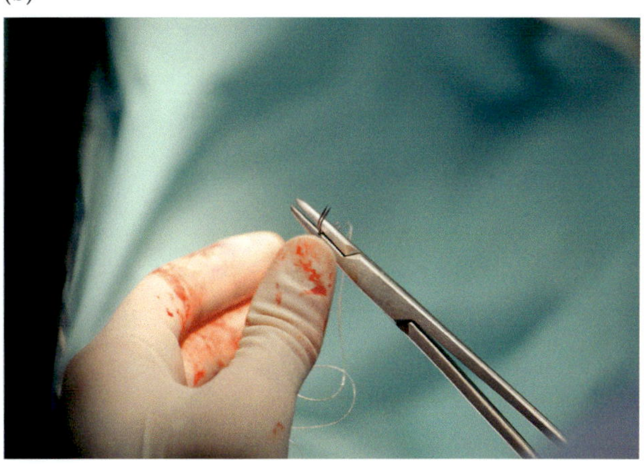

FIGURE 9.37 (a, b) Double-needle barbed thread.

POSTOPERATIVE CARE

The patient is advised to avoid physical exercises, swimming, and sexual intercourse for 6–8 weeks. Cleaning and drying the area are mandatory as some patients are reluctant to clean the area. Washing with tap water without using unique products protects the sutures from early dissolution. Drying by tapping the area with a clean towel, followed by using the hair dryer for a few minutes, sounds very helpful. The patient is advised to leave the area free and not covered. Avoid touching the wound with nails or naked fingers. A course of oral antibiotics, NSAIDs, and topical antibiotic ointment (Fucidin Oint) are prescribed. Estradiol cream can also be

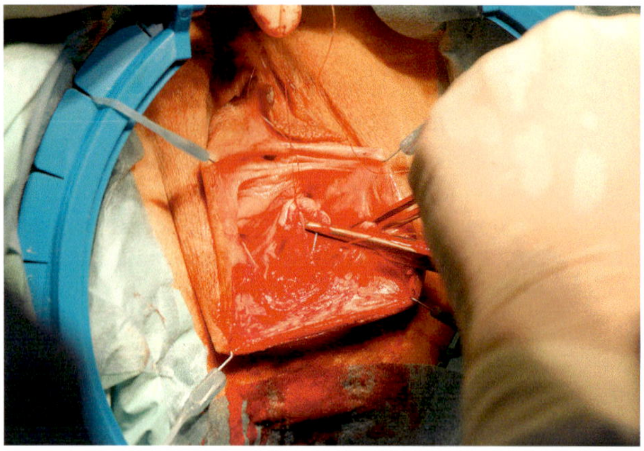

FIGURE 9.39 Rectovaginal approximation continuous unlocked.

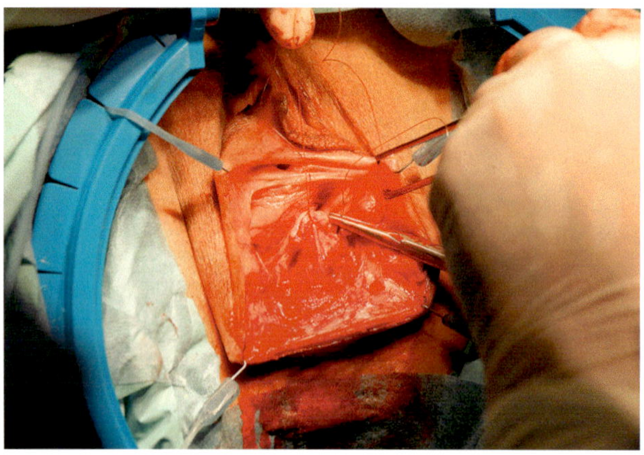

FIGURE 9.40 Rectovaginal approximation continuous unlocked.

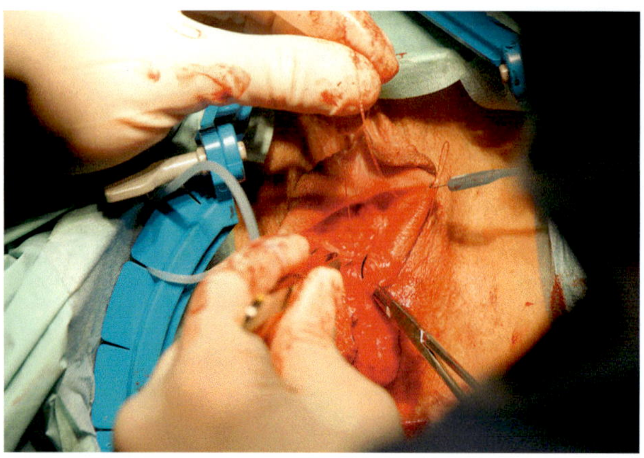

FIGURE 9.41 Introitus approximation.

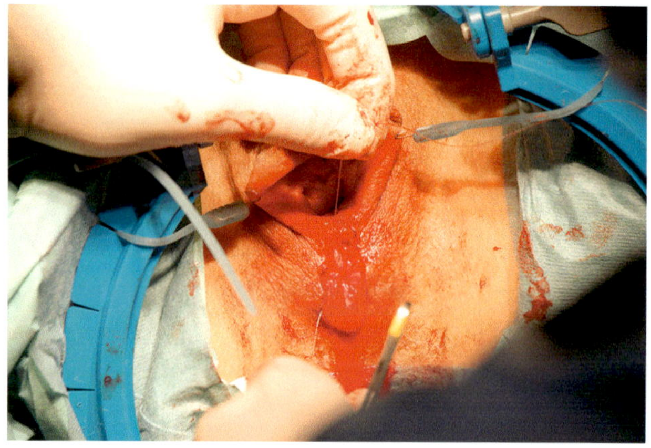

FIGURE 9.42 Introitus approximation.

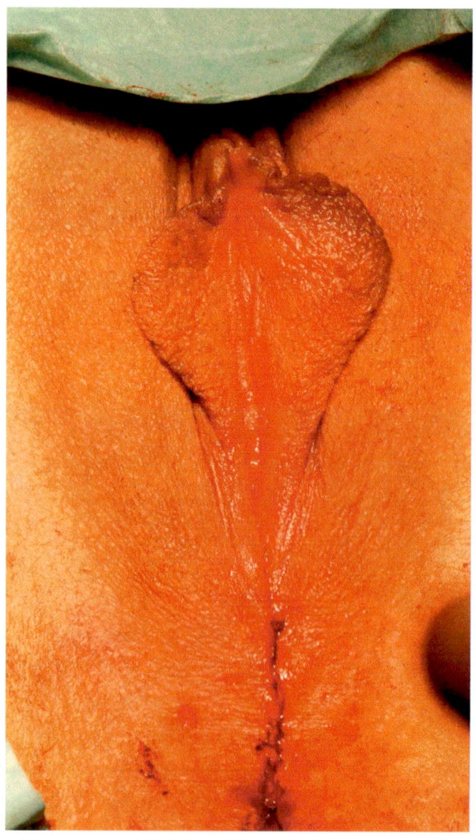

FIGURE 9.43 Perineum subcutaneous and subdermal closure.

(a) (b)

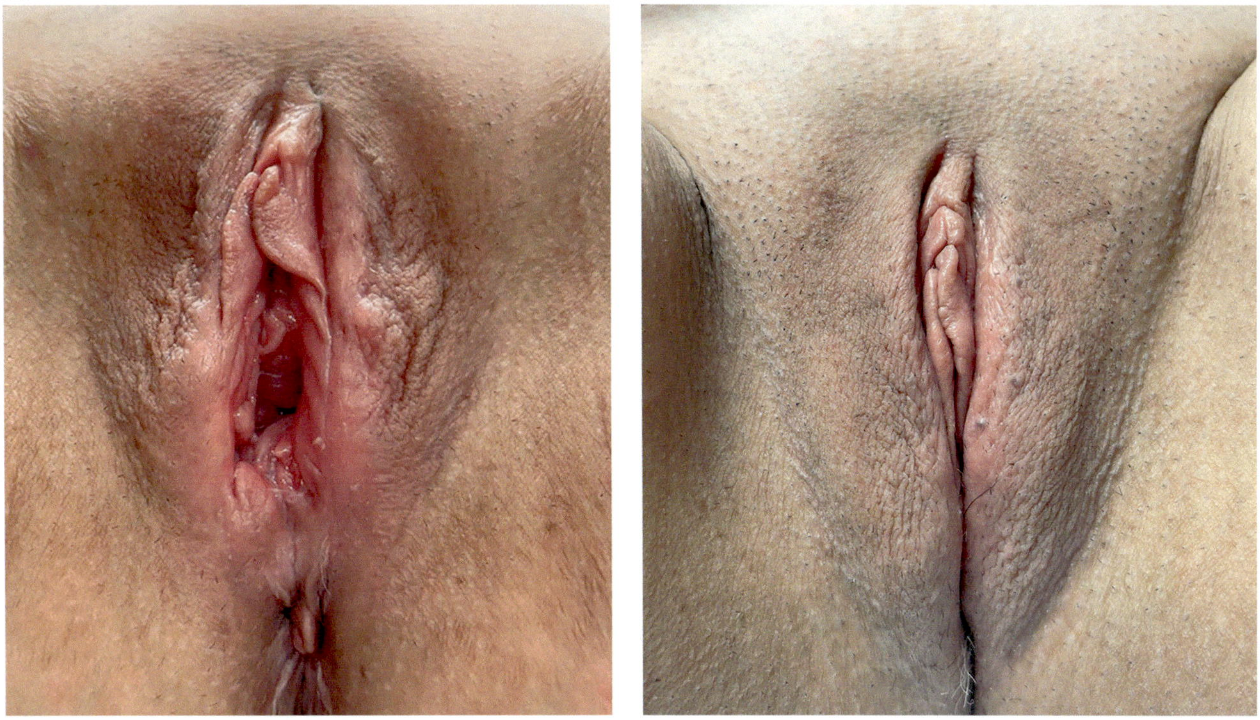

FIGURE 9.44 Case 1: (a) before and (b) after surgery.

(a) (b)

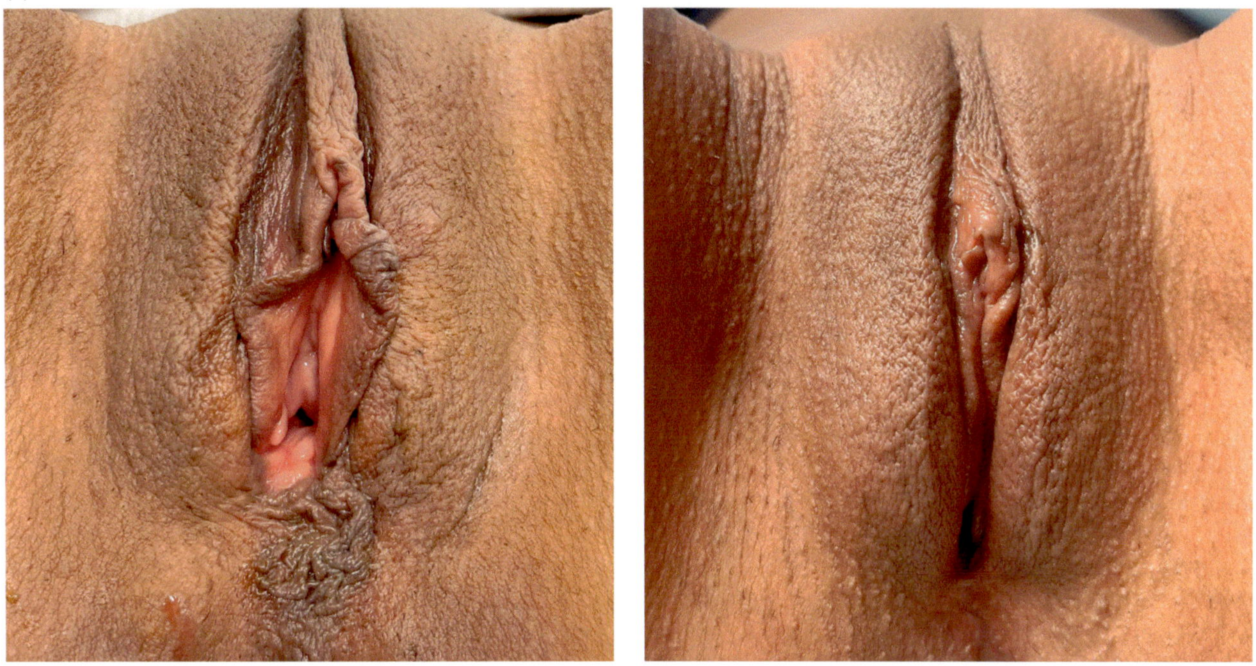

FIGURE 9.45 Case 2: (a) before and (b) after surgery.

(a) (b)

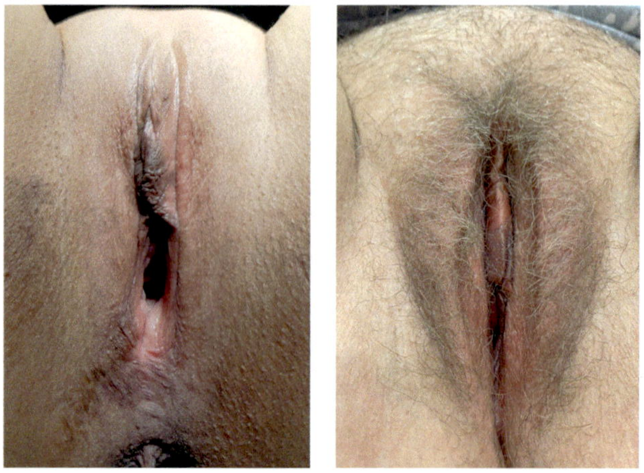

FIGURE 9.46 Case 3: (a) before and (b) after surgery.

COMPLICATIONS

Generally, the procedure rarely has complications. However, intraoperatively, the most common complication is rectal perforation, and the surgeon must know how to recognize it when it happens and deal with it. Postoperatively, a few complications might occur:

- Infections (these can be re-empted by giving antibiotics after the surgery)
- Cystitis and urethritis
- Partial wound dehiscence
- Pain from over-tight perineum
- Pain from levator ani over-correction
- Dyspareunia
- Bleeding
- Rectovaginal fistula [27,28]

(a) (b)

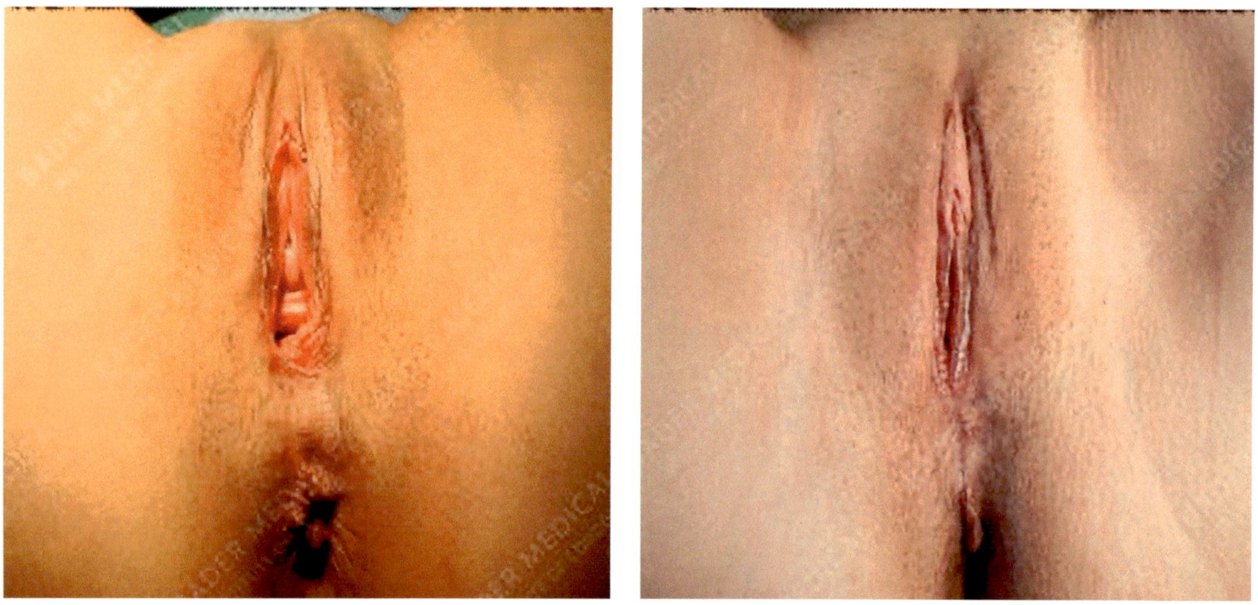

FIGURE 9.47 Case 4: (a) before and (b) after surgery.

prescribed as it helps in the healing process. Platelet-rich plasma (PRP) also can be used to improve the speed and quality of the healing. PRP can be applied immediately after the surgery and be repeated when the patient comes after 2 months for her third follow-up visit. Cessation of smoking is advisable before the surgery takes place. However, we need to clarify that their healing quality might be affected. The standard postoperative follow-up schedule is a visit 1 week after the surgery, 1 month after, and one more visit 2 months after. This might be modified based on the progress of the healing and recovery.

REFERENCES

1. Basson R, Berman J, Burnett A, et al. Report of the international consensus development conference on female sexual dysfunction: definitions and classifications. *J Urol* 2000;163(3):888–893.
2. Pauls RN, Segal JL, Silva WA, et al. Sexual function in patients presenting to an urogynecology practice. *Int Urogynecol J* 2006;17(6):576–580.
3. Ghanavatian S, Leslie SW, Derian A. *Pudendal Nerve Block*. StatPearls Publishing; Treasure Island, Florida, USA: 2020.
4. Chaturvedi R, Reddy R, Chakravarthy K. Neuropathic pain: pudendal nerve block. In: Banik RK (ed.),

Anesthesiology In-Training Exam Review. Springer, Champagne, Illinois, USA. 2022; 319–322.
5. Vancaillie T, Eggermont J, Armstrong G, et al. Response to pudendal nerve block in women with pudendal neuralgia. *Pain Med* 2012;13(4):596–603.
6. Choi SS, Lee PB, Kim YC, Kim HJ, Lee SC. C-arm-guided pudendal nerve block: a new technique. *Int J Clin Pract* 2006;60(5):553–556.
7. Bellingham G, Peng WHP. Pudendal nerve blockade. In Jankovic D, Peng WHP, (eds.), *Regional Nerve Blocks in Anesthesia and Pain Therapy: Traditional and Ultrasound-Guided Techniques 5E*. Springer, Champagne, Illinois, USA. 2022; 737–751.
8. Kim SH, Song SG, Paek OJ, et al. Nerve-stimulator-guided pudendal nerve block by pararectal approach. *Colorectal Dis* 2012;14(5):611–615.
9. Ricci P, Wash A. Pudendal nerve block by trans gluteal way guided by computed tomography in a woman with refractory pudendal neuralgia expressed like chronic perineal and pelvic pain. *Arch Esp Urol* 2014;67(6):565–571.
10. Ploteau S, Perrouin-Verbe MA, Labat JJ, et al. Anatomical variants of the pudendal nerve observed during a transgluteal surgical approach in a population of patients with pudendal neuralgia. *Pain Physician* 2017;20(1):E137–E143.
11. Levesque A, Bautrant E, Quistrebert V, et al. Recommendations on the management of pudendal nerve entrapment syndrome: a formalised expert consensus. *Eur J Pain* 2022;26(1):7–17.
12. Zador G, Lindmark G, Nilsson BA. Pudendal block in normal vaginal deliveries. *Acta Obstet Gynecol Scand Suppl* 1974;(34):51–64.
13. Kalava A, Pribish AM, Wiegand LR. Pudendal nerve blocks in men undergoing urethroplasty: a case series. *Rom J Anaesth Intensive Care* 2017;24(2):159–162.
14. Scudamore JH, Yates MJ. Pudendal block – a misnomer? *Lancet*. 1966;1(7427):23–24.
15. Schierup L, Schmidt JF, Torp Jensen A, Rye BA. Pudendal block in vaginal deliveries. Mepivacaine with and without epinephrine. *Acta Obstet Gynecol Scand* 1988;67(3): 195–197.
16. Antolak S, Antolak C, Lendway L. Measuring the quality of pudendal nerve perineural injections. *Pain Physician* 2016;19(4):299–306.
17. Ford JM, Owen DJ, Coughlin LB, Byrd LM. A critique of the current practice of transvaginal pudendal nerve blocks: a prospective audit of understanding and clinical practice. *J Obstet Gynaecol*. 2013;33(5):463–465.
18. Leslie SW, Antolak S, Feloney MP, Soon-Sutton TL. *Pudendal Neuralgia*. StatPearls Publishing; Treasure Island (FL): 2022.
19. Anderson D. Pudendal nerve block for vaginal birth. *J Midwifery Women's Health*. 2014 Nov–Dec;59(6): 651–659.
20. Saloheimo AM. Paracervical block anaesthesia in labor. *Acta Obstet Gynecol Scand* 1968;47(S5):1–21.
21. Aksoy H, Aksoy U, Ozyurt S, et al. Comparison of lidocaine spray and paracervical block application for pain relief during first-trimester surgical abortion: a randomised, double-blind, placebo-controlled trial. *J Obstet Gynaecol* 2016;36(5):649–653.
22. Chanrachakul B, Likittanasombut P, O-Prasertsawat P, Herabutya Y. Lidocaine versus plain saline for pain relief in fractional curettage: a randomised controlled trial. *Obstet Gynecol* 2001;98(4):592–595.
23. Gad C. Paracervical block. *Acta Obstet Gynecol Scand* 1967;46(1):7–18.
24. Nyirjesy I, Hawks BL, Hebert TJE, et al. Hazards of the use of paracervical block anesthesia in obstetrics. *Am J Obstet Gynecol* 1963;87:231–235.
25. Palomäki O, Huhtala H, Kirkinen P. A comparative study of the safety of 0.25% levobupivacaine and 0.25% racemic bupivacaine for paracervical block in the first stage of labour. *Acta Obstet Gynecol Scand* 2005;84(10): 956–961.
26. Basol G, Kale A, Gurbuz H, Gundogdu EC, et al. Transvaginal pudendal nerve blocks in patients with pudendal neuralgia: 2-year follow-up results. *Arch Gynecol Obstet* 2022;306(4):1107–1116.
27. Goodman MP, Placik OJ, Benson III RH, et al. A large multicenter outcomes study of female genital plastic surgery. *J Sex Med* 2010:7(4 pt 1):1565–1577.
28. Iglesia BC, Yunteri-Kaplan I, Alinsod R. Female genital cosmetic surgery: a review of techniques and outcomes. *Int Urogynecol J* 2013:24(12):1997–2009.

10 Perineoplasty

Piotr Kolczewski

INTRODUCTION

A normal vaginal delivery can result in widening of the vagina by stretching the tissues and separating the adjacent muscles. Postpartum vaginal laxity can create a gaping perineum and reduce friction sensation, diminishing sexual satisfaction [1,2]. This gaping also creates several functional concerns, including increased/excessive vaginal secretions due to mucosa exposure and vaginal air entrapment resulting in embarrassing sounds during sexual intercourse [3]. Not without significance is the fact of deterioration of vulvar aesthetic. Little wonder is that 80.4% women urogynecologists would choose elective cesarean section [4].

Although surgical vaginal tightening procedures are not new, historically they have been performed for repairs after delivery, rather than for sexual or aesthetic concerns [5]. The few studies that have been done show that vaginal tightening procedures, including vaginoplasty and perineoplasty, are associated with improved sexual function with low complication rates [1–3,5].

Surgical increasing of the height of the perineum and reduction of its width is called the perineoplasty. In most cases, perineoplasty is combined with posterior colporrhapy as a posterior repair (colpoperineoplasty), because isolated rectoceles are relatively uncommon and are found in approximately 7% of women who present for surgical repair [6].

A perineoplasty narrows the genital hiatus length, increases the functional length of the posterior vaginal wall, removes redundant perineal skin and tightens the introitus with approximation of the superficial transverse perineal and bulbocavernosus muscles as well as restores the integrity of the perineal body. This procedure is ideal for patients with complaints of loosened introitus who are interested in improving the appearance and sexual function of a postpartum perineum [5,7–9].

Although perineoplasties have been performed for a long time and are associated with very low complication rates, there are no established or uniform surgical methods for performing the procedure. Additionally, there are no published guidelines on patient selection criteria for perineoplasty [3].

According to Pelosi, the most common misapplication of the perineoplasty is its use without vaginoplasty in the presence of vaginal canal laxity [10]. However, some authors think otherwise. Taking into account that in vaginal mucosal excision procedures, fibrosis and scar tissue lead to decreased blood flow to the vagina resulting in vaginal dryness and dyspareunia [7], Ulubay in 2016 performed perineoplasty in a group of 38 women with the sensation of wide vagina. Following perineoplasty, the patient satisfaction rate was 87.9%, and the satisfaction rate (positive sensation) of their male partners was 92.6%. The number of patients who said they would recommend the procedure to friends was also very high (87.9%). The authors believe that perineoplasty alone, particularly fortifying the perineal body, not only reshapes and reinforces the perineum, but also provides extra support for the posterior vaginal wall. Although insightful, this study is limited by the small sample size of 38 women and the lack of validated quality of life questionnaires [7].

In urogynecology, perineoplasty is performed as a therapeutic procedure to maintain level 3 pelvic support in cases of pelvic organ prolapse, according to De Lancey [11]. More often, however, the procedure is performed for cosmetic and sexual reasons at the patient's request or to excise perineal scatrises or for vulvar vestibulitis and vulvar lichen sclerosis treatment with stenotic vaginal introitus [12–14]. Perineoplasty may also be performed to improve sexual satisfaction and decrease dyspareunia caused by incorrect episiotomy repair [15].

HISTORY

Vaginal and perineal plastic surgery began with the repair of complete obstetrical perineal tears. Based on available data, this operation was first suggested by Ambroise Pare in the 16th century, and first carried out successfully by his pupil Guillemeau [16].

Although the French School initiated the operation, called perineauxesis, perineosynthesis and perineorrhaphy, it was the Germans led by Dieffenbach, professor of surgery in Berlin, and his successor, Langenbeck, who gave it a firm basis [17,18].

At that time, the supports of the genital organs were a mystery. Causes of prolaps were unknown. Partial closure of the vagina was devised as a purely empirical method of treatment. With a similar objective, small areas of the vaginal wall were denuded with a knife. One of the earliest to do this was Fricke of Hamburg in 1831 [16,19].

Strips of different shapes and sizes were taken from various aspects of the vagina by Diffenbach, Friecke, Ireland, Velpeau, Roux, Stolz and others. All these operations received the name of elytrorrhaphy (Greek origin, a stitching of the sheath or cover) [16].

DOI: 10.1201/9780429353079-10

Among the many who developed posterior colpoperineorrhaphy in the second half of the 19th century are Sims, Emmet, Lawson, Martin, Schroder, Dolores and Hegar. They each modified the shape of incision, the method of suturing, and other details. Hegar (1870) was responsible for the classic triangular denudation. At the beginning of the 20th century, colpoperrineorrhapphy was frequently referred to as the Hegar's operation [16,20,21].

Historically, in the 1880s – Emmet – and in the 1910s – Kelly – described the posterior repair and perineorrhaphy that are still performed today. They emphasized performing a perineorrhaphy as an important component of posterior prolapse repair [22,23].

SURGICAL ANATOMY OF THE REGION: CONSIDERATIONS AND CONTROVERSY

Perineoplasty is not just about narrowing the vaginal introitus by excising and sewing perineal skin. This quite common approach results in creating a non-anatomical skin band leading to dyspareunia. Similarly, narrowing vaginal introitus by threads may produce good aesthetic results but is not capable of rebuilding perineum because it does not refer to the essence of perineoplasty, which is reinforcing the perineal muscles and perineal body.

The perineal muscles form the floor of the anterior perineum and are subjected to continuous variations in intra-abdominal pressure. They respond by contraction, an action mediated through the straining–perineal reflex [24]. The perineal muscle contraction protects the perineum against the increased intra-abdominal pressure with a prolonged increase of intra-abdominal pressure that exceeds normal physiological limits (pregnancy, vaginal delivery). The perineal muscles weaken, subluxate and sag, with resulting perineal descent [24] (Figs. 10.1 and 10.2).

The key objective of perineoplasty is a restoration of the perineal body.

The perineal body is the confluence of perineal muscles and the external anal sphincter. It is possible that when put under strain from other structural changes, such as levator ani injury or collagen fascial compromise, the confluence of muscles is slowly pulled apart. This possibility is supported by cadaver dissection work showing subluxation of the muscles that would normally attach on the perineal body [25]. Of note, traditionally, the perineal body has been thought of as being the central tendon of the perineum. However, it has been shown that this is a misnomer, because the perineal body is a confluence of muscles and histologically, it is not a tendon [26].

It is possible to obtain clear images of the posterior compartment of the pelvic floor by using 2D transperineal ultrasound. The perineal body can be measured on 2D ultrasound in its length, height, perimeter and area. A small perineal body (less than 2.4 cm^2) is strongly associated with posterior compartment prolapse [27].

These findings are in support of Emmet's and Kelly's thinking, in which they emphasized the importance of perineorrhaphy, i.e., perineal body reconstruction in vaginal prolapse repair [22,23].

It is also necessary to clarify some nomenclatural confusion regarding the so-called recto-vaginal fascia whose reinforcement is also a part of perineoplasty and vaginoplasty. Reports in the gynecologic literature are varied, but indicate a growing consensus that there is no true "rectovaginal fascia,"

(a) (b)

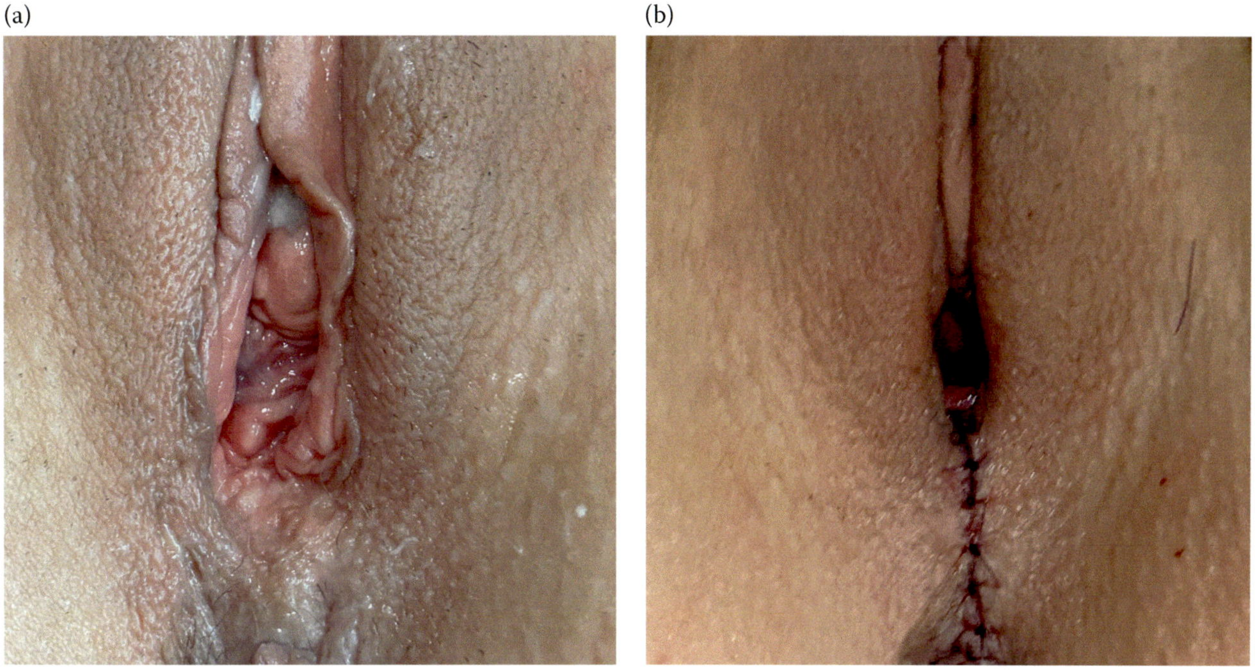

FIGURE 10.1 (a) Before and (b) after operation.

(a) (b)

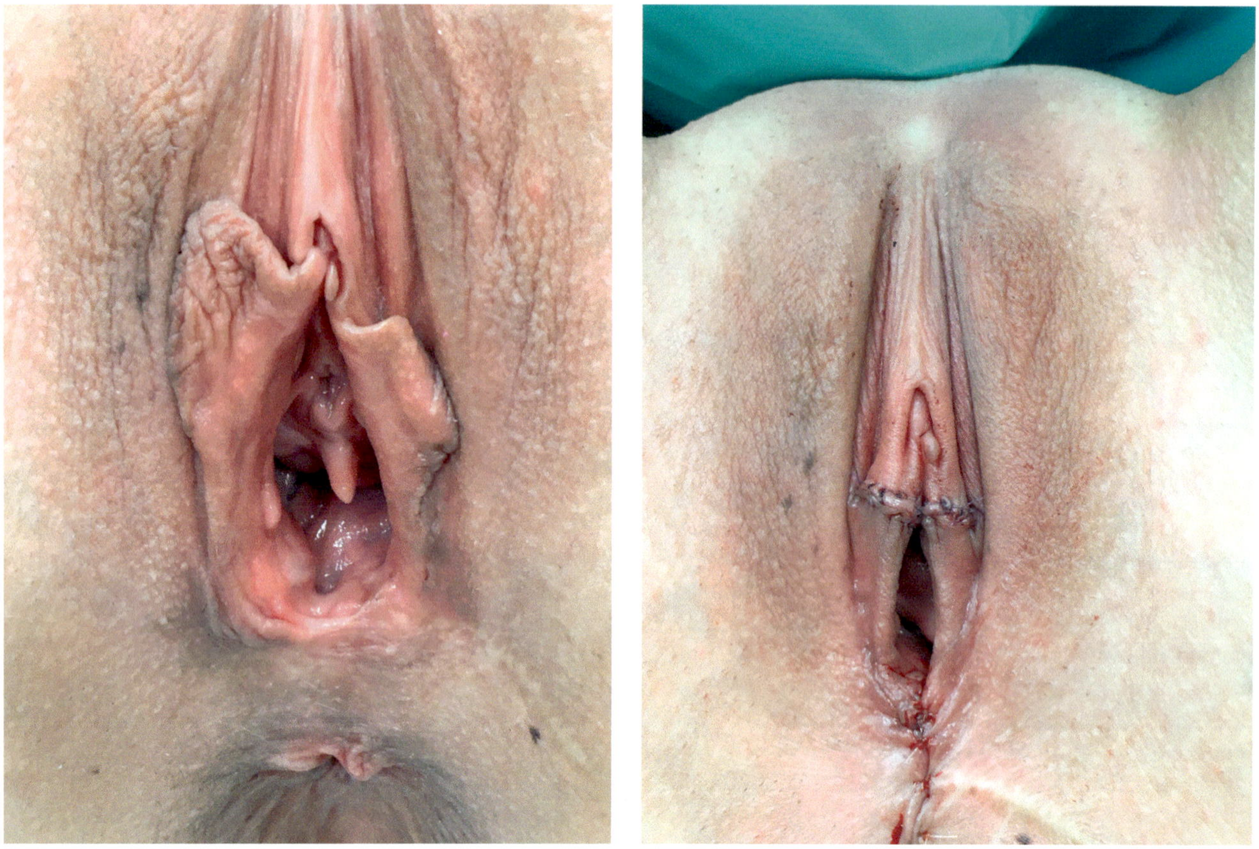

FIGURE 10.2 (a) Before and (b) after operation.

"rectovaginal septum," or Denonvilliers' fascia, and that these terms should be abandoned. Histologically, what textbooks refer to as a fascia, is a fibro-muscular layer of the vaginal wall [28].

Similarly, the pubovesicocervical fascia has not been identified as a separate histologic layer from the vaginal muscularis. With respect to the rectovaginal fascia (septum), the consensus is that there is no such layer between the posterior vaginal wall and the anterior rectal wall [29].

INDICATIONS

The lower part of the posterior vagina and perineum are closely related both in terms of anatomy and function; therefore, perineoplasty is an inherent part of colpoperineoplasty in the treatment of most cases of prolapse of the posterior vaginal wall and perineum.

Aside from prolapse repair, perineoplasty, as a single procedure, is commonly performed to improve sexual function by narrowing and reinforcing on a muscular level a relaxed introitus, as well as to address cosmetic concerns of the patient. Excising sensitive scars after episiotomy repair is also a quite common indication [15].

CONTRAINDICATIONS

Perineoplasty should be postponed in women who are planning to have a vaginal delivery. Active infections and undiagnosed pathology of the vulvar skin should be clarified and cured before planned perineoplasty [10].

Vulvodynia is a relative contraindication as it can be exacerbated by genital surgery. Problems with defecatory dysfunction should be consulted by a colorectal surgeon prior to surgery.

PATIENT EVALUATION

Cosmetic patients looking to improve their appearance and, as in the case of perineoplasty, sexual function, should also be completely healthy.

Regardless of the aesthetic considerations and expectations of the patient, the doctor should take a thorough medical and sexual history and, in particular, determine whether there are any dysfunctions in the bladder, bowel, or pelvic floor that may affect the planned surgery. Very clear questions should be asked about sex life, the presence or absence of orgasms, sexual comfort, vaginal laxity and lubrication during vaginal intercourse.

The perineum, its height, width, tension of the perineal and levator ani muscles as well as the perineal body should be evaluated in great detail. To fully assess the potential pelvic organ prolaps, the examination should be carried out in the gynecological and standing position. The patient is asked to cough to assess for urethra hipermobility, and during Valsalva manoeuvre we can evaluate the behaviour of the vagina and perineum under the strain. Digital rectal examination is required to assess the presence of rectocele, perineocele and thickness of rectovaginal junction and perineal body. Neurology of the area is evaluated by checking the clitoral, bulbocavernosus and straining–perineal reflex [10,24].

Using mirrors, fingers, and dilatators, as well as taking pictures, are useful to help patients understand the issue and visualize the degree of planned surgery.

All the data taken should be recorded, and the doctor should describe the planned procedure in a way that is understandable to the patient.

PHOTODOCUMENTATION

In plastic surgery, photographic documentation is essential. Standardized settings and lighting conditions with photos in the same position before and after the procedure allow the surgeon to show the effects of the planned procedure as objectively as possible. Follow-up photographs after 6 weeks and 6 months are excellent for full evaluation of the process of healing and changing the appearance of the operated area.

PATIENT INFORMED CONSENT

Under the law, the patient is to be given time to review and discuss detailed informed consent for the procedure.

MEDICATION AND PREPARATION

Operations on the external genitalia can be carried out easily as outpatient procedures, because they are usually performed under local anesthesia. An overnight stay is not required, even after general anaesthesia. It goes without saying that the patient should be able to contact the surgeon or designated staff at all times in case of emergency.

Perineoplasty and surgery of external genitalia can be performed under any type of anesthesia, but given the scope of the procedure, local anesthesia seems to be most appropriate here.

In my practice, 30 minutes before the scheduled surgery, an ointment with 15% lidocaine is applied to the skin of the perineum and into the vagina, which makes local injection of anesthesia almost painless. Adequate analgesia should be prescribed before every surgical procedure and should be continued depending on the patient's needs. Paracetamol and ketoprofen are most commonly used for this purpose. When peripherally acting analgesics are not sufficient, it is worthwhile combining them with central-acting agents.

The routine administration of antibiotics is to some extent disputed, but most surgeons in practise give cephalosporine 1 hour before surgery as blanket antibiotic cover and continue for up to 3–5 days.

PERINEOPLASTY: TECHNIQUE

The patient is placed in the lithotomy position; 10% povidone-iodine is applied to the skin, and the patient is draped in a sterile fashion. Care is taken during positioning to pad all pressure points to prevent iatrogenic injury. Compression stockings during the perioperative period and intermittent pneumatic compression devices are optional and should be considered in patients with a risk factors or history of VVTA.

The incision can be made with any instrument of the surgeon's choice. The author of the chapter prefers a hgh-radiofrequency unit (2.2 MHZ), which allows cutting without burning and also mono and bipolar coagulation.

In plastic surgery, marking is an important part, and a principle derived from carpentry – "measure twice cut once" – fits perfectly here. The procedure starts with marking the perineal V flap and introital inverted V flap using sterile permanent marker filler ink, which will not run on moist skin, to indicate incision lines. The triangles should meet, giving the overall excision pattern a diamond-shape at the border of the skin of the perineum and the mucosa of vaginal introitus maintaining the continuity of Hart's line. Care must be taken to also maintain the level of desired contact between labia majora. This transition point must be carefully selected as it will define the new position of the posterior fourchette. The tip of the introital V flap should be placed at the level of hymenal remnants and the perineal flap on the anterior margin of the external anal sphincter. To assess the lateral limits of the V flap, the surgeon inserts two fingers of the non-dominant hand into the vagina. The width of the resection can be confirmed by approximating the planned margins with tissue forceps to ensure they can be approximated with minimal tension. If there is any doubt as to the width of the planned resection, it is better to perform under-resection to avoid overtightening and the risk of introital stenosis and dyspareunia.

Resecting the perineal skin and introital mucosa exposes the underlying perineal musculature, often separated as a result of prior vaginal delivery. Identification of bulbospongiosus, transverse perineal superficial muscles, external anal sphincter and perineal body defects are essential to obtain the desired result. The identification of the fibro-muscularis layer of the vaginal wall is not necessary and even impossible because at this level there are no separate layers but rather a firm confluence of distended muscles and vaginal wall.

After bilateral identification of bulbospongiosus muscles, they are reapproximated using multiple deep interrupted delayed-absorbable sutures. Again, care must be taken to prevent overtightening to minimize the risk of dyspareunia. Next, transverse superficial perineal muscles and external anal sphincter are approximated with two or three delayed-absorbable sutures. The subdermal is closed with running or interrupted 3-0 absorbable sutures and the skin and mucosa with fine 4-0 or 5-0 absorbable sutures.

See further Figures 10.1 and 10.2.

POSTOPERATIVE CARE

Patients are provided with a postoperative prescription for Senna glycoside or plantago ovata to prevent constipation.

All patients return for follow-up on postoperative day one. Patients are instructed to gently rinse the perineum with soapy water four times daily and after every bathroom visit, they have to keep the area clean, minimize the risk of infection, and prevent scabs from forming along the incision. Soaking in the tub is discouraged. Patients return for follow-up appointments at the 1-week, 6-week and 3-month time points. Patients are instructed to refrain from strenuous physical activity for 4 weeks, and to avoid tampon use and sexual intercourse for 6 weeks.

INTRAOPERATIVE COMPLICATIONS

Intraoperative complications with a perineoplasty alone are extremely rare. The potential injury of the rectum or anal canal can be easily avoided by thorough rectal examination before the procedure, which allows the surgeon to evaluate the proximity of the rectal wall and anal canal. Particular care must be taken if perineocele is present.

POSTOPERATIVE COMPLICATIONS

Of the possible complications, delayed wound healing and superficial partial separation of the skin are the most common. Superficial separation does not require surgical repair, and some surgeons, including the author, recommend platelet-rich plasma to precipitate healing of the wound. Deeper dehiscence requires surgical repair by refreshing and approximation the edges. If the tension after refreshing the edges is too high, the wound should be left to heal spontaneously. Cleansing the area with 10% saline and applying a dressing with argosulfan or other agents for hard-to-heal wounds precipitate the formation of healthy granulation tissue. Swelling sometimes occurs and can be easily treated with cold compress. If prolonged, low doses of oral steroids are helpful.

If introital stenosis occurs, it should be first managed with vaginal dilators and massage.

In the case of ineffective conservative treatment, surgical perineal release is necessary. It can be easily made in local anaesthesia by vertical incision through the middle of a cramped perineum and suturing the incision transversely with interrupted sutures.

REFERENCES

1. Dobbelair JMLCL, Van Landuyt K, Monstrey SJ. Aesthetic surgery of the female genitalia. *Semin Plast Surg*. 2011;25:130–141.
2. Jamali S, Abedi P, Rasekh A, et al. The long term effect of elecive colpoperineoplasty on sexual function in the reproductive aged women in Iran. *Int Sch Res Notices*. 2014:1–5.
3. Kanter G, Jeppson PC, McGuire BL, et al. Perineorrhaphy: Commonly performed yet poorly understood. A survey of surgeons. *IntUrogynecol J*. 2015;26(12):1797–1801.
4. Wu JM, Hundley AF, Visco AG. Elective primary cesarean delivery: Attitudes of urogynecology and maternal- fetal medicine specialists. *Obstet Gynecol*. 2005;105(2):301–306.
5. Goodman MP. Female genital cosmetic and plastic surgery: A review. *J Sex Med*. 2011;8:1813–1825.
6. Olsen AL, Smith VJ, et al. Epidemiology of surgically managed pelvic organ props and urinary incontinence. *Obstet Gynecol*. 1997;89:501–506.
7. Ulubay M, Keskin U, Fidan U, et al. Safety, efficiency, and out-comes of perineoplasty: Treatment of the sensation of the wide vagina. *Biomed Res Int*. 2016;2495105:1–5.
8. Pardo JS, Solà VD, Ricci PA, Guiloff EF, Freundlich OK. Colpoperineoplasty in women with a sensation of a wide vagina. *Acta Obstetricia et Gynecologica Scandinavica*. 2006;85(9):1125–1127.
9. Kudish BI, Iglesia CB. Posterior wall prolapse and repair. *Clin Obstet Gynecol*. 2010;53:59Y71.
10. Hamori CA, Banwell P, Alinsod R. *Female Cosmetic Genital Surgery*. p. 165, 2017 Thieme.
11. DeLancey OL. Anatomic aspects of vaginal eversion after hysterectomy. *Am J Obstetr Gynecol*. 1992;166(6): 1717–1728.
12. Adamoand C, Corvi M. Cosmetic mcuosal vaginalt ightening (lateral colporrhaphy): Improving sexual sensitivity in women with a sensation of wide vagina. *Plastic Reconstr Surg*. 2009;123(6):212–213.
13. Rouzier R, Haddad B, Deyrolle C, Pelisse M, Moyal-Barracco M, Paniel B-J. Perineoplasty for the treatment of introital stenosis related to vulvar lichen sclerosus. *Am J Obstetr Gynecol*. 2002;186(1):49–52.
14. Goodman MP. Female cosmetic genital surgery. *Obstetr Gynecol*. 2009;113(1):154–159.
15. Woodward AP, Matthews CA. Outcomes of revision perineoplasty for persistent postpartum dyspareunia. *Female Pelvic Med Reconstr Surg*. 2010;16(2):135–139.
16. Jeffcoate TN. Posterior colpoperineorrhaphy. *Am J Obstet Gynecol*. 1959;77:490–502.
17. Dieffenbach JF. *Dublin J. M. Sc*. 12: 481, 183.
18. Dieffenbach JF. *Lancet*. 1838;1:810.
19. Fricke JCG. Ann. der Chirurg. Abtheil des allgemeinen Krankenha.uses. *Hamburg*. 2:142, 1R33.
20. Sims TM. *Clinical Notes on Uterine Surgery*, London, 1866, Robert Hardwicke. Hect. V.
21. Shaw WF. In: Munro Kerr JM, Johnstone R, Phillips HM, editors: *Historical Review of British Obstetrics and Gynaecology 1800–1950*, Edinburgh, 1954.
22. Kelly HA. *Operative Gynaecology*, London, 1898, Henry Kimpton.
23. Emmet TA. A study of the etiology of perineal laceration, with a new method for its proper repair. *Gynecological Transactions*, 1883.

24. Shafik A, El-Sibai O, Shafik AA, et al. Effect of straining on perineal muscles and their role in perineal support. Identification of the straining–perineal reflex. *J Surg Res*. 2003;112:162–167.
25. Shafik A, Ahmed I, Shafik AA, El-Ghamrawy TA, El-Sibai O. Surgical anatomy of the perineal muscles and their role in perineal disorders. *Anat Sci Int*. 2005;80(3):167–171.
26. Shafik A, Sibai OE, Shafik AA, Shafik IA. A novel concept for the surgical anatomy of the perineal body. *Dis Colon Rectum*. 2007;50(12):2120–2125.
27. Asfour V, Digesu GA et al. Ultrasound imaging of the perineal body: A useful clinical tool. *Int Urogynecol J*. 2020 Jun;31(6):1197–1202.
28. Kleeman SD, Westermann C, Karram MM. Rectoceles and the anatomy of the posterior vaginal wall: Revisited. *Am J Obstet Gynecol*. 2005;193:2050–2055.
29. Farrell SA, Dempsey T, Geldenhuys L. Histologic examination of "fascia" used in colporrhaphy. *Obstet Gynecol*. 2001;98:794–798.

11 Reconstructive Treatment of Female Genital Tract Anomalies

Elvira Bratila and Diana-Elena Coamdasu

INTRODUCTION

Congenital anomalies of the female genital organs are defined as deviations from the normal anatomy of the female genital tract, resulting from embryological defects of the Mullerian ducts or paramesonephrotic ducts. Compared to other malformations, they are relatively less common and constitute a rate of 5.5% in the general population, 8% in the group of women affected by infertility, 13.3% in patients with miscarriages and 24.5% in patients suffering from infertility and miscarriage.

Currently, the ESHRE/ESGE classification is the most commonly used for describing and diagnosing female gynecological congenital anomalies, while their surgical correction techniques are being constantly perfected [1–3].

DIAGNOSIS

Gynecological Examination

Gynecological examination is essential in the clinical evaluation of the patient. It is a non-invasive, simple, easy, and low-cost method. It provides us with useful information in the case of vaginal or cervical abnormalities. Certain congenital anomalies of the female genitals can be objectively diagnosed by inspection: aplasia, double cervix, longitudinal vaginal septum, and imperforate hymen.

Palpation (by bimanual examination or rectal examination in the case of vaginal aplasia) does not offer information about the integrity of the uterine cavity and the uterine wall, but it can provide information about the uterine body (in the case of the bicornuate uterus). Palpation offers details on the dilatation secondary to the obstruction of the menstrual flow in the case of hematocolpos or hematometry.

In the case of primary amenorrhea, the inspection of the external genitalia should be done carefully in order to detect distal vaginal aplasia, to distinguish the complete longitudinal vaginal septum from the incomplete one. The speculum or valves examination can objectify the double uterine cervix.

In the case of chronic pelvic pain with or without primary amenorrhea, palpation may reveal a pelvic mass secondary to the accumulation of menstrual blood (hematocolpos) [4,5].

Clinical examination is difficult in adolescent virgo patients; that is why the clinical exam does not bring many diagnostic details.

Ultrasound Examination

Ultrasound is a method often used in the clinic because it is accessible, simple, does not irradiate and provides valuable diagnostic information. We can measure the size of the uterine cavity and the cervix, we can observe the uterine contour, and we can detect associated pathologies (ovarian, tubal, fluid accumulation in the Douglas cul de sac, benign uterine pathologies – fibroids, polyps, adenomyosis).

Transperineal ultrasound is used especially in women who have not initiated sexual activity or in those with imperforate hymen or hematocolpos.

3D ultrasound provides much higher quality information than 2D ultrasound, with superior accuracy in measuring uterine and cervical dimensions and identifying possible pathologies [6].

MRI Examination

An MRI examination is superior to ultrasound, providing images in the three planes (sagittal, coronal and transverse) (Fig. 11.1). It is able to detect lesions or abnormalities that

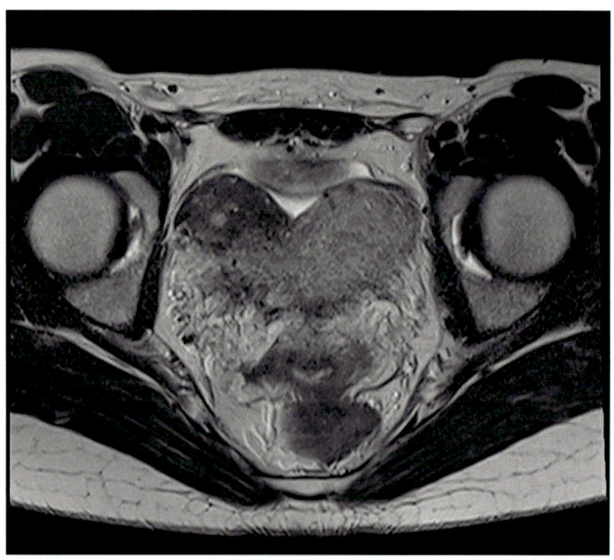

FIGURE 11.1 Unilateral uterine agenesis. Hemiuterus is to the left, while on the opposite side the Mullerian matrix is represented by a rudimentary canaliculated uterine horn.

DOI: 10.1201/9780429353079-11

cannot be visualized at a routine ultrasound examination. It is the gold standard examination in utero-cervical obstructive abnormalities [7].

Hysteroscopy

Hysteroscopy is a diagnostic and therapeutic method often used. It provides information on the vaginal walls, cervical canal, uterine cavity and tubal ostia. Pathologies such as the "T" -shaped uterus, septate uterus, and bicornuate uterus can be diagnosed and treated hysteroscopically [8].

Laparoscopy

Diagnostic laparoscopy is the method that provides the most valuable information about the uterine contour, ovaries and adjacent intraperitoneal organs, as well as the condition and patency of the fallopian tubes. Instead, the thickness of the uterine wall or the existence of a septum or intracavitary pathology cannot be estimated without opening the cavity [9].

MANAGEMENT

Surgical management of congenital anomalies of the female genitals depends on the type of malformation, its complexity, symptoms and the patient's desire to maintain or regain fertility. Most non-severe malformations can be treated hysteroscopically, but in advanced cases laparoscopy or sometimes laparotomy is required, and in complex cases a combined approach by vaginal and laparoscopic route is necessary.

Imperforate Hymen

Imperforate hymen is the consequence of the lack of canalization of the lower pole of the vaginal plateau and has an incidence of 1 in 1000 to 2000 women.

Symptomatology is caused by the lack of hymeneal orifice, producing pseudo-amenorrhea with crypto-menorrhea (present also in the case of complete transverse vaginal septa and cervical canal agenesis). The clinical onset is at puberty, consisting in intense cyclic pain, with perineal and abdominal location.

Clinical examination reveals a distended, purplish hymeneal membrane, suggesting hematocolpos. In neglected cases, it leads to hematometry and hematosalpinx, with symptoms of acute abdomen and difficulty in urinating and defecating.

The standard treatment for imperforate hymen is surgical. It is recommended to perform simple vertical incisions, "T-", "X-" or cross-shaped, in order to evacuate the menstrual blood collection. Blackened, modified, abundant blood is usually evacuated. "X" -shaped incisions have the lowest risk of intercepting the urethra and are therefore the most recommended. Performing pressure on the uterus is not recommended during surgery [10].

Vaginal Septum

The vaginal septum can be divided into transverse or longitudinal vaginal septum.

Transverse vaginal septum is diagnosed by inspection (narrowed vagina, which does not allow visualization of the cervix, hematometry) and by MRI.

The treatment of the transverse vaginal septum consists of an incision at the middle point of the septum, with the enlargement of the initial incision in order to evacuate the blood. Patients with transverse vaginal septum usually associate segments of vaginal agenesis. (See Video 11.1: Patient with normal uterus, partial cervical agenesis and superior vaginal agenesis [U0C4V3]. Surgery was done laparoscopically – excision of aplastic cervix and the part of vaginal aplasia, followed by utero-vaginal anastomosis.) In these cases more laborious interventions, such as laparoscopic resection of the vaginal septum, are needed with the entire part of the vaginal agenesis to realize the continuity of the genital tract – between the cervix and vagina [11].

Longitudinal vaginal septum is often associated with other genital malformations: complete uterine septum, didelphys uterus or bicornuate uterus.

The diagnosis is established by speculum examination, with the help of which the longitudinal septum is visualized directly, with/without palpation of a pelvic mass due to obstruction of the hemi-vagina. Patients experience difficulties during intercourse, having important dyspareunia. Usually these patients present in adolescence, with physiological menarche, complaining of progressive, monthly, pelvic or vaginal unilateral pain during menstruation.

The treatment is surgical. The excision of the vaginal septum is practised, with running absorbable sutures in order to face the edges and control the haemostasis (sometimes it can lead to scar retraction of the vaginal walls, with secondary dyspareunia). The uterine septum, if associated, can be resected hysteroscopically [12].

Vaginal Agenesis

Congenital absence of the vagina is present in 90% of cases as part of a more complex congenital anomaly, most frequently in the case of Mayer–Rokitanski–Kuster–Hauser syndrome. It is characterized by the congenital absence of the vagina; a rudimentary bicornuate, not channelized uterus; and normal fallopian tubes and ovaries. Patients present normal female phenotype, secondary sexual characteristics, and normal karyotype and endocrine functions (embryological development abnormalities appear after week 9).

The local examination reveals a normal or hypoplastic vulva, with the urethral orifice visible. Under the urethral orifice there is a small depression similar to a cul de sac (vaginal introitus). In incomplete forms, the short vagina has a length of 1–3 cm and is ended in a "glove finger".

Bimanual examination confirms the absence of the uterus or sometimes two small oblique, paramedian solid formations can be palpated, connected by a horizontal band, consisting in a rudimentary, bicornuate uterus.

Laparoscopy is the gold standard investigation, both diagnostic and therapeutic, and reveals complete rudimentary Mullerian horns, proximal to a median endopelvic band. Distally they continue with normal fallopian tubes and usually normal ovaries.

Ultrasound examination may detect associated abnormalities of the kidneys and urinary tract, most often single kidney, horseshoe kidney, and uni- or bilateral intrapelvic renal ectopia.

Treatment is recommended after puberty, a few months before the onset of sexual life. Constructing an artificial neovagina/vagina through a vaginoplasty or neocolpopoesis technique is required [13].

The Frank vaginoplasty method, most commonly used in the past, consists of progressive dilations of the rudimentary vagina during 3–4 weeks, creating finally a channel of 6–7 cm length, maintained by local self-application during the night of mold aplicators. In order to achieve the best results for this technique, an initial 1–3 cm channel length of the rudimentary vaginal wall is usually necessary.

Wharton's vaginoplasty consists of wide cleavage of the rectovaginal space, careful hemostasis and placement in the newly formed space of a guide, which is maintained until the vaginal vestibule epithelium slides into the newly formed canal and completes epithelialization. The risks are very high and include damage to the rectum and bladder, infections, decubitus necrosis, scar retraction and failure of the procedure.

McIndoe vaginoplasty is characterized by the cleavage of the intervesico-rectal space, in which a 8–12 cm long and 3 cm in diameter cylinder, with a flat lower extremity, is inserted, on top of which a free skin graft, collected from the thigh, is applied. Two weeks later the guide is removed, and the patient is counselled to continue to use daily an elastic cylinder for another 5–6 months, after which regular sexual intercourse is recommended. Intraoperative complications are frequent and include lesions of the urethra, bladder and rectum, hemorrhage, and accidental opening of the peritoneal cavity. Postoperative complications include decubitus fistulas, graft rejection infections, urinary tract infections, vicious scars, and late scar retraction of the newly created vagina.

Williams vulvovaginoplasty consists of the construction of an artificial vagina with tissues collected from the labia and perineum [14].

Other surgical vaginal reconstruction procedures include the use of skin, bowel and peritoneum as grafts or different biological prefabricated grafts.

Total Vaginal Agenesis with Functional Uterus

Symptomatology consists of blood retention into the uterine cavity and fallopian tubes, and possible reflux into the peritoneal cavity.

The treatment is represented by hystero-vestibulostomy (vesico-rectal cleavage up to the cervix) and incision of the uterus with the evacuation of accumulated blood. The cervix is lowered to the anterior cleaved space and opened vaginally, its edges being fixed to the vestibular mucosa.

Partial Vaginal Agenesis

Symptoms of partial vaginal agenesis include the appearance after puberty of hematometry, and hematocolpos causing lower abdominal and perineal pain.

The treatment consists in the transverse incision of the vestibular mucosa (in cases of low aplasia) or of the mucosa of the vagina (in cases of medium or high aplasia), with wide dissection of the inter-vesical-rectal space, the identification of the cervix and its anastomosis at the mucosal edges [15].

Cervical Agenesis

Bilateral Symmetrical Agenesis

The anomaly consists in two rudimentary, not tunnelled Mullerian horns attached to normal fallopian tubes, while the cervix and vagina are absent (Mayer-Rokitanski-Kuster-Hauser syndrome).

Bilateral Asymmetric Agenesis

This type of anomaly is very rare. In this case, part of a uterine horn or both are tunnelled until uneven and varied levels, while the cervix is absent or the cervical canal is missing.

Clinically, it manifests after puberty by primary amenorrhea and cyclic pain due to menstrual blood reflux through the fallopian tubes to the peritoneum. The treatment consists of surgical removal of rudimentary horns.

Unilateral Agenesis

In this type of anomaly, on one side there is a hemiuterus (unicornuate), while on the opposite side is variable Mullerian agenesis.

- True unicornuate uterus completely lacks the contralateral Mullerian canal
- Pseudo-unicornuate uterus consists in a hemiuterus on one side while on the opposite side the Mullerian matrix is represented by a rudimentary canaliculated uterine horn, without cervix or a uterine horn and cervix canaliculated, but not connected with permeable uterine vagina or a rudimentary uterine body with canaliculated cervix, connected to an isolated vagina, without the lower portion

Clinically, it manifests at puberty through intense dysmenorrhea, sometimes with signs of peritoneal irritation, while between menstruations there is usually permanent pelvic pain caused by reflux peritoneal endometriosis.

Vaginal examination establishes the presence of permeable hemiuterus and a formation of variable size, fluctuating and painful in the case of hemi-hematocervix or hemi-hematocolpos, which increases in size during menstruation [16].

Congenital Malformations of the Uterus

Didelphys Uterus

Didelphys uterus appears through the separate development of the two Mullerian canals, causing the formation of two independent uteri, with two cervixes and two vaginal cavities separated by a sagittal septum. The fallopian tubes are attached to the outer portion of the horns. Usually, the didelphys uterus is accompanied by a double vagina and the uterine cavities are independent (both can support a pregnancy, but the incidence of miscarriages is high). Less often a vagina can be obstructed, with hematocolpos on that side, hematometry and cyclic hemoperitoneum. Hysterosalpingography performed successively in the two cervical canals shows two independent uterine cavities and the corresponding fallopian tubes. Diagnostic laparoscopy confirms the two uteri separated by a rectal-bladder septum.

The treatment in the case of hematometry by cervical aplasia in one uterus consists of its anastomosis with the permeable uterus or its removal. In the case of an impermeable vagina a hemi-histerectomy can be performed on the obstructed side [17].

Unicornuate Uterus

It occurs due to the absence of the development and elongation of a Mullerian duct. Frequently, there is a contralateral rudimentary uterine horn, which may or may not communicate with the unicornuate uterus. The active endometrium in the case of a closed horn may become symptomatic with unilateral cyclic pain. Patients with unicornuate uterus have a higher rate of infertility and endometriosis. It also associates with cervico-isthmic incontinence and a high rate of miscarriages, premature births or abortions in the second trimester.

Clinical examination reveals an obviously deviated uterus. Hysterosalpingography shows a deviated, tubular cavity with a single fallopian tube. Ultrasound best shows the development of a rudimentary horn.

From a treatment point of view, there are no surgical approaches for enlarging the unicornuate uterus. In the case of a pregnancy obtained on the unicorn uterus, prophylactic cerclage or pessary insertion may be recommended [18].

Bicornuate Uterus

Bicornuate uterus is characterized by symmetrical abnormality (horns are not always equal), produced by muscular tissue filling in the space between the uterine horns and lack of resorption of the sagittal septum between the two cervical canals, causing a bicervical bicornuate uterus (with a single or double vagina, through a longitudinal septum; both vaginas can be permeable or only one, causing hematocolpos and sometimes the agenesis of the kidney on the obstructed side). If the resorption of the septum between the two cervical canals occurs, a unicervical bicornuate uterus is formed.

Diagnosis is established by first intention through hysterosalpingography, showing an unique cervical canal, continued with two divergently oriented fusiform cavities, at an obtuse angle. In the case of bicervical bicornuate uterus, if the two cavities are injected simultaneously, the aspect is similar to the unicervical one. If only one cervix is injected, the image resembles that of a unicornuate uterus. Vaginal examination shows a single vagina and cervix or a septate vagina and two unequal in size cervixes. If the two uterine horns are uneven, the small one may be confused with a fibroid or an adjacent tumour.

Symptomatology includes dyspareunia in the case of a septate vagina, repeated miscarriages at increasing ages of pregnancy and premature births with abnormal presentations.

Surgical treatment is indicated only if the woman is diagnosed with primary infertility with no other identified cause [19].

The three categories of patients described above require surgical intervention only if they associate a history of recurrent pregnancy loss or premature births.

Metroplasties by different procedures (Strassman, Jones, TeLinde, etc.), possibly with retrograde drainage and antibiotic prophylactic therapy, have been described. Pregnancy is allowed starting one year after surgery, as a prophylactic measure, although the rates of uterine rupture are low [20].

Hysteroscopic metroplasties are usually indicated in the case of septate uteruses with the base of the implantation of the septum not very thick. In recent years, hysteroscopic metroplasties have become the gold standard surgical treatment of any type of septate uterus. Double-control, hysteroscopic, and laparoscopic metroplastsy may also be performed for superior safety [21].

Septate Uterus

It is formed by lack of resorption or incomplete resorption of the median septum, resulting from the attachment of the two Mullerian canals, causing a totally septate uterus (from the fundus of the uterus to the exernal os and frequently associated with longitudinal vaginal septum) or a corporeal septate uterus (uterine cavity only) or a sub-septate uterus. The cervix is not double, but is possibly divided in two by a longitudinal vaginal septum.

Symptoms include dysmenorrhea, recurrent abortions and abnormal presentations at birth. Gynecological examination reveals a total vaginal septum, dividing the cervix into two halves, sometimes uneven or a partial one. If the uterus is septate, it can be accidentally identified during a curettage, a cesarean section or any uterine inspection.

At hysterosalpingography with simultaneous injection of the two cervical canals (in the case of totally septate uterus), the two cervical and isthmic hemi-channels with parallel trajectory are identified, continuing with a uterine cavity, which forms a sharp angle. Hysterosalpingography in the case of corporeal septate uterus shows a single cervical canal with two horns spaced by the thickness of the septum, but always at a sharp angle. Laparoscopy identifies a single uterus, with medio-sagittal groove on the uterine fundus, of variable depth [8].

A variety of incomplete septate uterus, with resorption of the median septum at the isthmic level, thus causing the two cavities to communicate with each other, was previously known as communicating uterus. In this case, hysterosalpingography reveals an "X" -shaped image, with divergence of the two cervical canals and uterine hemi-cavities at a sharp angle. It is frequently associated with complete or incomplete vaginal longitudinal septa. Rarely one of the vaginas is obstructed, causing hematocolpos, and there is renal aplasia on the same side [20].

PERSONAL EXPERIENCE IN RECONSTRUCTIVE TREATMENT OF COMPLEX UTERO-VAGINAL CONGENITAL MALFORMATIONS

From our point of view, the goals of reconstructive gynecologic surgery in the case of congenital anomalies must be the restoration of the vulvovaginal and uterine function and also the restoration of the normal appearance for an optimum cosmetic aspect.

Our clinical experience with the diagnosis and surgical treatment of gynecologic congenital anomalies includes successfully treating complex utero-cervico-vaginal malformations. The most difficult to manage are the malformations that associate to cervical anomalies C3/C4 and vaginal aplasia V3/V4.

When addressing complex utero-cervical-vaginal malformation, the objectives of the treatment are restoration of the menstrual function and preservation of fertility, given the fact that we are addressing young nulliparous women. Because of our experience with treating these types of complex and varied malformations, we don't usually have a standard operative procedure. This allows us to personalize each approach according to a particular patient. Even so, we usually set some standard steps of the procedure preoperative in order to best prepare the surgery.

Vaginal reconstruction techniques are multiple and vary, and have been described above.

The use of acellular biological grafts for reconstructive gynecologic purposes is frequent in our practise. Acellular grafts can be used in any procedure where there is a lack of substance that needs restoration. That is why it has good results in creating a neovagina after careful dissection of the rectal-bladder space. It is placed with absorbable sutures, and in term of days, it starts colonizing with fibroblasts into its mesh, stimulating the formation of new vaginal mucosa. During this time, the patient is instructed to use a vaginal expander during the night and partly during the day. Results in terms of sexual function are very good in these patients. (See Video 11.2: Neocolpopoesis with acellular graft in a case [U5C4V4].)

Another surgical intervention addressing vaginal agenesis is a procedure imagined by us; the principle of these procedures consists of the gradual traction of the aplastic vaginal walls.

The continuous traction on the aplastic vaginal wall is made by aplastic Mullerian structures or by uterus, depending on the uterine malformation associated. In different cases, we have a normal uterus or abnormal uterus – unicornuate, bicornuate with rudimentary horn or cervical agenesis (Fig. 11.2).

It is a pressure method in which the aplastic vagina is gradually lengthened by applying increased traction to the vaginal vault by Mullerian structures. Regardless of the uterine or cervical malformation present, the principle of the intervention consisted in reanastomosis of the cervix or, depending on the case, the Mullerian structure to the vaginal mucosa. Also, regardless of the extent of the vaginal agenesis area, by continuous traction of the Mullerian remnants during time, there was achieved a length of 7 to 9 centimetres of the vagina in 45 days. In order to maintain a normal vaginal calibre the patients are advised to use postoperative silicone expanders, daily in the first month and then just during the night for 4–5 months.

When operating on complex congenital gynecologic anomalies, the surgeon must have a set of steps in mind. Firstly, the manner of approach must be established: vaginal combined with laparoscopy, laparoscopic or robotic only or by laparotomy, depending on the characteristics of each case.

After entering the peritoneal cavity and exploring the appearance for a detailed diagnosis of the anomaly, it is very important to identify and dissect the ureters bilaterally. In these cases with altered anatomy, often presenting with severe pelvic adhesions or endometriosis lesions by retrograde menstruation, it is crucial to identify and dissect the ureter because we have to dissect the bladder from agenetic conjunctive tissue until we will reach the vaginal mucosa. The ureters may have different anatomy also by association with urologic congenital anomalies, frequent in this category of patients, making their identification even more important.

The next surgical step is represented by the careful dissection of the bladder and the rectum away from the conjunctive tissue found in the aplastic area. These spaces are frequently difficult to dissect, being very adherent due to abnormal anatomy. The laparoscopic approach has the advantage of the pneumoperitoneum in the dissection, which enhances the finding of the cleavage plane and uses CO_2 for gas dissection guiding the surgeon.

The next surgical step represents reconnecting the uterus or cervix to the vagina, in order to establish normal

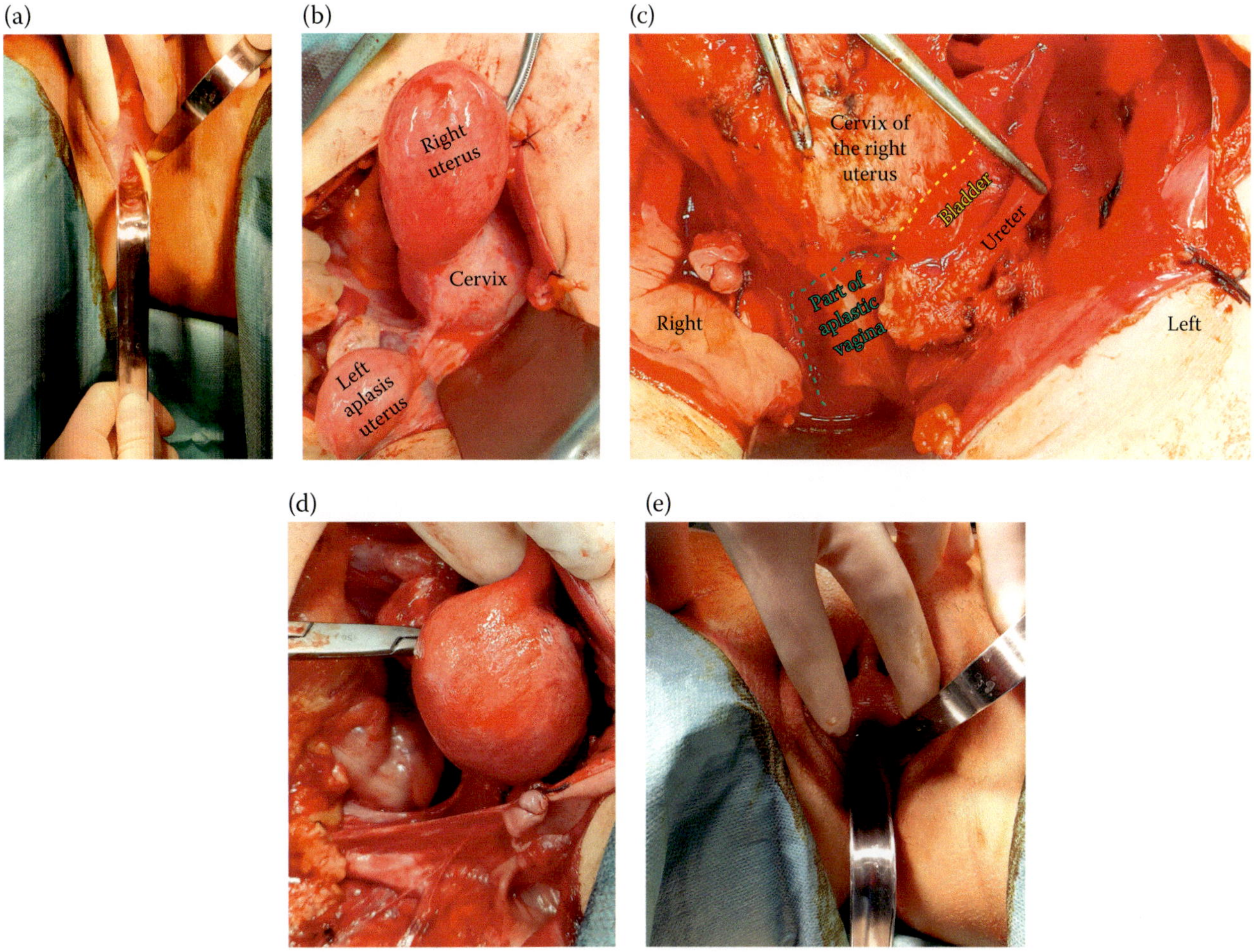

FIGURE 11.2 Intraoperative aspect in a case with right hemiuterus and rudimentary left horn, unilateral cervical aplasia, vaginal aplasia (U4C3V4). (a) Initial aspect: of agenesis vagina; (b) initial aspect bicorporeal uterus; (c) bilateral dissection of the ureters, dissection of the bladder from the agenesis part of vagina; (d) final aspect: reanastomosis of the right hemiuterus with inferior part of agenesic vagina; (e) final intraoperative vaginal aspect.

continuity. It is very important that in this anastomosis we always insert the vaginal mucosa inside the cervix or uterus in order to avoid stenosis.

After the surgery is performed, the patient is instructed to have intercourse at 6–8 weeks postoperative or use a vaginal expander (Fig. 11.3).

In the most severe and complex cases of utero-cervical-vaginal congenital anomalies, classified as C4, V3, or V4, the principles of reconstructive surgery must address the restoration of the continuity of the genital tract. The reconstruction in these cases may be realized using different types of grafts as described above or continuous traction of Mullerian structures on the aplastic vagina. Our technique involves in most cases, vaginal reconstruction by constant and continuous traction of Mullerian remnants. This causes the elongation of the vaginal walls, creating in time a normal length vagina. We consider this option superior to using grafts in order to create a neovagina, as it avoids most of the specific complications. Because the dissection is not as extensive as in the case of grafting, the bleeding, infection and visceral damage risks are lower with superior results for the patient in the long term. That is why we consider our technique optimum in addressing this category of patients.

In conclusion, we believe that complex utero-cervico-vaginal malformations must be treated by specialized personnel, with experience in this pathology and high surgical skills. Congenital gynecologic anomalies can be addressed by the paediatric surgeon as they manifest at puberty, the gynecologist, the plastic surgeon as they most frequently distort normal appearance of the vulvo-vaginal anatomy or the urologist as they associate frequently urinary tract and renal anomalies. However, we consider that a supra-specialized surgeon on this pathology as urogynecologist or aesthetic gynecologic surgeon is needed in order to offer optimum care to these patients and standardize care in the future.

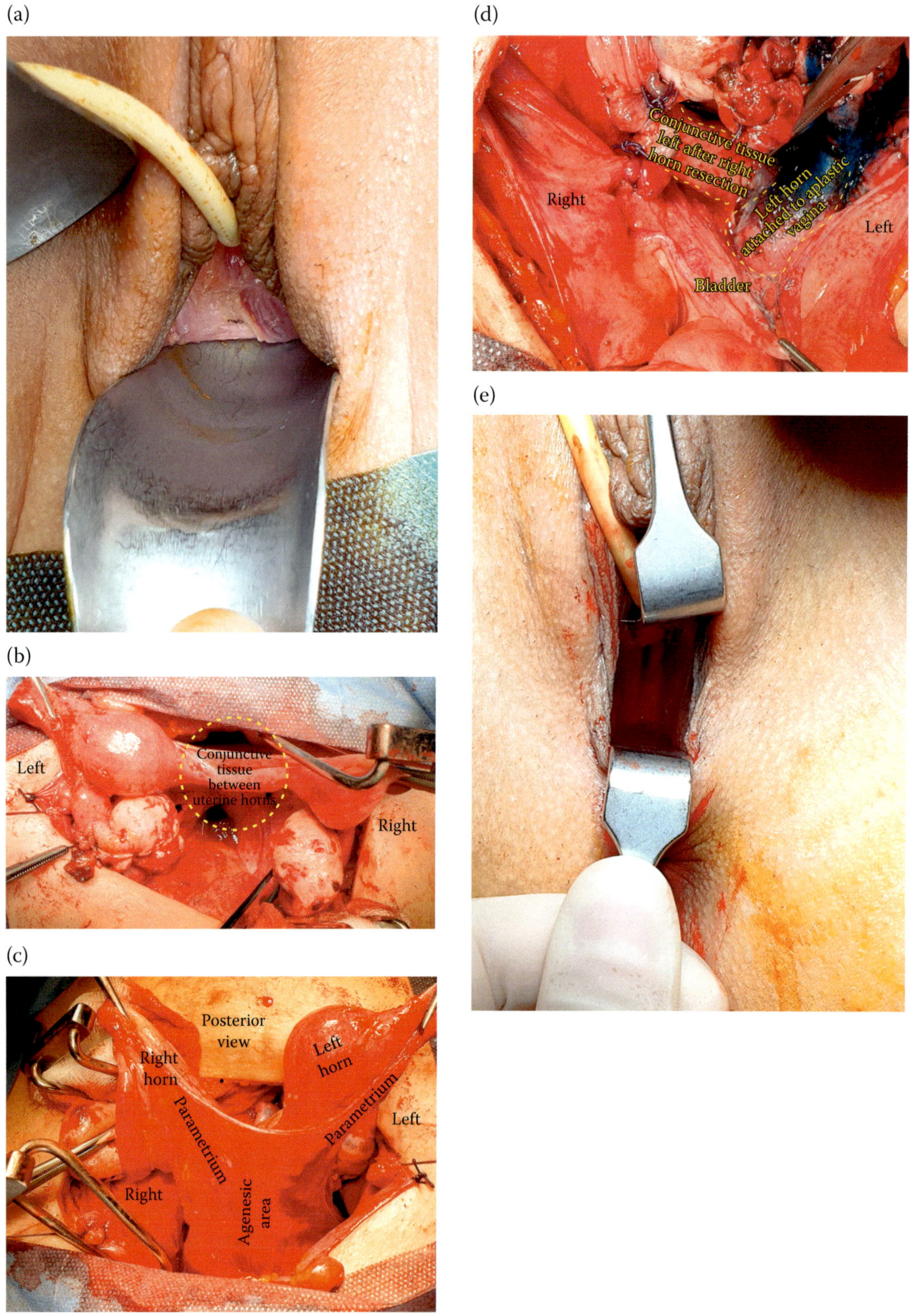

FIGURE 11.3 Intraoperative aspects in a case (U5C4V4). (a) Initial vaginal aspect; (b) initial intra-abdominal aspect; (c) posterior view – two uterine horns, bladder and rectum dissected from agenesis area; (d) final intra-abdominal aspect: reanastomosis of left horn to aplastic vagina; (e) final vaginal aspect.

REFERENCES

1. The ESHRE/ESGE consensus on the classification of female genital tract congenital anomalies, Grigoris F. Grimbizis, et al. *Hum Reprod.* 2013;28(8):2032–2044
2. The Thessaloniki ESHRE/ESGE consensus on diagnosis of female genital anomalies, Grigoris F. Grimbizis, et al. *Hum Reprod.* 2016;31(1):2–7.
3. Grimbizis GF et al. Clinical approach for the classification of congenital uterine malformations. *Gynecol Surg.* 2012;(9):119–129.
4. Saravelos SH, Cocksedge KA, Li T-C. Prevalence and diagnosis of congenital uterine anomalies in women with reproductive failure: a critical appraisal. *Human Reprod Updat.* 2008;14:415–419.
5. Acien P, Acien MS-FM. Complex malformations of the female genital tract. New types and revision of classification. *Hum Reprod.* 2004;19:2377–2384.
6. Rock JA, Roberts CPJH. Congenital anomalies of the uterine cervix: lessons from 30 cases managed clinically by a common protocol. *Fertil Steril.* 2010;94:1858–1863.
7. Ludwin A, Pityński K, Ludwin I, et al. Two- and three-dimensional ultrasonography and sonohysterography versus hysteroscopy with laparoscopy in the differential diagnosis of septate, bicornuate, and arcuate uteri. *J Minim Invasive Gynecol.* 2013;20(1):90–99.
8. Ledele L, Dorta M, Brioschi D, Massari CCG. Magnetic resonance evaluation of double uteri. *Obs Gynecol.* 1989;74(6):844–847.
9. Letterie GS. Management of congenital uterine abnormalities. *Reprod Biomed Online.* 2011;23(1).
10. Fedele L, Bianchi S, Zanconato G, Berlanda NB. Laparoscopic removal of the cavitated noncommunicating rudimentary uterine horn: surgical aspects in 10 cases. *Fertil Steril.* 2005;83.
11. Trawbrigde LC, Crough NS, Cutner ASCS. Obstructive Mullerian anomalies and modern laparoscopic management. *J Pediatr Adolesc Gynecol.* 2007;20:195–200.
12. Garcia RF. Z plasty for correction of congenital transverse vaginal septum. *Am J Obs Gynecol.* 1967;99(8).
13. Rall K, Barresi G, Wallwiener D, Brucker SYSA. Uterine rudiments in patients with Mayer-Rokitansky-Kuster-Hauser syndrome consist of typical uterine tissue types with predominantly basalis-like endometrium. *Fertil Steril.* 2013;99(5):1392–1399.
14. Mayer MRRDL. Rokitansky Kusher Hauser syndrome – fertility and treatment. *Fertil Steril.* 2010;94(5).
15. Edmonds DK et al. Congenital malformations of the genital tract and their management. *Best Pract Res Clin Obs Gynaecolo.* 2003;17(1).
16. Grimbizis GF, Campo R. Congenital malformations of the female genital tract: the need for a new classification system. *Fertil Steril.* 2010 Jul;94(2):401–407.
17. Dhar H, Razek YA, Hamdi I. Uterus didelphys with obstructed right hemivagina. *Oman Med J.* 2011;26(6).
18. Khati NJ. Frazier AA. Brindle KA. The unicornuate uterus and its variants. *J Ultrasound Med.* 2012;31(2).
19. Kcgme MH. Metroplasty versus expectant management for women with recurrent miscarriage and a septate uterus. *Cochrane Database Syst Rev.* 2011;6.
20. Gmgaf EJ. Treatment of twenty two patients with complete uterine and vaginal septum. *Minim Invasive Gynecol.* 2012;19(1).
21. Mollo A, De Franciscis P, Colacurci N, et al. Hysteroscopic resection of the septum improves the pregnancy rate of women with unexplained infertility: a prospective controlled trial. *Fertil Steril.* 2009;91:2628–1631.

12 Microfat and Nanofat Grafting in Genital Rejuvenation

Sophie Menkes

INTRODUCTION

The aesthetics and function of female genitals have become a particular concern for women over the past decade. Women choose to alter their genital anatomy to achieve sexual pleasure, reduce discomfort, and overcome functional difficulties. Genitourinary syndrome of menopause (GSM) is a very common disorder that is mostly related to the natural ageing process, particularly after menopause [1] ("GSM" has replaced the prior term "vulvovaginal atrophy"). GSM is defined as an array of signs and symptoms associated with a decrease in the levels of estrogen and other sex steroids, causing changes to the vulva, vagina, urethra, and bladder [1].

The symptoms of GSM are vaginal dryness, burning, irritation, loss of lubrication, laxity, discomfort, and pain. The consequences include vaginal infections, cystitis, dysuria, and dyspareunia. The physical effects of GSM include decreased epithelial proliferation, decreased glycogen synthesis, elimination of normal pelvic flora (*Lactobacillus*) due to very high pH levels, and decreased vascularity. These effects ultimately lower transudation and vaginal secretions [1]. The function of the labia majora, which are large and fleshy during youth, is to enclose and protect the other external reproductive organs. However, the labia majora lose volume and flatten with age, causing changes in the vulva; the labia minora, vagina, and urethra are thus no longer protected, leading to vaginal infections, cystitis, pain, and discomfort [2]. In postmenopausal women, the prevalence of vaginal dryness, dyspareunia, and urinary tract infections ranges between 27% and 55%, 32% and 42%, and 4% and 15%, respectively. Such changes may have a significant negative impact on quality of life [1]. There also seems to be a general dissatisfaction among women about the appearance of their genital area, which has been reinforced by the popularity of hair removal, fashion trends, and nude photographs throughout social media. The issues related to this dissatisfaction, however, may not only be limited to women; they may affect both individuals in a relationship [1].

Up to 50% of menopausal women suffer from at least one of the clinical symptoms associated with GSM and are affected in terms of their quality of life and sexual activity [3]. This subject remains taboo [1]. The only conventional treatments, apart from using creams and lubricants during sexual intercourse, are hormone replacement therapies, which are prescribed when there is no contraindication, and topical estrogens [4]. The goal of our treatment is to regenerate the vulvovaginal area and restore the trophicity and function of the labia majora, aiming to increase hydration and stimulation of the vaginal mucosa, normal pelvic flora (*Lactobacillus*), optimal transudation, and acidic pH. To achieve this, various tools are available that involve the use of hyaluronic acid, platelet-rich plasma (PRP), or lasers [5]. Microfat and nanofat grafting techniques were introduced at the Forever Institut a few years ago.

The nanofat grafting technique seeks to increase vascularization, neocollagenesis, and tissue regeneration. Adipose tissue-derived stem cells (ADSCs) play a vital role in rejuvenation, and their multipotent nature may not be the only advantage [6]. These cells also secrete stimulatory factors, such as cytokines, chemotactic factors, extracellular remodelers, growth factors, and their inhibitors. These factors have very complex functions, and it has been reported that bioactive factors produced by ADSCs are responsible for the regenerative effect [7].

MATERIALS AND METHODS

A total of 50 women were included in this study between January 2017 and June 2018. Menopausal women with the absence of menstruation for ≥12 months were included in this study. Women were excluded if they had used vaginal estrogen creams/tablets or vaginal moisturizers/lubricants within 1 month of study enrolment. This study was conducted according to the standards of good medical practise (ICH-E6) and the principles of the Declaration of Helsinki. All the patients taking part in the study signed a detailed consent form.

The microfat and nanofat grafting procedure was performed under local anesthesia. Anesthesia was induced via infiltration with Klein solution (500 mL normal saline, 50 mL 2% lidocaine, 1 mL 1:1000 adrenaline, and 15 mL 8.4% sodium bicarbonate). Briefly, following disinfection with povidone–iodine, fat was aspirated at the most superficial level possible to recover the maximum number of stem cells from the medial thigh, inner face of the knee, or lower abdomen. For fat collection, we used the HAPI FAT® kit (Benew Medical, Geneva, Switzerland); a 14 G 130 mm cannula was connected to a 10 cc Luer-lock syringe, and small adipocyte lobules were harvested under

DOI: 10.1201/9780429353079-12

low negative pressure via a fat lock connector valve system and a tube attached to a PureGraft® 50 pocket.

PURE GRAFT PROCEDURE

This procedure was conducted in a closed system, and the quantity of fat harvested ranged from 30 mL to 50 mL. Each 10 mL sample of fat that was aspirated and flushed into the PureGraft® pocket was washed with 10 mL of sterile saline. At the end of the procedure, 40 mL of fat were collected to obtain approximately 20 mL of microfat tissue.

Emulsification of the microfat to obtain a suspension of nanofat was achieved using the Tulip® kit (Tulip Medical Products, San Diego, CA); this process included three connectors (2.4, 1.4, and 1.2 mm) and involved shifting between two 20 cc syringes connected to each other by a female-to-female Luer-lock connector for >30 passes for each filter. The final filter included a Tulip NanoTransfer 600/400 μm device, and only one pass was used to obtain a pure product with the least number of fibres possible; the product can be easily injected through a 25 G cannula or 30 G needle.

A total of 8 mL of nanofat suspension was expected to be recovered from 10 mL of microfat. To this suspension, 20% PRP was added, which was prepared with patient blood, followed by two-step centrifugation using a Duografter II (Fidia®, Trento, Italy). The platelets were counted using a Horiba ABX Micro® ES60 Analyser (Axonlab, Baden, Switzerland) to ensure appropriate quality for nanofat grafting.

Twenty percent of PRP was added to the microfat suspension. PRP was mixed by one passage between two 20 cc syringes, then the emulsion immediately transferred using a 1 cc syringe. This microfat–PRP suspension was then injected into each labia majora. An 18 G cannula (80 mm) was used; one point of entry at the top of each labia majora was used, and a retrograde technique was applied. Local anesthesia was administered with 2% 2 mL docaine–epinephrine, which was injected into each labia majora with a 34 G needle. A total of 12 mL of the microfat–PRP suspension was injected under the dartos in the subcutaneous fat layer.

After administering local anesthesia 1 h before with lidocaine urethral gel 5 mL, 9.6 mL of the nanofat–PRP suspension was injected in the vagina with a 30 G needle (13 mm): the vestibule, the lateral and posterior walls, and the G-spot area on either side of the urethra were injected with a multipoint technique. These injections were performed very superficially, approximately 0.5–1 mm deep, at an angle of 10°, not to be too superficial and lose the product, but not to be too deep to inject into the rectum.

The procedure lasted for approximately 2 h and was painless. Only minor complications were noted, which included redness and edema between days 2 and 4, as well as bruising and pain at the donor site. No antibiotics were used. The patients were advised to avoid the use of aspirin and anti-inflammatory medication for 1 week; refrain from swimming, sauna, and hammam for 1 week; avoid sports such as cycling and horse back riding for 5 days; and abstain from sexual activities for 5 days.

CLINICAL ASSESSMENT AND PATIENT FOLLOW-UP

The impact of symptoms was measured using two scales. First, the Vaginal Health Index VHI (see appendix), which is a vaginal dryness index [8]. The VHI measures vaginal pH, elasticity, secretion volume, epithelial integrity, and hydration levels with a five-item rating scale (ratings between zero and five). The Female Sexual Distress Scale–Revised (FSDS-R) measures sexual distress in women [9]. The FSDS-R consists of 13 items, and every item requires an answer that is then rated as 0–4 (never [0], rarely [1], occasionally [2], frequently [3], or always [4]). For the VHI, the variation in scores ranges from 0 to 25; a score of >15 is normal. For the FSDS-R, the variation in scores ranges from 0 to 52; a score >11 can effectively discriminate between women with and without sexual distress. The pertinent questionnaires were anonymously completed on paper, under the supervision of an assistant at the Forever Institut. Examination for VHI scoring was performed by an independent doctor. Questions were asked to evaluate whether patients had greater self-esteem and reduced functional discomfort and difficulties, and improvement in orgasm and sexual desire post-treatment. After examination with a speculum, measurement of pH was made (Ellen® pH-Control, Stockholm, Sweden). The volume of secretion, integrity of the epithelium, hydration, and elasticity were measured by visual inspection and with palpation of the vaginal mucosa using the index finger.

STATISTICAL ANALYSIS

Values are presented as the mean ± standard deviation. The averages were compared using Student's *t*-test. $p < 0.05$ indicated statistical significance. Graphical representation of data and statistical analyses were performed with GraphPad software version 7.0.

RESULTS

The average age of patients in this study was 53 (45–63) years, the average number of pregnancies was 2.6 ± 1.2, and the average number of vaginal deliveries was 1.8 ± 1.2. Follow-up was conducted 1, 3, 6, 12, and 18 months post-treatment. After approximately 4 weeks, the patients started to experience better hydration at the level of the mucosa. A significant change was noted in the VHI (Fig. 12.1) and FSDS-R (Fig. 12.2) scores.

The VHI measures vaginal pH, elasticity, secretion volume, epithelial integrity, and hydration levels. The average VHI score increased from 3.35 ± 1.46 pretreatment to 6.35 ± 1.53 1-month post-treatment ($p < 0.0001$);

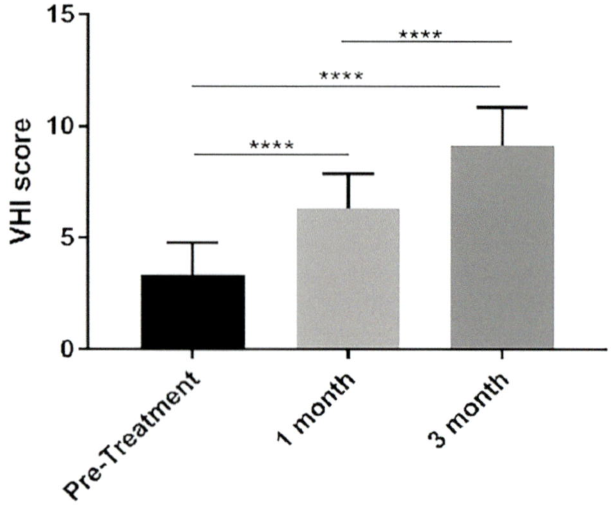

FIGURE 12.1 Mean VHI change from pretreatment to 1 and 3 months after treatment. Results represent mean ± standard deviation. ****$P < 0.0001$.

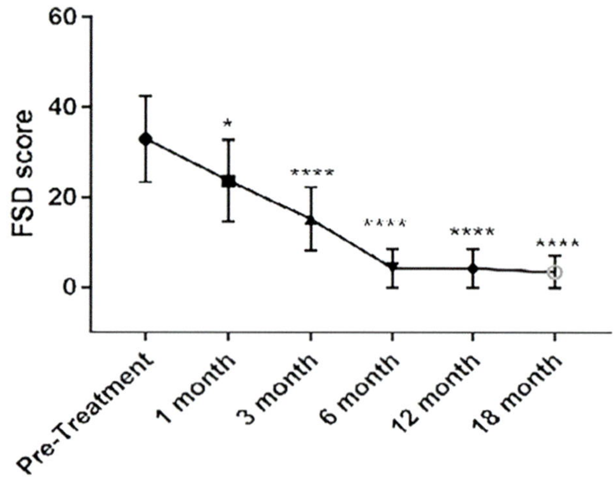

FIGURE 12.2 Female Sexual Distress (FSD) score from baseline pretreatment to 1, 3, 6, 12, and 18 months after treatment. Results represent mean ± standard deviation. *$P < 0.05$; ****$P < 0.0001$.

at 3 months post-treatment, the VHI score further increased, to 9.15 ± 1.73 ($p < 0.0001$) (Fig. 12.1).

FSDS-R scores also showed a significant change in the sexual health of the patients. The average pretreatment FSDS-R score was 32.9 ± 9.5; at 1 month post-treatment, the score significantly decreased (23.7 ± 9.05, an improvement of 28%; $p < 0.05$), and at 3 and 6 months post-treatment, the score significantly decreased even further (15.2 ± 7.02, an improvement of 53%, and 4.2 ± 4.28, an improvement of 87%, respectively, $p < 0.0001$). The score was stable from 6 to 12 months (4.2 ± 4.28, $p < 0.0001$), but at 18 months post-treatment, it further decreased (3.4 ± 3.65, $p < 0.0001$) (Fig. 12.2). At 6 months post-treatment, for both scales, data pertaining to 80% of patients appeared normalized.

There was a particular benefit of the treatment noted for dryness and dyspareunia. The patients experienced an improvement in the symptoms of GSM, sexual function, and vaginal sensation, as portrayed by the FSD-R questionnaire.

Analysis of pre- and post-procedure images indicated the achievement of a lifting effect in the vulval region. All patients confirmed changes in texture, elasticity, firmness, fine wrinkles, and skin hydration, along with a regenerative effect. The results of four cases are reported in Figures 12.3–12.6.

No major side effects were observed in the present study. Minor complications, including redness and edema, were noted between days 2 and 4. All the patients had bruises and pain at the donor site, but only one patient (2%) had redness and edema of the labia majora. Side effects were assessed by an independent doctor. No infections, fat cysts, or granulomas were observed after treatment or during the follow-up period.

DISCUSSION

As with skin elsewhere, due to the lack of hormones, ageing of the labia majora manifests by decreased volume, wrinkles, lost elasticity, and dyschromia. Volume loss may also expose the labia minora, leading to discomfort, dryness, and cosmetic distress. The results of this study showed that the injection of microfat and nanofat changed the symptoms of vulvovaginal dryness. The VHI score significantly increased at 1–3 and 6 months after treatment, showing an improvement in vaginal trophicity. Furthermore, the FSDS-R score significantly improved by 28%, 53%, 87%, 87%, and 89% at 1, 3, 6, 12, and 18 months, post-treatment, respectively, indicating that the effects lasted over time. Although the VHI score is prone to subjectivity regarding hydration and elasticity, the FSD-R score works well regarding sexual distress. With one treatment, patients benefited from significant changes that lasted over time. The treatments described in this study may be a helpful approach for managing GSM.

Since its introduction, lipofilling has become increasingly popular. Several changes have been made to the procedures for harvesting, processing, and injecting fat. Many techniques have been proposed for the removal of fat tissue. Coleman et al. [10] described a technique to minimize fat cell trauma. In 2013, Tonnard et al. introduced a nanofat grafting technique, wherein emulsification was used to mechanically dissociate adipose tissue while retaining the extracellular matrix with all nucleated cells, including the already present stem cells [11]. While macrofat is characterized by fat lobules with a diameter of 2.4 mm, microfat is characterized by those with a diameter of 1 mm [12]. The cannula used for microfat grafting in the Alharbi et al. study is 2 mm in diameter with a blunt tip and four 600 μm gauged orifices to harvest small lobules [13].

(a) (b)

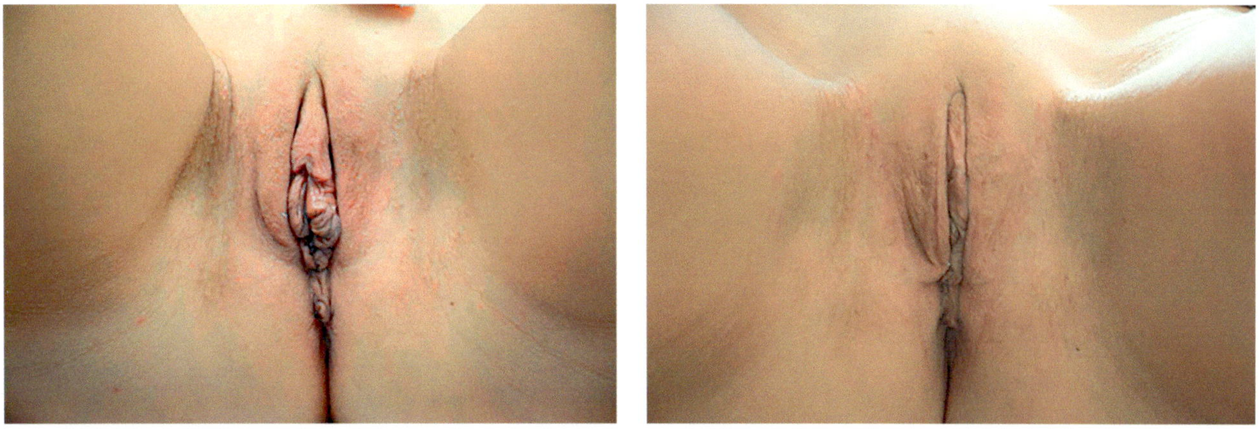

FIGURE 12.3 (a) A 55-year-old woman before treatment with 6 mL of microfat–PRP injected in each labia majora and 9.6 mL nanofat–PRP injected in vaginal walls. (b) Result 18 months after treatment.

(a) (b)

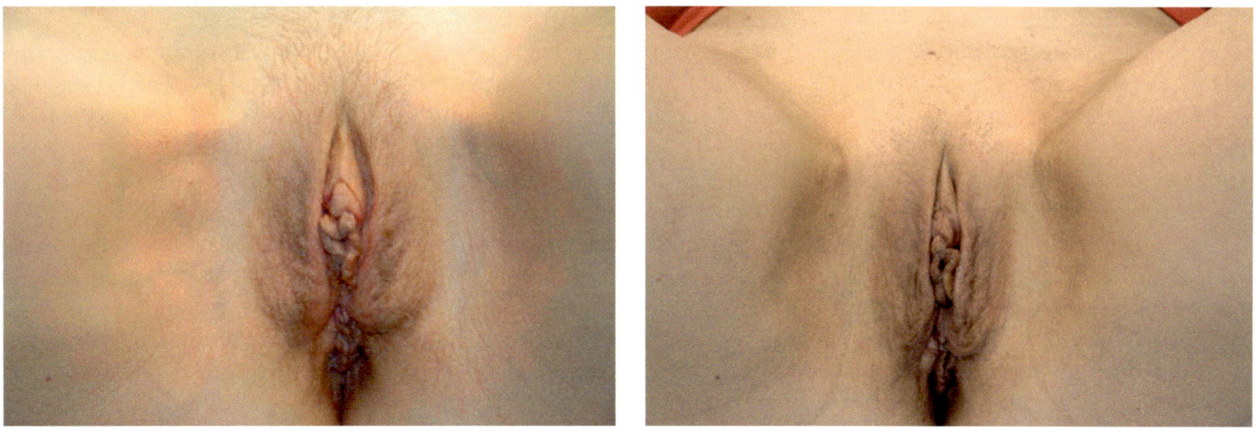

FIGURE 12.4 (a) A 58-year-old woman before treatment with 6 mL of microfat–PRP injected in each labia majora and 9.6 mL nanofat–PRP injected in vaginal walls. (b) The result 18 months after treatment.

(a) (b)

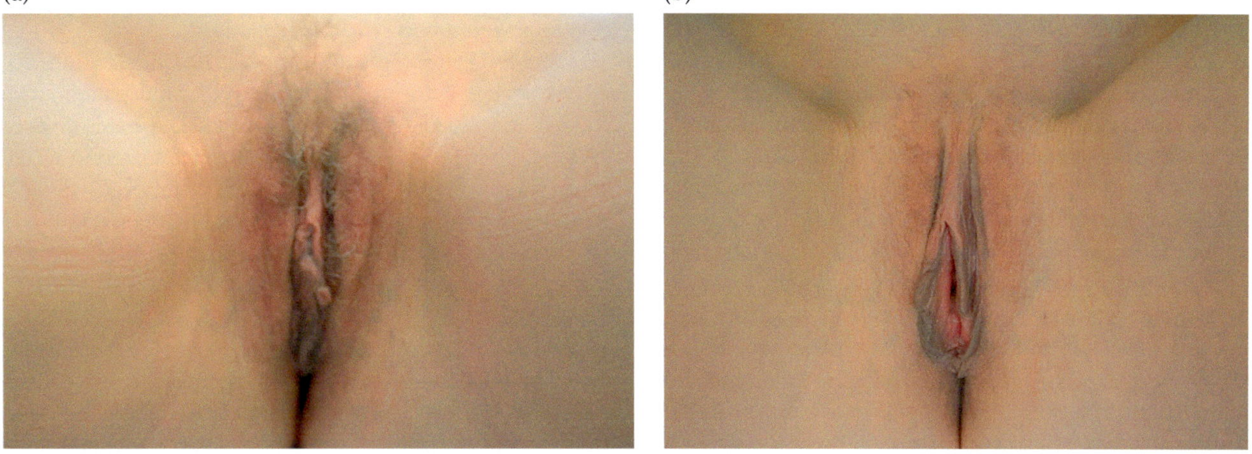

FIGURE 12.5 (a) A 53-year-old woman before treatment with 6 mL of microfat–PRP injected in each labia majora and 9.6 mL nanofat–PRP injected in vaginal walls. (b) The result 18 months after treatment.

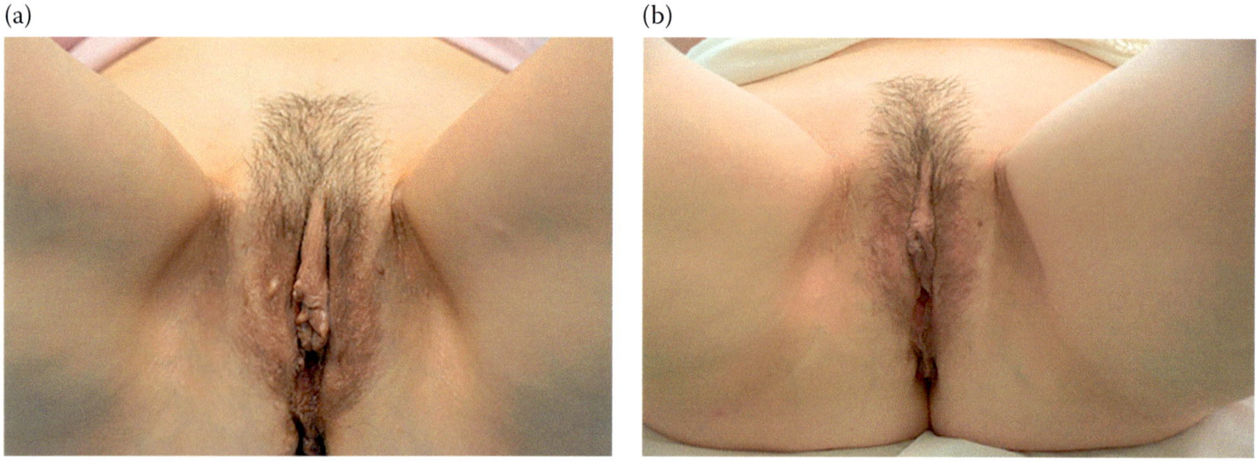

FIGURE 12.6 (a) A 54-year-old woman before treatment with 6 mL of microfat–PRP injected in each labia majora and 9.6 mL nanofat–PRP injected in vaginal walls. (b) The result 18 months after treatment.

Microfat is used to enhance trophicity as well as for filling. Nanofat is obtained by passing emulsified microfat between two syringes. After 30 passages for each connector, the fat becomes emulsified and appears whitish. The emulsified fat is then filtered through a superfine filter to obtain nanofat [14]. Nanofat transplants are devoid of mature fat cells, and the native architecture is disrupted. However, nanografts were observed to maintain a rich supply of adipose stem cells, and many other progenitor cells with a resilient phenotype. Trivisonno et al. showed that the aspiration of adipose tissue with a microcannula can be a minimally invasive method to obtain clinically relevant numbers of stromal and vascular cells that can be used for autologous transplant procedures and for promoting tissue regeneration and neovascularization [15]. In this study, ADSCs were collected from the lipoaspirate of the abdomen and hip regions of six healthy female donors. For adipose tissue harvest, two options were compared: (1) a rounded-tip cannula with a length of 170 mm, a diameter of 3 mm, and a single elliptic suction port on the side near its distal end (port diameter: 3 × 9 mm); or (2) a rounded-tip infiltration cannula with a length of 170 mm, a diameter of 2 mm, and 5 round ports placed spirally along the sides of the distal cannula shaft (each port diameter: 1 mm)

It was also shown in a recent study that >90% of cells remained viable after the mechanical disruption procedure. Total nucleated cells counts are also in the range of what is obtained by regular stromal vascular fraction (SVF) extraction without the nanofat procedure; with >300 samples processed using good manufacturing practises guidelines, a comparable mean value was found. Finally, the number of ADSCs is also similar to that obtained without the nanofat procedure. Overall, the data confirm that the nanofat procedure does not damage cells contained in the adipose tissue, maintaining cell viability, and the number of ADSCs. In this same study, skin biopsy performed on the posttreatment zone showed an increase in collagen (denser and broader collagen fibres) and elastic fibres (control: 171 ± 9.5; nanofat: 266 ± 17.3; $P < 0.005$) in the superficial dermis. Treated zones also displayed an increased dermal cellularity (mainly fibroblasts; control: 59.6 ± 6.8; nanofat: 90.6 ± 3.05; $P < 0.03$) and vascular density (control: 15.6 ± 0.5; nanofat: 26.6 ± 3.05; $P < 0.01$) in the superficial dermis [14].

In a patient with episiotomy sequelae and an impact on their sexual life, it was previously reported that lipofilling and injecting PRP–HA were effective for vulvovaginal rejuvenation. Moreover, the results of this study showed changes in vaginal trophicity [16]. A study by Kim et al. reported similar results; they found injecting PRP and lipofilling to be effective in a patient with vulvovaginal atrophy and lichen sclerosus [17]. Wei et al. also showed that in several clinical cases, nanofat grafts led to an improvement in skin quality 6 months postoperatively [18]. Mesguich et al. reported an improvement in fine lines after treatment with the nanofat process. In addition, tolerance results confirmed the safety of the intradermal injection of emulsified fat. No erythema or inflammatory reactions were observed in patients [19].

There was an interesting study on lipofilling with PRP to restore the labia majora in a 67-year-old patient with vaginal atrophy and lichen sclerosus [17]. A total of 40 cc of autologous fat mixed with PRP were transferred to the labia majora. Lipofilling with PRP relieved clinical symptoms. Missing fullness and tone were corrected, and the augmented volume was well maintained. White patchy lesions of lichen sclerosus on the labia minora also improved.

The effectiveness of microfat and nanofat grafting for vulvovaginal rejuvenation has not previously been assessed. Here, good results were achieved using microfat and nanofat with PRP with significant changes in the genital area. Microfat and emulsified fat such as nanofat seems to be a simple alternative to cell therapy processes and SVF preparation. Mechanical disaggregation offers a better cell inoculum than conventional enzymatic dissociation methods, using 10 times less fat tissue as starting material and delivering a higher cell yield [20]. The injection of fragmented adipocytes present in emulsified fat and released cytokines could have a stimulatory effect on tissue differentiation and regeneration [21]. Furthermore, an increase in elastin synthesis and dermal remodelling may be induced by the secretory activity of stem cells mechanically stimulated by the emulsion process [22–24].

The addition of autologous PRP to adipose tissue has been shown to result in better preservation of adipocyte structure, providing a strong blood supply, creating an optimal *in vivo* microenvironment for the proliferation of stem cells derived from adipose tissue, and promoting cellular interactions and the growth and differentiation of adipose tissue [25]. PRP has recently emerged as a new matrix to improve fat graft survival. PRP is an autologous biological product derived from patient blood, in which, after centrifugation, a plasma fraction is obtained with a higher platelet concentration than that in circulating blood. This process is gaining popularity in regenerative medicine because of its potential to stimulate and accelerate tissue healing [26–28]. Autologous PRP can thus be used as a delivery system for *in vivo* tissue engineering applications. Indeed, many active substances are present in the α-granules of platelets; these substances can stimulate the revascularization of a gel enriched with adipocytes and constitute a three-dimensional matrix, allowing the arrangement of adipocytes in an adequate spatial organization. Thus, PRP stimulates the proliferation of adipose stem cells and adipose tissue *in vitro*. These stem cells are generally present in the removed fat tissue and therefore are usually present in fat grafts [29,30]. Kakudo et al. showed that activated PRP contains large amounts of PDGF-AB and TGF-β1, which promote the proliferation of human stem cells derived from adipose tissue and human dermal fibroblasts *in vitro* [31].

At 6 months post-treatment, 80% of our patients scored >15 for VIH and <11 for FSD-R, but the limit of these scoring systems is their subjectivity. Even if patient-reported outcomes are the most relevant factor (i.e., criteria such as patient satisfaction, comfort, and resumption of a fulfilling sex life), we also need objective measurements. The results from the two scales showing changes in hydration, secretions, and pH are indirect signs that the treatment was effective. However, additional studies need to be conducted to validate our results. The process of grafting should include objective skin quality tests with a cutometer to measure improvement, elasticity, and firmness of the labia majora, and biopsies of the vaginal mucosa to histologically confirm the increase in the fibrillar components of the extracellular matrix and vaginal epithelial thickness.

But is the regenerative effect related to the differentiation and proliferation capacity of the cell or due to its paracrine activity? Several studies indicate that the mechanism of therapeutic action of mesenchymal stromal stem cells (MSCs) is mainly mediated by paracrine factors that are released by MSCs, such as exosomes. Exosomes are nanosized extracellular vesicles that are transferred to target cells for cell-to-cell communication.

These extracellular microvesicles released from cells appear to be the key components of the cellular secretome [32]. Even more recently the functional roles of exosomes are being investigated. Mesenchymal stem cell exosomes seem to be interesting treatment options for hair growth, but also for skin improvement, in terms of wrinkles, spots, inflammation, scars, etc.

Topical washing buffer is an autologous product, which was applied morning and evening on the skin for 3 months; it shows very promising results. New studies are underway, tending to prove that even after stopping the application of the cream, the regenerative effect continues. Although MSC-derived exosomes (MSC exosomes) are being proposed as novel cell-free therapies for various human diseases, studies evaluating the safety and toxicity of MSC exosomes are limited [33].

The results on skin and hair have just been published and are also very promising. A clinical study, after approval from the ethics committee, in the indication of post chemotherapy vaginal atrophy after breast cancer, will start at Nescens Clinic.

CONCLUSIONS

There are now many ways to rejuvenate the vulvovaginal area, but microfat and nanofat grafting seems to offer significant and long-lasting improvement with one treatment and an autologous procedure. Moreover, microfat and nanofat naturally integrate into host tissues, and there are no major side effects. The long-term effects need to be further evaluated, but the initial results appear very promising. Exosomes have several beneficial capabilities for tissue regeneration, such as angiogenic capacity, collagen synthesis, and regulation of inflammation. By using exosomes, the current limitations of skin and mucosal treatments can be overcome. In addition, these extracellular vesicles can be integrated into various fields such as cancer treatment and vaccines. Hopefully, exosomes will provide a new platform to cure various diseases and cancers soon.

FUNDING

The authors received no financial support for the research, authorship, and publication of this article.

The authors declare that they have no conflict of interest.

REFERENCES

1. Farrell AE. Genitourinary syndrome of menopause. *Aust Fam Physician*. 2017;46(7):481–484.
2. Palacios S, Mejía A, Neyro JL. Treatment of the genitourinary syndrome of menopause. *Climacteric*. 2015; 18(Supp 1):23–29.

3. Van der laak JA, De Bie LM, De Leeuw H, et al. The effect of Replens on vaginal cytology in the treatment of post-menopausal atrophy: cytomorphology versus computerized cytometry. *J Clin Pathol*. 2002;55:446–451.
4. Cumming GP, Herald J, Moncur R, et al. Women's attitudes to hormone replacement therapy, alternative therapy and sexual health: a web-based survey. *Menopause Int*. 2007;13:79–83.
5. Wańczyk-Baszak J, Woźniak S, Milejski B, et al. Genitourinary syndrome of menopause treatment using lasers and temperature-controlled radiofrequency. *Prz Menopauzalny*. 2018 Dec;17(4):180–184.
6. Charles-de-Sa L, Gontijo-de-Amorin NF, Maeda Takiya C, et al. Antiaging treatment of the facial skin by fat graft and adipose-derived stem cells. *Plast Reconstr Surg*. 2015 Apr; 135(4):999–1009.
7. Crisan M, Yao S, Casteilla L et al. Perivascular origin for mesenchymal stem cells in multiple human organs. *Cell Stem Cell*. 2008;3:301–313.
8. Bachmann G. Urogenital ageing: an old problem newly recognized. *Maturitas*. 1995;22:S1–S5.
9. Derogatis L, Clayton A, Lewis-D'Agostino D, et al. Validation of the female sexual distress scale-revised for assessing distress in women with hypoactive sexual desire disorder. *J Sex Med*. 2008;5:357–364.
10. Coleman SR. Structural fat grafts: the ideal filler? *Plast Reconstr Surg*. 2006 Sep;118(3 Suppl):108S–120S.
11. Tonnard P, Peeters G, Hamdi M, et al. Nanofat grafting: basic research and clinical applications. *Plast Reconstr Surg*. 2013;132:1017–1026.
12. Gause TM, Kling RE, Sivak WN, et al. Particle size in fat graft retention: a review on the impact of harvesting technique in lipofilling surgical outcomes *Adipocyte*. 2014 Oct–Dec;3(4):273–279.
13. Alharbi Z, Opländer C, Almakadi S, et al. Conventional vs. micro-fat harvesting: how fat harvesting technique affects tissue-engineering approaches using adipose tissue-derived stem/stromal cells. *J Plast Reconstr Aesthet Surg*. 2013 Sep;66(9):1271–1278.
14. Menkes S, Mariotta L, Soldati G, et al. Subcutaneous injections of nanofat adipose derived stem cell grafting in facila rejuvenation. *Plast Reconstr Surg Glob Open*. 2020;8:e2550.
15. Trivisonno A, Di Rocco G, Canistra C. Harvest of superficial layers fat with microcannula and isolation of adipose tissue-derived stromal and vascular cells. *Aesthet Surg J*. 2014;34:601–613.
16. Aguilar P, Hersant B, SidAhmed-Mezi M, et al. Novel technique of vulvo-vaginal rejuvenation by lipofilling and injection of combined platelet-rich-plasma and hyaluronic acid: a case-report. *Springerplus*. 2016 Jul 26;5(1):1184.
17. Kim SH, Park ES, Kim TH. Rejuvenation using platelet-rich plasma and lipofilling for vaginal atrophy and lichen sclerosus. *J Menopausal Med*. 2017 Apr;23(1):63–68.
18. Wei H, Gu SX, Liang YD, et al. Nanofat derived stem cells with platelet-rich fibrin improve facial contour remodeling and skin rejuvenation after autologous structural fat transplantation. *Oncotarget*. 2017 Jul 31;8(40):68542–68556.
19. Mesguich Batel F, Bertrand B, Magalon J, et al. Treatment of wrinkles of the upper lip by emulsified fat or "Nanofat": biological and clinical study about 4 cases. *Ann Chir Plast Esthet*. 2018 Feb;63(1): 31–40.
20. Sese B, Sammartin JM, Ortega B, et al. Nanofat cell aggregates: a nearly constitutive stromal cell inoculum for regenerative site-specific therapies. *Plast Reconstr Surg*. 2019;144:1079.
21. Bertheuil N, Chaput B. A novel and effective strategy for the isolation of adipose-derived stem cells: minimally manipulated adipose-derived stem cells for more rapid and safe stem cell therapy. *Plast Reconstr Surg*. 2015;135 (2):454–455.
22. Vezzani B, Shaw I, Lesme H, et al. Pericyte content and secretory activity of microfragmented human adipose tissue compared to enzymatically derived stromal vascular fraction. *Stem Cells Transl Med*. 2018 Dec;7(12): 876–886.
23. Banyard DA, Sarantopoulos CN, Borovikova AA, et al. Phenotypic analysis of stromal vascular fraction after mechanical shear reveals stress-induced progenitor populations. *Plast Reconstr Surg*. 2016;138(2): 237e–247e.
24. Osinga R, Menzi NR, Tchang LA, et al. Effects of intersyringe processing on adipose tissue and its cellular components: implications in autologous fat grafting. *Plast Reconstr Surg*. 2015;135(6):1618–1628.
25. Pires Fraga FM, Nishio RT, Ishikawa RS, et al. Increased survival of free fat grafts with platelet-rich plasma in rabbits. *J Plast Reconstr Aesthet Surg*. 2010;63(12): e818–e822.
26. Oh DS, Cheon YW, Jeon YR, et al. Activated platelet-rich plasma improves fat graft survival in nude mice: a pilot study. *Dermatol Surg*. 2011;37:619–625.
27. Nakamura S, Ishihara M, Takikawa M, et al. Platelet-rich plasma (PRP) promotes survival of fat grafts in rats. *Ann Plast Surg*. 2010;65:101–106.
28. Rodriguez-Flores J, Palomar-Gallego MA, Enguita-Valls AB, et al. Influence of platelet rich plasma on the histologic characteristics of the autologous fat graft to the upper lip of rabbits. *Aesthetic Plast Surg*. 2011;35:480–486.
29. Marx RE. Platelet-rich plasma (PRP): what is PRP and what is not PRP? *Implant Dent*. 2001;10:225–228.
30. Jin R, Zhang YG. Does platelet-rich plasma enhance the survival of grafted fat? An update review. *Int J Clin Exp Med*. 2013;6:252–258.
31. Kakudo N, Minakata T, Mitsui T, et al. Proliferation-promoting effect of platelet-rich plasma on human adipose-derived stem cells and human dermal fibroblasts. *Plast Reconstr Surg*. 2008;122(5):1352–1360.
32. Yang GH, Lee YB, Kang D, et al. Overcome the barriers of the skin: exosome therapy. *Biomaterials Research*. 2021;25:22.
33. Ha DH, Kim HK, Lee J, et al. Mesenchymal stem/stromal cell-derived exosomes for immunomodulatory therapeutics and skin regeneration. *Cells*. 2020;9(5): 1157.

13 Nanofat

O-Shot into the G-Spot Area

Claudio Catalisano and Mario Goisis

DEFINITIONS

Nanofat is a concentrate of stem cells and growth factors with an extraordinary ability to regenerate and repair tissues. It can be obtained through the use of a Dermal Graft (DG) and prepared with special filters. We can harvest DG from several parts of the human body, such as the abdomen (under the skin) and the lateral back (under the skin).

The G-spot (or Grafenberg spot) is a sensitive area of the vaginal wall that, if stimulated, can produce high sexual arousal. It was named by Grafenberg in 1950 [1], although perhaps in identifying that particular area of the vaginal canal he was not intending to revolutionize anatomy. However, is it a genuine anatomical part, present and recognizable in every woman? It is obviously difficult to demonstrate this concept, because sexual arousal is a private experience. However, many scientific trials and studies have now been published [2], including an anatomical study using echography that demonstrates that there is, in the anterior vaginal wall, an area that, during intercourse or autoerotism, can produce female orgasm [3]. It may be very difficult to prove with certainty that the G-spot exists, but many scientific studies in which groups of women have been questioned reveal that a high percentage of women are aware of it [4–10].

PRP O-SHOT

Psychosexual studies have also shown that more than 10% of women have never experienced orgasm [11]. From this starting point, Runels pioneered a particular new treatment, the platelet-rich plasma (PRP) O-Shot, whereby a patient's blood is harvested, centrifuged (first to separate red blood cells and then to concentrate platelets), and injected back into the patient in the form of platelet-rich plasma [12,13]. The rationale for this procedure is to introduce growth factors, present in platelet cells, into the clitoral erogenous zone and the paraurethral Skene glands in order to promote increased sexual pleasure.

Platelets are cell fragments in the blood that start the coagulation process by means of growth factors – proteins able to stimulate mesenchymal stem cells, which in turn can start or restart cellular production. The clitoris has usually about 8000 nerves, but has less in many women [14–16,17]. Skene glands produce a secretion during female sexual activity, which spreads out of the vagina, but the amount of secretion is not the same in all women. Some women do not have this "female ejaculation", and 10% are unable to have an orgasm at all (Figs. 13.1 and 13.2) [18–25]. So, Runels's procedure aims to produce new nerves in the clitoris and new cells into Skene glands to increase their secretions [26,27].

From 2014, Runels performed thousands of treatments, and a large percentage of patients developed significant enhancement of their sexual satisfaction [12,13]. However, it should be noted that the legislation covering PRP injection varies between territories and in some jurisdictions its use is not permitted in the private office of a medical professional, so the treatment may not be available as an option for all practitioners.

THE NANOFAT O-SHOT

From this starting point, the present authors developed a new type of G-spot injection of growth factors and mesenchymal stem cells – the nanofat O-Shot [28]. If the end result of the PRP O-Shot is better sexual satisfaction for the patient, this technique should have the same results because body fat (adipose tissue) contains similar high quantities of the same cell stimulators [29].

Video 13.1 shows the harvesting of fat. Our goal is to have a minimal quantity of dermal fat to prepare by filtration to obtain a more fluid preparation to inject. Klein's solution is a mixture of saline solution (500 mL), lidocaine (10 mL 2%), plus sodium bicarbonate. The patient is prepped, lying on the bed. We inject Klein's solution to obtain anesthesia. Using an aspiration cannula (the Va Clock system), we harvest a quantity of dermal graft (around 50 mL). This procedure is very easy and not uncomfortable for the patient.

Video 13.2 shows the infiltration process of turning fat into microfat and finally into nanofat. Our kit has three types of filters. The first fat harvested is macrofat (through the bigger filter), which is not useful to inject. By a second (finer) filter we produce microfat. A third filter commutes microfat into nanofat, a very fluid solution capable of being injected using a very small needle. Microfat is suitable for filling, and we can use this type if it is necessary for the cosmetic procedure of enlarging vulvar lips.

DOI: 10.1201/9780429353079-13

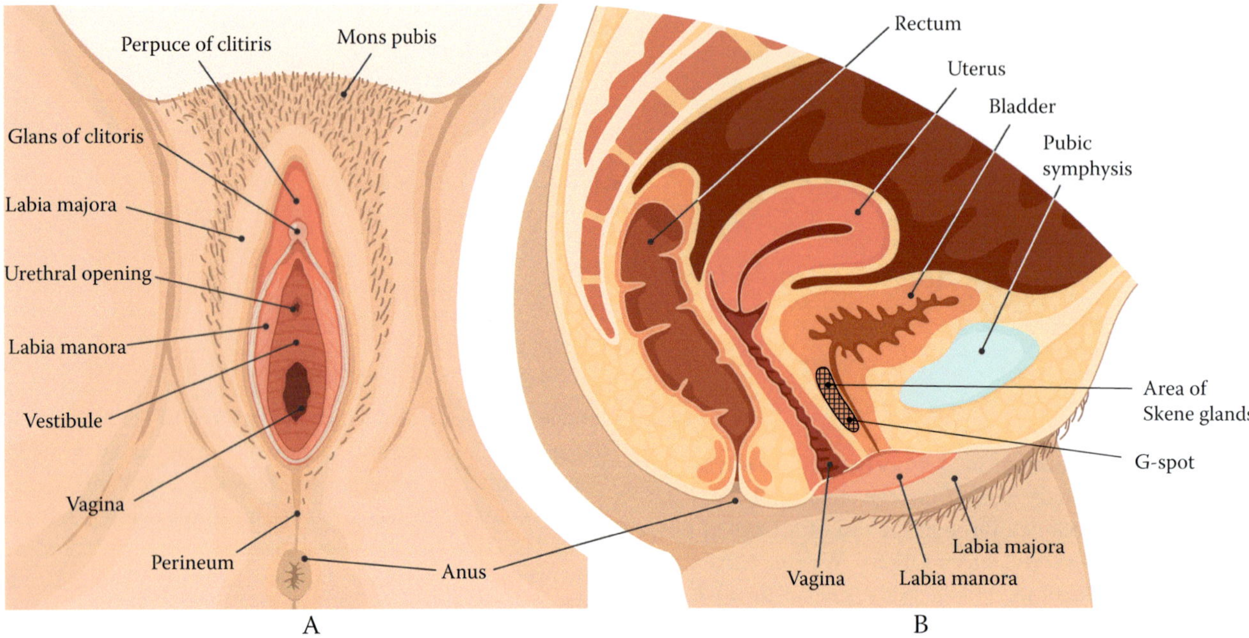

FIGURE 13.1 (A) The female external genital organs. (B) The female internal organs, showing the G-spot area, at the site of the Skene glands. We should consider the external genitalia, clitoris, small and big labia, and the Skene glands all comprise the Female Orgasm System [12] and are together responsible for the best sexual pleasure.

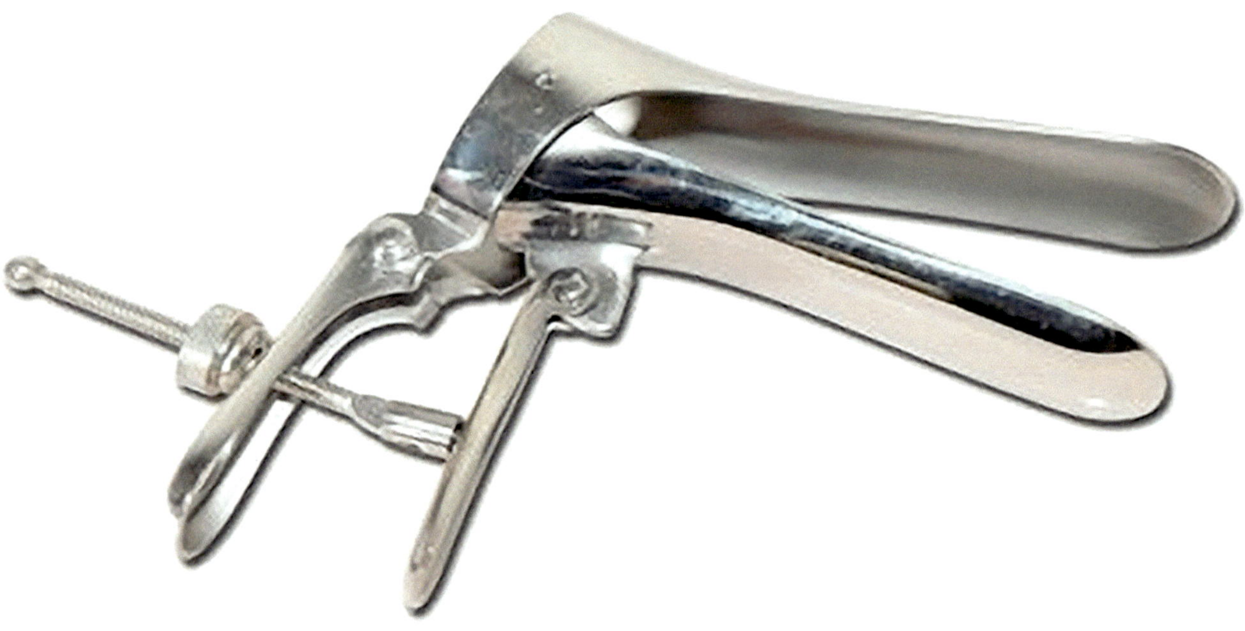

FIGURE 13.2 This grooved speculum has the advantage of not having to be rotated in the vagina to access the point where we want to inject.

The final stage is injection by syringe. A speculum is not always required but can be helpful. Several types of speculum can be used, but the type shown in Figure 13.2 is made of metal and can be modified by creating a groove in the upper valve, through which to introduce the needle.

Anesthesisa is not always required because the needle is very small, but many patients prefer anesthesia. When patients require anesthesia, they are asked to apply EMLA cream to the clitoris and upper vaginal wall 30 minutes before starting the procedure.

For the injection procedure (see Video 13.3), a syringe with a small needle is used. This procedure is not uncomfortable, but some patients prefer to have local topical anesthesia with lidocaine cream. Nanofat solution is injected into the right and the left side of clitoris (1 mL each side) and in the upper vaginal wall near the urethral meatus (2 mL each side) close to the Skene glands. To prevent an intraurethral injection it is possible to catheterize.

Growth factors present in the nanofat will stimulate mesenchymal stem cells to produce new sensitive nerves into the clitoris; nanofat also produces more muciparous cells in these glands, which produce female "ejaculation", so larger fluid production will result.

It is very difficult to say how much time is necessary to produce new nerves or more female ejaculation and thence finally the enhancement of sexual satisfaction. As with Runels's experience using PRP [12], we found a good response to this nanofat technique with regards to the absence of adverse side effects; however, after 3 months about 10% of patients report no improvement in their sexual pleasure (unpublished data). Further follow-up studies are needed with larger numbers of patients to establish more firmly the results for this safe and risk-free procedure.

REFERENCES

1. Grafenberg E, The role of urethra in female orgasm. *Int J Sexology*. 1950;3:145–148.
2. Puppo V, Anatomy and physiology of the clitoris, vestibular bulbs, and labia minora with a review of the female orgasm and the prevention of female sexual dysfunction. *Clin Anat*. 2013 Jan;26(1):134–152.
3. Jannini EA, Buisson O, Alberto Rubio-Casillas A, Beyond the G-spot: Clitourethrovaginal complex anatomy in female orgasm. *Nat Rev Urol*. 2014 Sep;11(9):531–538.
4. Ellibeş Kaya A, Çalışkan A, Women self-reported G-spot existence and relation with sexual function and genital perception. *Turk J Obstet Gynecol*. 2018;15:182–187.
5. Puppo V, Embryology and anatomy of the vulva: The female orgasm and women's sexual health. *Eur J Obstet Gynecol Reprod Biol*. 2011 Jan;154(1):3–8.
6. Emhardt E, Siegel J, Hoffman L, Anatomic variation and orgasm: Could variations in anatomy explain differences in orgasmic success? *Clin Anat*. 2016 Jul;29(5):665–672.
7. Maratos YK, Gombergh R, Cornier E, et al., The G-spot: An observational MRI pilot study. *BJOG*. 2016 Aug;123(9):1542–1549.
8. Herold C, Motamedi M, Hartmann U, et al., G-spot augmentation with autologous fat transplantation. *J Turk Ger Gynecol Assoc*. 2015 Jul 14;16(3):187–188.
9. Ostrzenski A, The G-spot anatomical structure spotted. *J Sex Med*. 2018 May;15(5):803.
10. Puppo V, Gruenwald I, Does the G-spot exist? A review of the current literature. *Int Urogynecol J*. 2012 Dec;23(12):1665–1669.
11. Symonds T, Kingsberg SA, James A Simon JA, et al., Symptoms and associated impact in pre- and postmenopausal women with sexual arousal disorder: A concept elicitation study. *J Sex Med*. 2023;27;20(3):277–286.
12. Runels C, *Activate the Female Orgasm System: The Story of O-Shot*. CreateSpace, Scotts Valley, CA, USA, 2013.
13. Runels C, Melnick H, Debourbon E, et al., A pilot study of the effect of localized injections of autologous platelet rich plasma (PRP) for the treatment of female sexual dysfunction. *J Women's Health Care*. 3:169. 10.4172/2167-0420.1000169.
14. Kamina P, *Anatomie Clinique: Organes Urinaires Et Génitaux, Pelvis, Coupes Du Tronc*, 3rd Edition. Maloine, Paris, 2008.
15. Ceccaroni M, Fanfani F, Ercoli A, Innervazione viscerale e somatica della pelvi femminile: Testo-Atlante di Anatomia Chirurgica con tavole anatomiche originali. *Il Giornale di Chirurgia – Journal of the Italian Association of Hospital Surgeons*. 2007;28(11):458.
16. Yeung J, Pauls RN, Anatomy of the vulva and the female sexual response. *Obstet Gynecol Clin North Am*. 2016 Mar;43(1):27–44.
17. Pan S, Leung C, Shah J, et al., Clinical anatomy of the G-spot. *Clin Anat*. 2015 Apr;28(3):363–367.
18. Pastor Z, Chmel R, Differential diagnostics of female "sexual" fluids: A narrative review. *Int Urogynecol J*. 2018 May;29(5):621–629.
19. Rabinerson D, Horowitz E, G-spot and female ejaculation: Fiction or reality? *Harefuah*. 2007 Feb;146(2): 145–147, 163.
20. Rodriguez FD, Camacho A, Bordes SJ, et al., Female ejaculation: An update on anatomy, history, and controversies. *Clin Anat*. 2021 Jan;34(1):103–107.
21. Dwyer PL, Skene's gland revisited: Function, dysfunction and the G spot. *Int Urogynecol J*. 2012 Feb;23(2): 135–137.
22. Hines TM, The G-spot: A modern gynecologic myth. *Am J Obstet Gynecol*. 2001 Aug;185(2):359–362.
23. Miller CE, G-spot: The facts to the fantasy. *BJOG*. 2014 Oct;121(11):1340.
24. Thabet SMA, New findings and concepts about the G-spot in normal and absent vagina: Precautions possibly needed for preservation of the G-spot and sexuality during surgery. *J Obstet Gynaecol Res*. 2013 Aug;39(8):1339–1346.
25. Pauls RN, Anatomy of the clitoris and the female sexual response. *Clin Anat*. 2015 Apr;28(3):376–384.
26. Aloe L, Rita Levi-Montalcini: The discovery of nerve growth factor and modern neurobiology. *Trends Cell Biol*. 2004 Jul;14(7):395–399.
27. Tocci A, Forte L, Mesenchymal stem cell: Use and perspectives. *Hematol J*. 2003;4(2):92–96.
28. Catalisano C, Enriched nanofat injection vs PRP injection (presentation). Focus: Regenerative medicine for the genital area, IMCAS World Congress 2020, Paris.
29. Miana VV, Prieto González EA, Adipose tissue stem cells in regenerative medicine. *Ecancermedicalscience*. 2018;12:822.

14 Hymenoplasty

Piotr Kolczewski

INTRODUCTION

Hymenoplasty, or the surgical restoration of the hymen, is one of the least described vulvovaginal procedures in plastic surgery, without any surgical standard that attempts to restore the hymen's ability to bleed during sexual intercourse on a couple's wedding night [1,2]. Although controversial from an ethical and social perspective, hymenoplasty is now offered in many countries [3], and its demand is increasing in Western countries, especially after successive waves of immigration. According to the BBC, hymenoplasty has gained popularity in recent years, especially among young women. Private clinics that offer the procedure, which is legal in the United Kingdom, do not collect data on the number of women who have undergone the procedure, but it is estimated that approximately 9000 women searched for the procedure on Google in 2019. Mohammad Masood, Director of MAS Gynecology Clinic in London, said in the British newspaper *Metro* that the number of women seeking the procedure had quadrupled compared to the previous 6 years [4].

ANATOMY AND HISTOLOGY

Named after the god of marriage in classical Greek mythology (Hymenaios), the hymen is a membrane-like structure that separates the vaginal canal from the vaginal vestibulum. It has two borders: an attached or adherent border and a free border around the hymenal orifice. The free border is usually irregular, festooned or dentel or divided into multiple fingers. The hymenal orifice may take different shapes. It may be semilunar, falciform, cubiform or septate. The main bulk of the hymen is formed of fibrous connective tissue covered on both vulvar and vaginal surfaces by stratified squamous epithelium. It is composed of vascular connective tissue covered on both vaginal and vulvar surfaces by stratified squamous epithelium [5].

The vascular supply of the hymen is rich, especially near the free edge, where vessels are dilated and engorged. Multiple capillaries were observed penetrating the covering epithelium and reaching its superficial layers. The vascularity is the cause of sometimes severe bleeding that occasionally accompanies defloration injuries [5]. The hymen is not richly supplied with nerve fibres. It was found that the nerve supply is relatively rich in the attached part, detected with difficulty in the middle part and absent in the free edge [5].

The amount of elastic fibres is variable. Some hymens were rich in elastic fibres, while others were mainly formed of collagenous fibres. This supports the clinical observation that the hymen is of variable consistency and elasticity. Sometimes it tears easily, while on certain occasion it is elastic, allowing sexual intercourse without being torn [5].

FUNCTION OF THE HUMAN HYMEN

According to most sources, human females are the only animal to possess a hymen [6–9].

The function of this structure is unknown [7,8]. Until late in a female's fetal life, the lumen of the vagina is separated from the cavity of the urogenital sinus by the hymen. During the perinatal period it ruptures and remains as a fold of mucous membrane around the entrance to the vagina. Failure of the inferior end of the vagina to perforate results in blockage of the vagina, and the condition known as imperforate hymen [9]. Some authors suggest that the hymen is an embryological structure that has been retained into the juvenile period [6].

With the greater helplessness of human infants relative to other great apes [10], infection due to inability to clean the vaginal area may be a significant cause of mortality. Thus, any structure that limited fecal or other material from entering the vagina would be favoured by natural selection. The hymen, persisting into infants, has thus been exapted to serve a protective function [11].

CULTURE, ETHICS AND LAW

The hymen is presumed to be broken during the first sexual intercourse, and its intact condition is believed to represent virginity. However, the hymen may be ruptured or torn unintentionally in several circumstances, including vaginal insertion of objects such as tampons, vigorous sporting activities, surgical procedures and falling on sharp objects [12].

In cultures in which assurance of a woman's virginity is a precondition to her marriage, lack of such evidence at first marital intercourse is a source of disgrace for the woman and her family and may lead to divorce and violence against her [13]. A bride's evidence may be shown, for instance, in public display of the blooded sheet from the wedding bed [14]. Even in modern times, unmarried girls suspected of lost virginity may be at risk in some communities of suffering "honour killing" at the hands of their family members.

DOI: 10.1201/9780429353079-14

A request for repair of a hymen, whether ruptured in voluntary, coerced, or forceful intercourse, such as by rape or without intercourse, is not necessarily a purely cosmetic choice analogous to breast enlargement and liposuction. It may serve purposes more worthy and protective than personal vanity [12].

On purely medical grounds, hymen reconstruction is not medically indicated. The procedure provides no medical benefit, so accordingly there is no favourable benefit-to-risk ratio. There may be a health benefit, bearing in mind the World Health Organization (WHO) description of "health" as a state of "physical, mental and social well-being and not merely the absence of disease or infirmity" [15].

Gynecologists with sufficient skills asked to perform the procedure should ethically take into account the consequences of their refusal. These include women's expulsion from their families and communities, terminated betrothal, divorce, personal violence and, at its most extreme, so-called "honour killing", usually by close family members. It has been reported, for instance, that almost 2000 Pakistani women were killed in the name of honour between 2004 and 2007, constituting more than nine murders every week [16]. It has been claimed, however, that the procedure has reduced the rate of honour killings by 80% in Egypt in recent years [17].

Practitioners able to perform the procedure who, however, object, for instance on grounds of conscience regarding deception, are bound by Guideline 14(4) of the FIGO Ethics Committee guidelines on appropriate referral [18], to "give priority to their patients' lives, health and well-being".

Although there is evidence that 40–50% of all women from different cultural backgrounds do not have any blood loss at first coitus [19], this does not seem to alter the importance attached to staining the nuptial bed. Thus, it is not just women who are not virgins anymore who fear the wedding night. The pursuit to hide lack of virginity has a long history. Therefore, in many cultures, women are secretly instructed by elderly women on how to use deception in case of a lack of blood loss, for example by hiding a little sac filled with animal blood or a needle in the wedding gown to give oneself a finger puncture, or by using a blood-stained sheet that the elderly women in the family saved for the younger ones [20–23]. A harsher method consists in applying nettles or other herbs a few days before marriage to make the vagina raw, dry and vulnerable. Women who have migrated to Western countries are often cut off from this transgenerational information on how to ensure nuptial bleeding or otherwise mimic virginity [24].

The faith in the myth that an intact hymen proves virginity is still so implicit, that in many countries parents decide to have their daughters "officially certified" as a virgin by a gynecologist [25]. In the scientific literature, however, there is a broad consensus that the archaic assumption that virginity is diagnosable by external genital examination [26] is yet another myth [27,28]. For example, in one study it was found that in 19% of sexually active female adolescents the hymen showed no tears, clefts or notches [28].

According to a very interesting analysis by Bianca R. Van Moorst [3], proper counselling and awareness of women seeking hymenoplasty is crucial. For most women participating in the study conducted by the team of Van Moorst, increased knowledge and self-confidence acquired during counselling meant that they could decide against surgery, even though at first they considered it was the only solution to the problem they were facing. The minority of women who still felt that the operation was necessary, were all very glad to have done it, despite the fact that they often had to resort to some "tricks" to mimic virginity. After extensive counselling, only 24 of the 82 women (29%) enrolled in the study decided to be operated upon.

In its recent positional statement, the RCOG (Royal College of Obstetricians & Gynecologists) strongly opposes the practises of virginity testing and hymenoplasty on the grounds that neither is medically required in any circumstance [29]. The RCOG stated, "We believe that both virginity testing and hymenoplasty should be banned in the UK. Neither procedure has any medical benefit and both are harmful practises that create and exacerbate social, cultural and political beliefs that attach a false value to women and girls in relation to whether or not they have a sexual history. However, we are clear that in no circumstances should clinical procedures be undertaken with the sole purpose of safeguarding a patient in this way. Instead, medical professionals should follow the appropriate protocols to refer women and girls perceived to be at risk of violence to police and social services. Wider public services must also be adequately resourced to safeguard these vulnerable individuals. The RCOG believes that the current availability of these procedures is contributing to entrenching the myths around virginity that are compelling individuals to seek virginity testing and hymenoplasty in the first place. By removing the availability of these procedures, by law, the ability for those currently seeking to infringe on the bodily autonomy and sexual freedoms of women and girls will be significantly limited."

SURGICAL TECHNIQUES

The aim of the surgery is to produce a narrowing of the introital opening with temporary tightening, which can be obtained in many ways.

Lumenal Reductions

This approach to the reconstruction of torn hymenal remnants seems to be more anatomical, intuitive and easier in execution and the most popular. The luminal reduction can be executed in several ways. Simple removal of the epithelial layer of the edges of the opposing hymenal fragments and stitching external (vestibular) and interna (vaginal) layer resulting in adhesions of hymenal fragments seems to be the most common approach [1,2].

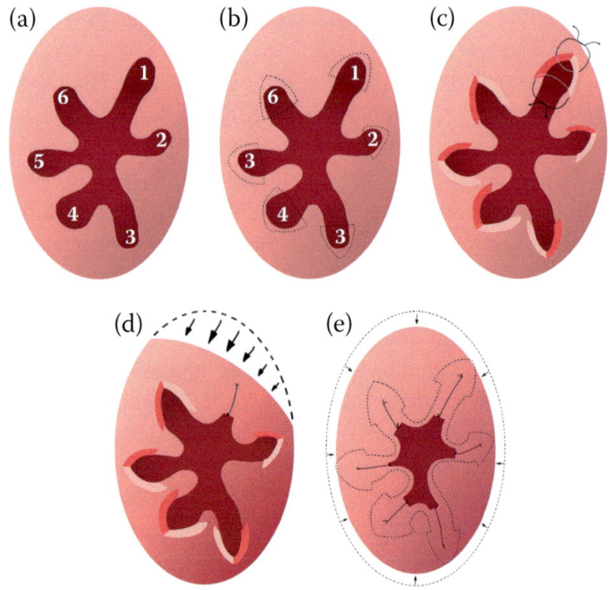

FIGURE 14.1 Lumenal reduction by Goodman technique: (a) clefts identified along periphery of hymenal ring; (b) small, diamond-shaped excisions at base of each cleft; (c) denuded tissues approximated with sutures; (d) closure of diamond-shaped excision decreases outer circumference and size of lumen; (e) closure of all excisions decreases lumen of vaginal introitus. (From Placik OJ, Hymenoplasty, in Hamori CA et al., *Female Cosmetic Genital Surgery*, Thieme, New York, 2017, with permission.)

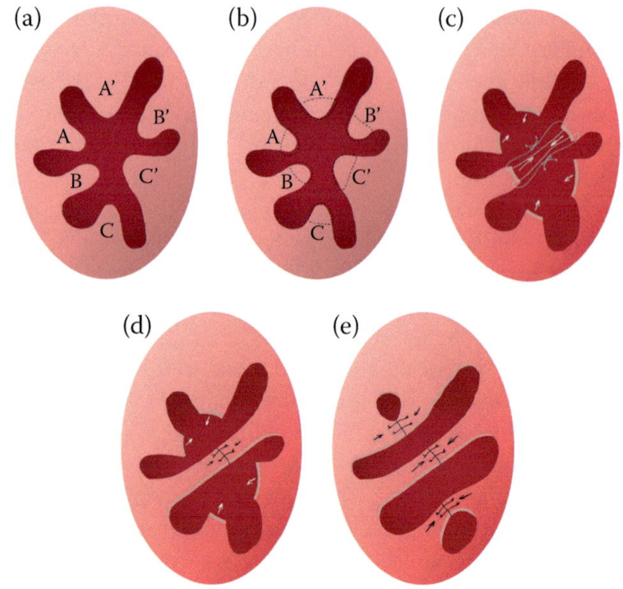

FIGURE 14.2 Lumenal reduction by denuding opposing remnants: (a) opposing fragments identified; (b) tips of remnants are surgically denuded by excising epithelium; (c) denuded tissues on opposing fragments are approximated with sutures; (d) first surgical adhesion completed; (e) after further surgical adhesions, lumen is obstructed but not increased in diameter. (From Placik OJ, Hymenoplasty, in Hamori CA, et al., *Female Cosmetic Genital Surgery*, Thieme, New York, 2017, with permission.)

Another option given by Goodman is to decrease in calibre the introitus by multiple diamond-shaped excisions of mucosa in the clefts between hymenal remnants followed by left to right approximation [30] (Fig. 14.1).

Lumenal reduction can also be achieved by just denuding epithelium and stitching the opposite hymenal remnants, creating transluminal adhesions [31] (Fig. 14.2).

Wei and colleagues [32] went a bit further, considering adhesions techniques as transient because of frequently occurring dehiscence, resulting from the bloodless nature of the hymen. This technique was used on 125 patients in a Chinese centre, and only one patient presented an early postoperative complication in the form of uncontrollable bleeding. In their method called STSI (suturing tree stratum of the introitus), the rim of the hymen is removed according to the designed line and resection is continued to a depth of 0.5–1.0 cm in the direction of the vagina to expose the fascia layer under the hymenal mucosa. The STSI method resects the hymen transversely and sutures the wound in a vertical direction, which increases the wound area and thus increases the blood supply. According to the authors, the high healing rate (91.9%) results from the additional fascia layer that can both increase the blood supply and bear most of the tension among the three layers. Another feature is that the hymenal mucosa (the first and third stratum) is sutured by mattress suture, which is generally considered to be a favourable technique for incision healing (Fig. 14.3).

Another technique was recently described by Eserdag et al. [33] called Vestibulo-Introital Tightening Technique (VITT), which includes a diamond-shaped incision to the vestibulum with the base in the posterior midline and superior corner, 2–3 cm higher above the hymen. The angles are accommodated according to the degree of tightening, and the submucosal layer is closed from the apex downwards involving the vaginal mucosa, and posterior and anterior aspects of hymenal carbuncles are sutured separately. The satisfaction rate of the patients was 99.3%. The authors state that the technique looks like "minor perineoplasty", but taking into account the anatomy involved, we can rather define it as vagino-vestibuloplasty. With this technique, approximately 69% of women reported bleeding with sexual penetration, whereas it has been reported that only 34% of virgins recall bleeding on first intercourse [34]. In the commentary to the VITT [35], Dr. Placik states: "[…] this method effectively doubles the occurrence of bleeding, which then begs the question: are we attempting to reproduce an event that would be expected but would not otherwise have occurred without our intervention? To the credit of the authors, this question can now be raised in light of their report, but further reinforces the need for preoperative counseling" (Fig. 14.4).

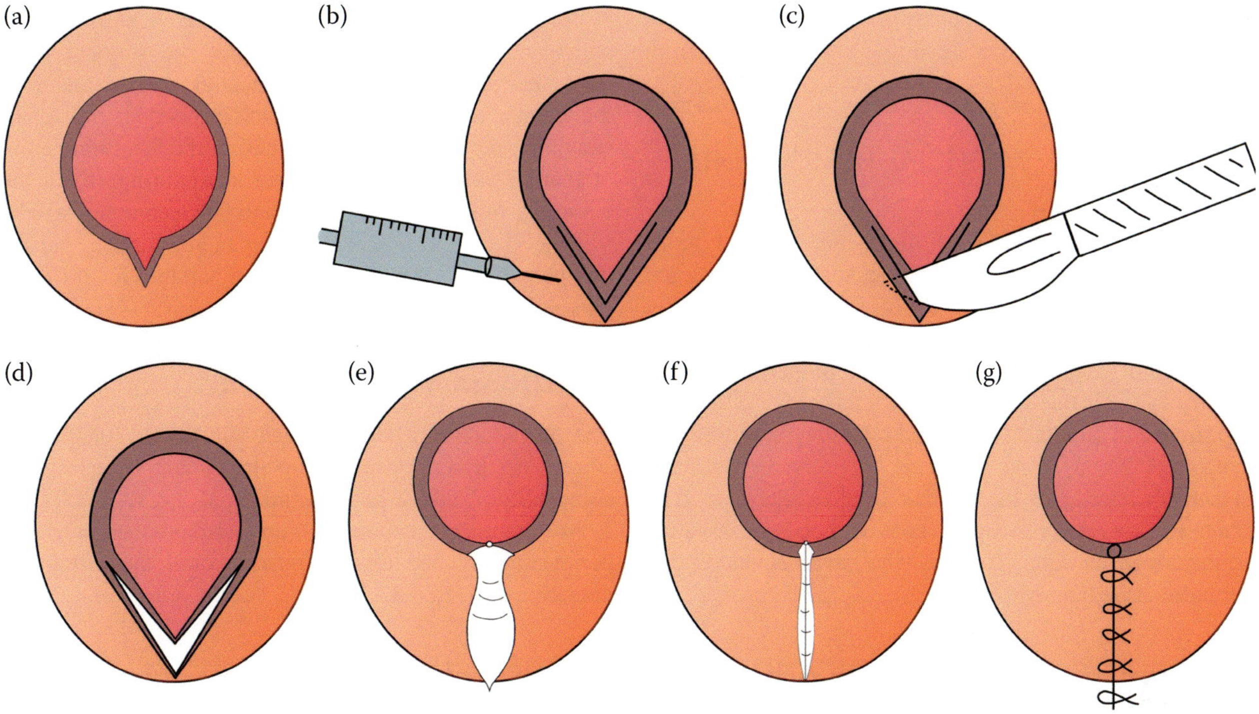

FIGURE 14.3 Lumenal reduction by STSI method: (a) cleft located; (b) local anaesthesia; (c) resection of rim of hymen; (d) resection continued to a depth of 0.5–1.0 cm in the direction of the vagina to expose fascial layer; (e) suture of the upper part of third stratum; (f) suturing continued until the hymenal opening is small enough; (g) end result after suturing completed. (From Ref. [32], with permission.)

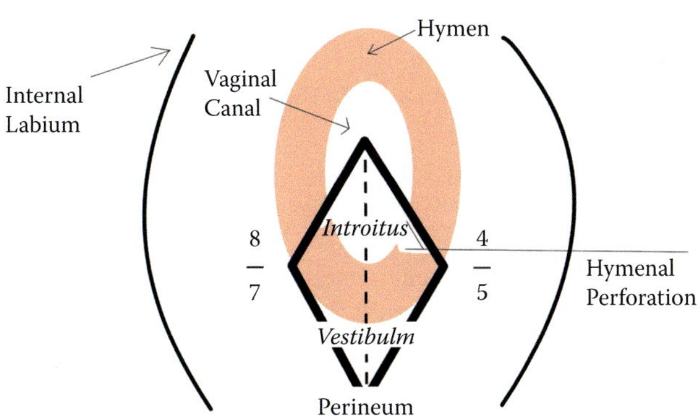

FIGURE 14.4 Vestibulo-introital tightening technique. (From Ref. [33], with permission.)

Suture-Only Techniques (Hymenorrhaphy)

The idea behind these techniques is to create a narrower vaginal orifice without removing the epithelial layer and creating durable adhesions of hymenal clefts; therefore, they should be considered shortly before marriage, in less than 15 days. It can be achieved by a simple suturing of the adjacent hymenal remnants [4] or by a submucosal cerclage method [36]. In this very clever approach described by Ou [36], the suture was run clockwise into the submucosa to the 12-o'clock position, where the needle was pulled out. The needle was then re-introduced into the same small pore where it came out, and the suture was run clockwise back to the original 6-o'clock position. The needle was then pulled through the original needle pore. The ends of the suture were tied together around a 12 mm Hegar dilator to form an annular hymen, and the tie was placed under the mucosa.

Given the temporal nature of the procedure, El Hennawy recommends simplifying the procedure by just placing a transluminal catgut suture, approximately 3–7 days before expected coitus [37].

FLAP TECHNIQUES

Vaginal flap hymenoplasty is based on vaginal mucosal flaps raised from the anterior vaginal wall just behind labia minora [38]. According to the author, having performed the flap method on 11 patients, two flaps were based proximally, and their two opposing flaps were based distally. These flaps were overlapped in a crisscross fashion. The flap method creates a network-like thickened mucosal structure in and around the introitus. The technique seems controversial, with a potential risk of iatrogenic vaginal stenosis and subsequent risk of dyspareunia. It should be considered rather as a second option when hymenal remnants are insufficient or absent in the case of vaginal agenesis [39].

Hymenal flap hymenoplasty is described by Dr. Placik as a "modified surgical adhesion" [31]. The goal of the method is to create a minimum of three flap adhesions of the opposite hymenal remnants. The idea is similar to the above vaginal flap hymenoplasty, but definitely more anatomical thanks to its recreating a "new" hymen from hymenal remnants.

NON-SURGICAL: ARTIFICIAL HYMENS AND RESERVOIRS

According to Wikipedia, an artificial hymen is a type of prosthetic often accompanied by reservoirs containing red liquid, created for the purpose of simulating an intact human hymen, usually to fake virginity. Artificial hymens are made of a material which, when properly inserted, adheres to the inside of the vagina, temporarily giving the appearance of an intact hymen and releasing red liquid that looks like blood when subjected to pressure. Artificial hymens ordered over the internet from retailers based in China by consumers in Egypt have outraged conservative politicians in the latter country, who have demanded that the product be banned [40–43].

PREPARING, COUNSELING, INDICATIONS AND CONTRADICTIONS

According to the WHO, on purely medical grounds hymen reconstruction is not medically indicated. The procedure provides no medical benefit, so accordingly there is no favourable benefit-to-risk ratio [15], but we should take into account the entire cultural background mentioned above and act in the best interest of the patient.

The patient should be educated that sometimes hymens of sexually active females show no tears, clefts or notches [28] as well that 40–50% of all women from different cultural backgrounds do not have any blood loss at first coitus [19]. The surgeon should also highlight that even if she regained an intact hymen, the possibility of bleeding during the first intercourse is approximately 50% [3,12,32].

Convincing evidence-based counseling can make the majority of women planning the procedure decide against surgery, even though at first they considered it was the only solution to the problem they were facing [3].

Indications

As stated above, the reconstruction of hymen is not medically indicated and is performed for cultural reasons only at the patient's request.

Contraindications

Contraindications to the surgery apply to patients who have active menstruation, delayed menses without blood pregnancy test, active genital infections, unrealistic expectations, and patients under 18 years of age who are unaccompanied by their parents. Vulvodynia or chronic pain in the area is a relative contraindication as this can be exacerbated by genital surgery [2].

A surgeon should also take into account timing of anticipated coitus, which determines the surgical technique. For patients who desire structural integrity and need the hymen to be intact on visual inspection, the repair should be performed 3 months before the "consummation of marital vows" [31]. To obtain an enduring effect, the variations of luminal reductions and flap techniques will be suitable [1,2,30,32,34]. Those demanding "quick" repair, just before their wedding night, are suitable for different versions of hymenorrhaphy [4,36,37].

ANESTHESIA AND ANTIBIOTICS

The procedure can be performed with local, general and spinal anesthesia depending on the patient's request and complexity of the surgical technique [1,2,4,31,36,38].

Most authors recommend an antibiotic administered perioperatively and its continuation until the fifth postoperative day [1,31,33,38].

POSTOPERATIVE CARE

Dr. Placik recommends using ice-packs for the first 24 to 48 hours and a standard analgesic regimen. Wound care consists in gentle irrigation after urination and defecation. Patients are encouraged to take showers, but they should not bathe [31].

After the intervention, patients should be advised to avoid the following [4]:

- Side or straddle splits
- Increased abdominal pressure
- Baths
- Tampons
- Self-examination to check the integrity of the hymen
- Penetrative sexual intercourse, which could compromise the results

FAILURES AND COMPLICATIONS

Most authors report that complications are minor; however, surgical risks of the procedure include wound dehiscence, infection, scarring, distortion of the external vaginal orifice, and creating overly small introitus leading to obstruction of vaginal outflow and hematocolpos, dyspareunia, and feelings of guilt [2].

In the presentation of the largest known series of patients undergoing different methods of hymenoplasty/hymenorrhaphy [4], among the 518 patients, only 3 (0.5%) presented an early complication in the form of active hemorrhage requiring surgical hemostasis. Of the 227 women who underwent a hymenorrhaphy, no failure was reported, and all the patients who had sexual intercourse within 15 days of the procedure experienced vaginal bleeding.

The following complications were documented among the 204 hymenoplasties using hymenal flaps: 5 failures

(0.025%), 20 cases of wound dehiscence before the wedding (0.1%), 5 cases of difficult vaginal penetration requiring surgical correction (0.01%), and 3 cases of hemorrhage requiring surgery due to tearing during vaginal penetration (0.025%) [4].

Of the 99 hymenoplasties using vaginal flaps, only one failure (0.1%) was reported; however, the patient did not follow post-surgical care recommendations. Five (0.05%) of the patients underwent a second procedure to resect tight scars, 10 women (0.1%) reported difficult vaginal penetration requiring surgical resection of the sutures, and 2 experienced vaginal bleeding due to a tear requiring a resumption of the procedure [4]. The author emphasizes that no obstetric complications were reported in the examined group [4].

REFERENCES

1. Prakash V. Hymenoplasty—how to do. *Indian J Surg*. 2009;71:221–223.
2. Vojvodic M et al. Luminal reduction hymenoplasty: a Canadian experience with hymen restoration. *Aesthet Surg J*. 2018;38(7):802–806.
3. Bianca R van Moorst et al. Backgrounds of women applying for hymen reconstruction, the effects of counselling on myths and misunderstandings about virginity, and the results of hymen reconstruction. *Eur J Contracept Reproduct Health Care*. 2012 Apr;17(2):93–105.
4. Abelelilah L et al. Hymen restoration: an experience from a Moroccan center. *Aesthet Surg J*. 2021;41(12): NP2053–NP2059.
5. Mahran M, Saleh AM. The microscopic anatomy of the hymen. *Anat Rec*. 1964:313–318.
6. Hobday AJ, Haury L, Dayton PK. Function of the human hymen. *Med Hypotheses*. 1997;49:171–173.
7. Bufley N. The evolution of concealed ovulation. *Am Nat*. 1979;114:835–858.
8. Smith RL. Human sperm competition. In: Smith RL, ed. *Sperm Competition and the Evolution of Animal Mating Systems*. New York: Academic Press, 1984:601–659.
9. Katchadorian HA. *Biological Aspects of Human Sexuality*, 4th edn. Fort Worth, Texas: Holt, Rinehart & Winston, 1990:453.
10. Leutenegger W. Encephalization and obstetrics in primates with particular reference to human evolution. In: Armstrong E, Falk D, eds. *Primate Brain Evolution: Methods and Concepts*. New York: Plenum Press, 1982:85–95.
11. Fisher HE. *The Sex Contract: The Evolution of Human Behavior*. New York: William Morrow, 1982.
12. Cook RJ, Dickens BM. Hymen reconstruction: ethical and legal issues. *Int J Gynecol Obstet*. 2009;107:266–269.
13. Welchman L, Hossain S, eds. *"Honour": Crimes, Paradigms and Violence against Women*. London: Zed Books, 2005.
14. Roberts H. Reconstructing virginity in Guatemala. *Lancet*. 2006;367(9518):1227–1228.
15. World Health Organization. Preamble to the Constitution, para. 1. Accessed from: https://www.who.int/about/governance/constitution.
16. Solberg KE. Killed in the name of honour. *Lancet*. 2009;373(9679):1933–1934.
17. Kandela P. Egypt's trade in hymen repair. *Lancet*. 1996;347(9015):1615.
18. FIGO Ethics Committee. Ethical guidelines on conscientious objection. *Ethical Issues in Obstetrics and Gynecology*. London: FIGO, 2006:24–26.
19. Loeber O. Over het zwaard en de schede; bloedverlies en pijn bij de eerste coïtus; Een onderzoek bij vrouwen uit diverse culturen. [About the sword and the sheet; blood loss and pain at first coitus. A study of women with different cultural backgrounds.] *Tijdschrift voor Seksuologie*. 2008;32:129–137.
20. Gomiddleeast.com. Afraid that you won't bleed on your wedding night? Accessed 13 August 2011 from: www.gomiddleeast.com/tag/bleeding-on-wedding-night/.
21. Blank H. *Virgin: The Untouched History*. New York: Bloomsbury, 2007: 89–91.
22. Medievalists.net. How to cheat on a virginity test. Accessed from: https://www.medievalists.net/2016/06/how-to-cheat-on-a-virginity-test/.
23. Islamicgarden.com. The myth of the hymen continues. Accessed 13 August 2011 from: www.islamicgarden.com/mythhymen.html.
24. Gürsoy E, Gülsen Vural G. Nurses' and midwives' views on approaches to hymen examination. *Nurs Ethics*. 2003;10:485–494.
25. Parla A. The 'honor' of the state: virginity examinations in Turkey. *Feminist Stud*. 2001;27:65–88.
26. Curtis E, Lazaro CS. Appearance of the hymen in adolescents is not well documented. *BMJ*. 1999;318:605.
27. Rogers DJ, Stark M. The hymen is not necessarily torn after sexual intercourse. *BMJ*. 1998;317:414.
28. Emans SJ, Woods ER, Allred EN, Grace E. Hymeneal findings in adolescent women: the impact of tampon use and consensual sexual activity. *J Pediatr*. 1994; 125:153–160.
29. RCOG position statement. Virginity testing and hymenoplasty. Accessed at: www.rcog.org.uk/media/qlxh3wro/rcog-virginity-testing-hymenoplasty-position-statement-august-2021.pdf.
30. Goodman MP. Female genital cosmetic and plastic surgery: a review. *J Sex Med*. 2011;8(6):1813–1825.
31. Placik OJ. Hymenoplasty. In: Hamori CA et al. Female Cosmetic Genital Surgery. New York: Thieme, 2017: 190–199.
32. Wei S-Y, Li Q, Li S-K, Zhou C-D, Li F-Y, Zhou Y. A new surgical technique of hymenoplasty. *Int J Gynaecol Obstet*. 2015;130(1):14–18.
33. Eserdag S. A new practical surgical technique for hymenoplasty: primary repair of hymen with vestibulo-introital tightening technique (VITT). *Aesthet Sur J*. 2021 Feb 12;41(3):333–337.
34. Paterson-Brown S. Should doctors reconstruct the vaginal introitus of adolescent girls to mimic the virginal state? Education about the hymen is needed. *BMJ*. 1998;316(7129):461.
35. Placik O. Commentary on: a new practical surgical technique for hymenoplasty: primary repair of hymen with vestibulo-introital tightening technique. *Aesthet Sur J*. 2021 Feb 12;41(3):338–343.
36. Ou MC, Lin CC, Pang CC, Ou D. A cerclage method for hymenoplasty. *Taiwan J Obstet Gynecol*. 2008;47: 355–356.
37. El Hennawy M. Hymenoplasty. Accessed from: www.powershow.com/view/3b58f5-MjAzZ

38. Saraiya HA. Surgical revirgination: four vaginal mucosal flaps for reconstruction of a hymen. *Indian J Plast Surg*. 2015;48:192–195.
39. Kimberley N, Hutson JM, Southwell BR, Grover SR. Vaginal agenesis, the hymen, and associated anomalies. *J Pediatr Adolesc Gynecol*. 2012;25:54–58.
40. Wikipedia. Artificial hymen. Accessed from: https://wikipedia.org/wiki/Artificial_hymen.
41. Hymen shop. Accessed from: https://hymenshop.com.
42. CNNGo. The unlikely Chinese product that could start a trade war. Archived October 10, 2009 at: https://profilpelajar.com/article/Artificial_hymen.
43. CBS News. Egyptian lawmakers want to ban fake hymen. Accessed from: www.cbsnews.com/news/egyptian-lawmakers-want-to-ban-fake-hymen/.

15 Psychological Implications in Aesthetic Gynecology

A Case of Body Dysmorphic Disorder

Stelios Kiosses

INTRODUCTION

Body Dysmorphic Disorder (BDD) is a severe mental health condition that often goes underrecognized. As the popularity of cosmetic procedures continues to rise, physicians are increasingly likely to encounter patients with BDD. Accurate identification, assessment, and appropriate selection procedures are essential, considering the ethical and legal considerations involved in these patients' aesthetic treatments.

It is true to say that when mental illness is related to body image, the conditions that we usually think of are anorexia or other eating disorders. However, five times more prevalent than anorexia, the lesser-known BDD is the cause of even higher psychological impairment levels. Described first by an Italian psychiatrist, Enrico Morselli, in 1891 [1], BDD was initially described as "dysmorphophobia", but this term is used less often nowadays: "The dysmorphophobic patient is miserable in the middle of his daily routines, everywhere and at any time, he is caught by the doubt of deformity".

Body image encompasses perceptions, thoughts, and feelings about the body influenced by development, perception, and sociocultural factors [2]. Patients who suffer from BDD have the feeling that they are ugly in some aspect of their appearance, despite usually being mostly regular in appearance. They may think some part of their body is too small, too large, or the wrong shape. Generally, other people will not see what the BDD patient sees, and if they do, they will notice only a minimal and unremarkable abnormality. BDD may be more prevalent in patients presenting for cosmetic surgery than often believed. A recent review in the psychology literature found the prevalence of BDD in cosmetic surgery patients to be 13.2%, despite the frequently underdiagnosed and underreported cases [3,4].

BDD was initially called "imagined ugliness syndrome" and has also been called a "dysmorphic syndrome", "dermatologic hypochondriasis", and "dysmorphophobia" [5]. The most common areas of concern for BDD sufferers are the ears, nose, shape of their mouth, size and shape of their breasts, buttocks, or genitalia. When somebody suffers from BDD, they are preoccupied continuously with how they look and are convinced that other people notice that they are deformed somehow. They will often attribute any other difficulties they have in their life with what they see as their glaring deformity.

While BDD is primarily a mental health condition, individuals affected by it frequently consult plastic surgeons, aesthetic practitioners, dermatologists, and other healthcare professionals in search of remedies for perceived physical deformities.

THE STATS

The estimated worldwide occurrence of BDD varies between 1.7% and 3.3%, and notably high prevalence rates have been documented among student populations [see further ref 3]. Approximately 8% to 15% of individuals consider undergoing cosmetic surgery, and plastic surgeons can reasonably anticipate encountering such patients. However, it is important to note that around 10% of healthcare practitioners may not recognize the presence of BDD in these patients.

In people with BDD, the rate of suicide is some 45 times higher than people in the general population. More than 90% of BDD patients will not be happy even after having had cosmetic surgery, and having surgical intervention can often make their condition worse. Unfortunately, most people who suffer from BDD lack full insight into the condition and will vehemently believe their problem to be physical rather than psychological, prompting them to seek surgical rather than psychiatric help with their condition. The existing literature on the relationship between BDD and cosmetic surgery indicates that BDD patients generally show impaired judgement regarding the psychological origin of their symptoms [22]. In such cases, the psychological disorder should be treated first because surgical treatment without prior psychological treatment can result in dangerous or even deadly consequences for the physician [6].

SIMILARITIES WITH OCD

BDD and OCD (obsessive-compulsive disorder) exhibit notable similarities in their underlying neurobiology, both stemming from irregular activity in the amygdala region of the brain, responsible for regulating emotions and alerting us to potential threats. This region, often referred to as the

DOI: 10.1201/9780429353079-15

brain's emotional center, plays a crucial role in sounding the alarm when something seems amiss, generally responding to various stressors. However, in the case of individuals with BDD, neuroimaging studies have shown that this amygdala activation appears to be random. Rather than responding to a specific threat or danger, those with BDD interpret this erratic amygdala activity as a signal that something is wrong with their appearance. This perception triggers a cascade of distressing thoughts and behaviors, driving them to focus relentlessly on perceived flaws. This fixation can lead to a range of debilitating issues, including severe anxiety, persistent depression, avoidance of social interactions, and even suicidal ideation.

Suicidal thoughts, suicide attempts, and instances of completed suicide are distressingly common among individuals diagnosed with body dysmorphic disorder (BDD). Research indicates that approximately 80% of those with BDD have grappled with suicidal ideation at some point in their lives, while between 24% and 28% have taken steps to end their lives [7]. Although data on completed suicides among BDD sufferers are limited and preliminary, the observed suicide rate is significantly higher within this group. These findings emphasize the critical importance of effectively addressing BDD.

Recognizing patients who are suffering from BDD and seeking aesthetic procedures is of utmost importance because:

- **Recognition of Prime Pathology:** It's crucial to acknowledge that the primary issue in individuals with BDD is psychological rather than physical. Their distress arises from the perception of flaws that may not be evident to others.
- **Psychosocial Co-Morbidities and Suicidal Tendencies:** BDD is often accompanied by psychosocial co-morbidities, including anxiety and depression. Additionally, the suicide risk among individuals with BDD is alarmingly high, with a significantly increased rate compared to the general population.
- **Dissatisfaction with Cosmetic Procedures:** Patients with BDD tend to be dissatisfied with the outcomes of their cosmetic procedures. Their fixation on perceived flaws may lead them to view even successful procedures as failures, exacerbating their distress.
- **Litigious Tendencies:** It's worth noting that individuals with BDD may become litigious following perceived "failures" to resolve their perceived "defects." This emphasizes the need for careful evaluation and ethical considerations in providing aesthetic treatments to such patients.

In 1980, Body Dysmorphic Disorder (BDD) was included in the Diagnostic and Statistical Manual of Mental Disorders (DSM) by the American Psychiatric Association as an a typical somatoform disorder. Subsequently, in 2013, BDD was reclassified and added to the obsessive-compulsive related disorders spectrum, characterized by the following four criteria:

1. Preoccupation with one or more perceived defects or flaws in physical appearance that are not observable or appear slight to others
2. Repetitive behaviours (i.e., mirror checking, excessive grooming, skin picking, reassurance seeking) or mental acts (i.e., comparing own appearance with that of others) in response to concerns with appearance
3. Preoccupation causing clinically significant distress or impairment in social, occupational, or other important areas of functioning
4. Preoccupation with appearance is not better explained by concerns with body fat or weight in an individual whose symptoms meet the diagnostic criteria for an eating disorder [see further Ref. 7]; however, the sine qua non of BDD is the obsessive fixation on some perceived defect in one's appearance

SYMPATHETIC APPROACH

Once the diagnosis of BDD has been made, a sympathetic dialogue must be established with the patient. It is crucial to acknowledge any visible difference in their appearance because completely dismissing their concern or trying to reassure them that they look excellent is not likely to work. The practitioner should listen patiently and with sympathy and allow plenty of time for discussion. One successful technique is to ask the patient to rate their defect on a scale of 1 to 10 (it would usually be a 10 for BDD patients). The practitioner's assessment of any deformity will likely be a lot less than this, and discussion should be held between the patient and practitioner to discuss this disparity. It is from this point on that the idea of BDD can be introduced.

THE MOST COMMON BODY DYSMORPHIC DISORDER COMPULSIONS

- Avoiding looking at photographs and often removing mirrors from the house
- Attempts to cover up the defect with using cosmetics or wearing baggy clothing, a hat or even adopting a particular posture
- Excessively skin-picking, combing hair, plucking eyebrows, shaving, etc.
- Touching the skin compulsively, especially to feel or measure the defect perceived
- Showing hostility to people without any apparent reason, often to people of the opposite gender
- Obsessively seeking to be reassured by loved ones
- Dieting and exercising excessively
- An unhealthy obsession with celebrities and other people that the sufferer wants to look like

- The use of distraction techniques: trying to draw people's attention away from what the sufferer sees as their defect by wearing bold or excessive jewellery or very extravagant, flamboyant clothing
- Compulsively reading books and looking at articles and websites related to whatever their perceived defect is
- A preoccupation with dermatology procedures or plastic surgery
- Attempts to perform cosmetic surgery on themselves, including liposuction or removal of unwanted blemishes with home kits
- Avoiding leaving home, or only leaving at certain times, for example, under the cover of darkness

THE COMMON SYMPTOMS OF BDD

- Preoccupation with the appearance of what they perceive as the "defect"
- Depression
- Delusions and skewed beliefs related to the appearance
- Suicidal tendencies
- Panic attacks and anxiety
- A chronic low self-esteem
- Social self-consciousness – imagining that other people notice and are mocking the perceived defect
- Strong feelings of shame
- Withdrawing from family and socially, social phobia, loneliness and self-imposed social isolation
- Overdependence on other people, such as a friend, partner or parents
- A preoccupation with appearance that leads to an inability to work or focus at work
- Impaired academic performance, not maintaining grades and problems with attendance
- Problems initiating and maintaining relationships (both friendships and intimate relationships)
- Abuse of alcohol or drugs and attempts to self-medicate

TREATMENT FOR BDD

The National Institute for Health and Care Excellence (NICE) recommends two treatments:

- **Cognitive Behaviour Therapy (CBT):** CBT is a form of psychotherapy that focuses on the connection between a person's thoughts, behaviors, and emotions. Through CBT, individuals with BDD work with a therapist to identify and modify thought patterns that exacerbate self-criticism, anxiety, and social withdrawal. Additionally, CBT can address body image concerns and help reduce repetitive behaviors, such as excessive mirror-checking or grooming.
- **Serotonergic Antidepressant Medications:** BDD can also be treated with antidepressant medications, typically serotonergic antidepressants. These medications are often taken at higher doses daily for approximately 3 months, with their effectiveness evaluated during this period. The medication may either significantly improve the condition or have no effect. If it proves effective, individuals may need to continue taking it for a year or more, as discontinuing the medication can lead to a relapse. Although the exact mechanism of action is not fully understood, these medications have been found to be effective even in the absence of depression. They can be used as a stand-alone treatment or in conjunction with CBT.

CBT is a form of psychotherapy that emphasizes the importance of our underlying thoughts on how we act and feel. A CBT therapist will help someone with BDD uncover their behaviour and thought patterns that make their self-criticism, anxiety, and social withdrawal worse. It can also be used to treat body image issues and reduce repetitive behaviour such as continually looking in the mirror or grooming excessively. Medication for this condition will be antidepressants. A higher dose of antidepressants will usually be taken daily for around 3 months and its effectiveness evaluated after that. The medication can produce a cure or not affect the condition at all. If the drug is found to work, then a sufferer may need to take it for a year or more because ceasing the medication can lead to a relapse. The exact way this medication works is unknown, but it may also work where there is no depression and can be used alone or combined with CBT.

RECOGNIZING THE CONDITION OF BDD

The vast majority of patients who have received an aesthetic procedure are satisfied with their results, care, and physician. Nevertheless, it can be challenging to turn away a patient, even with BDD, who feels that an aesthetic procedure will significantly improve their self-esteem. However, performing a cosmetic procedure on a BDD patient will most likely result in a catastrophic outcome for both the patient and the aesthetic practitioner. Surgical and even non-surgical interventions for these patients are usually the wrong course of action.

If physicians suspect that their patient might have BDD, they should refer the patient to a mental health professional for full evaluation and diagnosis. However, aesthetic practitioners should also be involved in their patients' initial screening to determine any adverse psychological issues; furthermore, if the physician wants to incorporate assessment tools for BDD with questionnaires that have been mainly produced to evaluate and to arrive at a diagnosis of this condition, that is also advisable. There are available general screening tools [8,9], such as the Body Dysmorphic Disorder Questionnaire (BDDQ) [10], which has been used to determine whether a person should seek a more formal diagnosis and is well-established. Existing measures, however, evaluate dysmorphia as a whole rather than just in one particular body part. Although dysmorphic preoccupation tends to focus on the nose, eyes, skin, and hair [11], Barbara argues that more focus should be placed on genital-specific dysmorphia in women because many young girls undergoing non-medically indicated genital surgery meet diagnostic criteria for BDD [12,13].

One of these questionnaires, the Bader-Kiosses–Defective Genital Appearance Questionaire (BK-DGAQ), or the Genital Dysmorphia Questionnaire (GDQ), asks specific questions but relates to a patient's genitals rather than their body image and is currently being developed at the University of Oxford under Professor Robin Murphy's supervision. It is hoped that this study will validate the BK-DGAQ (GDQ) to be used as a tool for screening for BDD in women who are seeking surgical alteration of their genitals. Several groups are studying BDD at the moment in the hope of gaining insight into the condition and into the best way of treating and assessing this devastating psychological disorder. The research in Oxford suggests that the GDQ can be both valid and reliable, allowing it to pave the way forward for potential future BDD screening in cosmetic surgery clinics. Use of this questionnaire in such establishments may help aesthetic practitioners to discuss with their patients what benefits (or lack thereof) they may see from going through with cosmetic surgery if they appear to be suffering from the symptoms of body dysmorphia.

In recent developments, a groundbreaking study conducted at the University of Oxford [15] has introduced a new tool known as the Genital Dysmorphia Questionnaire (GDQ), also referred to as the Bader-Kiosses–Defective Genital Appearance Questionnaire (BK-DGAQ). Unlike traditional assessments, the GDQ focuses specifically on concerns related to a patient's genital appearance rather than their overall body image. This innovative questionnaire aims to address the unique needs of women seeking surgical alterations in this area. It's important to note that this study is currently undergoing evaluation and has not yet undergone peer review. The Oxford research provides promising results, suggesting that the GDQ exhibits both validity and reliability. This discovery paves the way for potential future utilization of the GDQ as a screening tool for Body Dysmorphic Disorder (BDD) in women considering genital cosmetic surgery. Several research groups are currently dedicated to studying BDD, aiming to gain deeper insights into this complex psychological condition and to refine the most effective approaches for assessment and treatment. By incorporating the GDQ into cosmetic surgery clinics, aesthetic practitioners may facilitate more informed discussions with their patients, helping them assess the potential benefits and risks associated with cosmetic surgery, especially when symptoms of body dysmorphia are present.

Referral to a specialist in mental health will likely be necessary to manage their BDD for some patients. In this respect, the role of a surgeon, aesthetic practitioner or dermatologist should be to prepare a person for that referral. Without the necessary groundwork being done, the patient may refuse to have any psychological treatment and, convinced that their problem is physical, will turn to other cosmetic doctors. One suggestion to doctors is that they discuss how upsetting and distressing the condition is for the patient to see the value in a mental health referral. A patient should always be told that this is a recognized problem and that treatment can be successful. It is true, however, that many will be resistant to this idea.

The advice for those practitioners seeing a BDD patient is to allow them time to process the information and the ideas being posed to them while keeping an excellent professional relationship, allowing them to come back once they have had time to think things over. It is a well-accepted doctrine that operating on patients with BDD should be discouraged until first diagnosing and treating this psychological disorder.

Throughout my experience in treating BDD patients, it has become evident that external influences, such as the pervasive 'celebrity culture' and the widespread popularity of specific cosmetic procedures, can significantly impact and exacerbate the compulsions and obsessions associated with this condition.

CONCLUSIONS

There is no doubt that recognizing BDD early can help prevent the disease's progress and improve the quality of life of the sufferer and the people they live with. It may also save their life and the reputation and well-being of the aesthetic doctors who have been treating them. A therapist with CBT training is the ideal practitioner to offer help in treating patients with BDD and OCD, depression and eating disorders. To help people with BDD, the aesthetic practitioner and psychologist must collaborate to find the best way forward for that patient.

REFERENCES

1. Morselli E. Sulla dismorfofobia e sulla tafefobia. *Boll Reale Accad Med Genova*. 1891;6:3–14.
2. Sarcu D, Adamson P. Psychology of the facelift patient. *Facial Plast Surg*. 2017;33:252–259.
3. Veale D, et al. Body dysmorphic disorder in different settings: A systematic review and estimated weighted prevalence. *Body Image*. 2016;18:168–186.
4. Veale D, Boocock A, Gournay K, et al. Body dysmorphic disorder: A survey of fifty cases. *Br J Psychiatry*. 1996;169:196–201.
5. Franca K, Roccia MG, Castillo D, et al. Body dysmorphic disorder: History and curiosities, *Wien Med Wochenschr*. 2017;167(Suppl 1):5–7.
6. Sweis IE, Spitz J, Barry DR Jr, Cohen M. A review of body dysmorphic disorder in aesthetic surgery patients and the legal implications. *Aesthetic Plast Surg*. 2017;41:949–954.

7. *Diagnostic and Statistical Manual of Mental Disorders* (Fourth text revision ed.). American Psychiatric Association, Washington, DC. 2000. pp. 507–510.
8. Manusco SG, Knoesen NP, Castle DJ. The dysmorphic concern questionnaire: A screening measure for body dysmorphic disorder. *Australian and New Zealand Journal of Psychiatry*. 2010;44(6):535–542.
9. Rosen JC, Reiter J. Development of the body dysmorphic disorder examination. *Behaviour Research and Therapy*. 1996;34(9):755–766.
10. Phillips KA, Atala KD, Pope HG. Diagnostic instruments for body dysmorphic disorder. In New Research Program and Abstracts. *American Psychiatric Association 148th Annual Meeting*, American Psychiatric Press, Miami, 1995.
11. Phillips KA, Menard W, Quinn E, et al. A 4-year prospective observational follow-up study of course and predictors of course in body dysmorphic disorder. *Psychological Medicine*. 2013;43(5):1109–1117.
12. Barbara G, Facchin F, Meschia M, Vercellini P. "The first cut is the deepest": A psychological, sexological and gynecological perspective on female genital cosmetic surgery. *Acta obstetricia et gynecologica Scandinavica*. 2015;94(9):915–920.
13. Veale D, Bewley A. Body dysmorphic disorder. *BMJ*. 2015;18(350):1–4.

FURTHER READING

14. Cororve MB, Gleaves DH. Body dysmorphic disorder: A review of conceptualisations, assessment, and treatment strategies. *Clinical Psychology Review*. 2001;21(6): 949–970.
15. Fang A, Hofmann SG. Relationship between social anxiety disorder and body dysmorphic disorder. *Clinical Psychology Review*. 2010;30(8):1040–1048.
16. Fornaro M, Gabrielli F, Albano C, et al. Obsessive-compulsive disorder and related disorders: A comprehensive survey. *Annals of General Psychiatry*. 2009;8:13.
17. Grant J, Kim SW, Crow S. Prevalence and clinical features of body dysmorphic disorder in adolescent and adult psychiatric inpatients. *J Clin Psychiatry*. 2001;62(7):517–522.
18. Harrison A, Fernández de la Cruz L, Enander J, et al. Cognitive-behavioral therapy for body dysmorphic disorder: A systematic review and meta-analysis of randomised controlled trials. *Clin Psychol Rev*. 2016;48:43–51.
19. Hunt TJ, Thienhaus O, Ellwood A. The mirror lies; body dysmorphic disorder. *Am Family Physician*. 2008;78(2): 217–222.
20. Mufaddel A, Osman Ossama T, Almugaddam F, Jafferany M. A review of body dysmorphic disorder and its presentation in different clinical settings. *Primary Care Companion for CNS Disorders*. 2013;15(4).
21. Phillips KA. *The Broken Mirror: Understanding and Treating Body Dysmorphic Disorder* (2nd edn). Oxford University Press, 2005.
22. Phillips KA, Dufresne RG Jr, Wilkel CS, Vittorio CC. Rate of body dysmorphic disorder in dermatology patients. *J Am Acad Dermatol*. 2000;42:436–444.
23. Phillips KA, Hart, AS, Simpson HB, Stein DJ. Delusional versus nondelusional body dysmorphic disorder: Recommendations for DSM-5. *CNS Spectrums*. 2013; 19(1):10–20.
24. Phillips KA, Hollander E, Rasmussen SA, et al. A severity rating scale for body dysmorphic disorder: Development, reliability, and validity of a modified version of the Yale-Brown Obsessive Compulsive Scale. *Psychopharmacol Bullet*. 1997;33(1):17–22.
25. Rosen JC, Reiter J, Orosan P. Cognitive-behavioral body image therapy for body dysmorphic disorder. *J Consult Clin Psychol*. 1995;63:263–269.
26. Phillips KA. *Understanding Body Dysmorphic Disorder: An Essential Guide*. New York: Oxford University Press, 2009.
27. Vats M. Selfie syndrome: An infectious gift of IT to health care. *J Lung Pulm Respir Res*. 2015;2:48.
28. Veale D, Gournay K, Dryden W, et al. Body dysmorphic disorder: A cognitive behavioural model and pilot randomised controlled trial. *Behaviour Research and Therapy*. 1996;34(9):717–729.
29. Veale D. Outcome of cosmetic surgery and 'DIY' surgery in patients with body dysmorphic disorder. *Psychiatric Bulletin*. 2000;24(6):218–221.
30. Veale D, De Haro L., Lambrou C. Cosmetic rhinoplasty in body dysmorphic disorder. *British Journal of Plastic Surgery*. 2003;56(6):546–551.
31. Veale D, Anson M, Miles S, et al. Efficacy of cognitive behaviour therapy versus anxiety management for body dysmorphic disorder: A randomised controlled trial. *Psychother Psychosomat*. 2014;83:341–353.
32. Veale D, Gledhill LJ, Christodoulou P, Hodsoll J. Body dysmorphic disorder in different settings: A systematic review and estimated weighted prevalence. *Body Image*. 2016;18:168–186.

Index

Note: Locators in *italics* represent figures and **bold** indicate tables in the text.